Laboratory and Diagnostic Testing in Ambulatory Care

A GUIDE FOR HEALTH CARE PROFESSIONALS

THIRD EDITION

Laboratory and Diagnostic Testing in Ambulatory Care

A GUIDE FOR HEALTH CARE PROFESSIONALS

THIRD EDITION

Marti Garrels, MSA, MT (ASCP), CMA (AAMA)
Medical Assisting Program Consultant
Retired Medical Assisting Program Director
Lake Washington Institute of Technology
Kirkland, Washington

Carol S. Oatis, MSEd, MT SM (ASCP)
Microbiology Adjunct Instructor
Lake Sumter State College
Leesburg, Florida

ELSEVIER

ELSEVIER
SAUNDERS

3251 Riverport Lane
St. Louis, Missouri 63043

Notice

Knowledge and best practice in this field are constantly changing. As new research and experience broaden our understanding, changes in research methods, professional practices, or medical treatment may become necessary.

Practitioners and researchers must always rely on their own experience and knowledge in
evaluating and using any information, methods, compounds, or experiments described herein.
In using such information or methods they should be mindful of their own safety and the safety
of others, including parties for whom they have a professional responsibility.

With respect to any drug or pharmaceutical products identified, readers are advised to check
the most current information provided (i) on procedures featured or (ii) by the manufacturer of
each product to be administered, to verify the recommended dose or formula, the method and
duration of administration, and contraindications. It is the responsibility of practitioners, rely-
ing on their own experience and knowledge of their patients, to make diagnoses, to determine
dosages and the best treatment for each individual patient, and to take all appropriate safety
precautions.

To the fullest extent of the law, neither the Publisher nor the authors, contributors, or editors
assume any liability for any injury and/or damage to persons or property as a matter of products liability, negligence or otherwise, or from any use or operation of any methods, products,
instructions, or ideas contained in the material herein.

Library of Congress Cataloging-in-Publication Data
Garrels, Marti, author.
  [Laboratory testing for ambulatory settings]
  Laboratory and diagnostic testing in ambulatory care : a guide for health care professionals /
Marti Garrels, Carol S. Oatis. -- Third edition.
      p. ; cm.
  Preceded by Laboratory testing for ambulatory settings : a guide for health care professionals /
Marti Garrels, Carol S. Oatis. 2nd ed. 2011.
  Includes bibliographical references and index.
  ISBN 978-1-4557-7246-9 (pbk. : alk. paper)
  I. Oatis, Carol, author. II. Title.
  [DNLM: 1. Clinical Laboratory Techniques--methods. 2. Ambulatory Care--methods. 3. Clinical
Laboratory Techniques. QY 25]
  RB37
  616.07'56--dc23
                                                           2014028075

Executive Content Strategist: Jennifer Janson
Content Development Manager: Luke Held
Senior Content Development Specialist: Jennifer Bertucci
Publishing Services Manager: Jeffrey Patterson
Senior Project Manager: Jeanne Genz
Designer: Brian Salisbury

Printed in China

Last digit is the print number: 9 8 7 6 5 4 3 2 1

Reviewers

Sandra Alexander, MPA, BA/S, CMA (AAMA)
Program Director/Coordinator
El Centro College
Dallas, Texas

Pamela A. Audette, MBA, MT (ASCP), RMA
Assistant Professor; Medical Assisting Program Director
Finlandia University
Hancock, Michigan

Julie A. Grassel, MSN Ed, BSN, RN
Allied Health Instructor
Medical Assistant Program
Waukesha County Technical College
Pewaukee, Wisconsin

Diana Lee-Greene, RMA (AMT), MT (ASCP), MBA
Program Director, Medical Assisting
Columbia Gorge Community College
The Dalles, Oregon

Tonya M. Lloyd, CMA (AAMA), BAS
Medical Assisting Program Director and
    Patient Care Technician Coordinator
EHOVE Adult Career Center
Milan, Ohio

Debra J. Paul, BA, CMA (AAMA)
Medical Assisting Program Chair
Ivy Tech Community College
South Bend, Indiana

Paula Phelps, MBA with an emphasis in
Healthcare Administration
Allied Health Program Director
National American University
Wichita, Kansas

Cathy D. Soto, PhD, MBA, CMA (AAMA)
MA Program Director, Retired
El Paso Community College
CEO, Global Education Company
El Paso, Texas

Carolyn A. Zolnoski, BS-HCA, MS-HCA
Instructor, Adjunct Faculty
Department of Health and Science
Macomb Community College
Clinton Township, Michigan

Preface

This text is designed to provide students with a thorough understanding of the most common procedures and techniques of the current CLIA-waived tests and of cardiopulmonary diagnostic tests as they apply to the ambulatory care setting. The first two chapters provide an introduction to the clinical laboratory and the government regulations for setting up a CLIA-waived laboratory. The remaining chapters, 3 through 10, present a consistent "triad" organization by first focusing on the *fundamental concepts* related to the procedures presented in each chapter, followed by the *application of the procedures,* and then concluding with *advanced concepts* to stimulate critical thinking. Procedure boxes are integrated throughout with step-by-step instructions that are reinforced with numerous full-color photographs or illustrations. Throughout the text there is also a strong emphasis placed on proper patient interactions, specimen collections, safety, and government compliance. Written exams are provided to measure cognitive (conceptual) competency. Measurable outcome-based procedure sheets and evaluation forms are provided in the workbook to measure psychomotor and affective (behavioral) competencies.

When writing the workbook and instructor materials, our intention was to provide instructors and health care practitioners with many customizable tools that will help them produce well-trained, qualified allied health professionals who are able to effectively work in the CLIA-waived laboratory setting, and in ambulatory settings where cardiopulmonary tests are performed.

Outstanding Features

More than 600 full-color photographs, illustrations, and tables provide powerful visual learning tools that are reinforced in the PowerPoint lectures and in the workbook. Each of the testing chapters is organized into three sections to bring the reader through progressive levels of learning:

- Fundamental Concepts
- Procedures
- Advanced Concepts

This organization allows students and instructors to move from "seeing and understanding" the basic concepts to "performing the procedures" to "problem solving and more difficult concepts."

NOTE: In general, the first two sections of each chapter consist of material students must know and be able to perform, whereas the last section, "Advanced Concepts," allows instructors to determine the level of information the students will need to learn.

Laboratory and diagnostic terms are presented at the beginning of each chapter and are boldfaced throughout the chapter. The terms are also reinforced via the workbook and Evolve resources exercises. Ambulatory medicine has an abundance of terms that must be mastered to understand and communicate the testing concepts and procedures effectively.

Included with the purchase of this book is access to interactive web resources, located at **http://evolve.elsevier.com/Garrels/laboratory,** which provides a variety of exercises and activities to reinforce learning, including the following:

- *Comprehensive printable "structured notes"* outlines for each chapter. Students are able to print chapter outlines with fill-in-the-blanks that can be found in their text or during the PowerPoint lecture. The filled-out "structured notes" outline provides an excellent source of review for each chapter.
- *PowerPoint lectures* that are enhanced with corresponding text images and that provide the answers to the fill-in-the-blanks structured notes.
- *Drag-and-drop terminology,* which quizzes students on essential key terms and topics learned in the chapters.
- *Labeling exercises* that give students a chance to practice key concepts learned in the textbook (e.g., labeling the parts of a microscope).
- *Animations, videos, and lessons* that complement the content in the textbook and give students a chance to interactively engage in learning the material.
- *Clinical skills videos* that show various skills essential to students' success. Topics of the videos range from asepsis, infection control, and sterilization; to collecting and testing urine, blood, and microbiological specimens; to performing hematology, blood chemistry, immunology, toxicology, and cardiopulmonary tests. The videos provide students with a great tool to visualize concepts learned in the textbook chapters.
- *Log sheets and forms,* taken from the appendix in the workbook, are available to print and/or edit as needed. These additional log sheets and forms

include laboratory forms, record-keeping logs, generic procedure sheets (if a student's program uses a method other than what is presented in the textbook), a sample health assessment form, a student professionalism evaluation form (for measuring behavioral competencies), and much more.

New to This Edition

In this new and exciting third edition, the text has been updated and expanded to provide better coverage on a multitude of topics. This additional material will help students and instructors to work together as a team in order to discover and learn about the most up-to-date procedures and concepts. The reader will find that every chapter has been updated for this new edition, and that each chapter incorporates new information to assist in the learning process. Important additions include the following:

- More than 70 new pictures and drawings.
- Updates on government regulations in Chapters 1 and 2.
- Updates on proper collection and processing of urine specimens, microbiology specimens, blood capillary and venipuncture specimens, which include nasal swab for influenza specimen collections, and an expanded blood draw complications section.
- Six new CLIA-waived laboratory procedures with corresponding skill check sheets—30-minute ESR test using the Streck method, iFOB test for fecal occult blood, i-STAT chemistry procedure, oral and blood testing methods for HIV, rapid urine culture testing.
- A new chapter on cardiopulmonary diagnostic tests (Chapter 10) with fundamental concepts on heart and lung function, and the following five new procedures with corresponding skill check sheets—performing a *12-lead ECG* using a three-channel instrument and/or a computerized method, *Spirometry testing* using a computerized method, *Peak Expiratory Flow Monitoring* with patient instructions and setup, and *Holter Monitoring* with patient instructions and setup.

Workbook for *Laboratory and Diagnostic Testing in Ambulatory Care* (ISBN 978-1-4557-7248-3)

This valuable learning tool for the student contains measurable outcomes for all the conceptual and competency-based objectives in each chapter in order to fulfill national accreditation standards. Accreditation agencies now require measurable outcomes along with competency-based objectives.

It contains *Skill Competency Check Sheets* for specimen collections and patient instructions, and *Diagnostic Testing Check Sheets* for each of the laboratory and diagnostic tests performed. The testing procedures are organized into *preanalytical*, *analytical*,

and *postanalytical* testing phases. These sheets can be used in the classroom and clinical laboratory settings to verify individual competency that meets the "Good Laboratory Practice" criteria for quality assurance. In this new edition, 11 new procedure sheets have been added (to correspond with the 11 new procedures in the text).

The appendix includes useful quality control log sheets, lab maintenance log sheets, report forms, a sample health screening assessment form, and a sample student/employee professional evaluation form. These forms provide the necessary documentation needed to prove laboratory quality assurance, safety compliance, and proper charting of test results.

TEACH Instructor's Resources for *Laboratory and Diagnostic Testing in Ambulatory Care,* located on the Evolve site at http://evolve.elsevier.com/Garrels/laboratory

The *TEACH Instructor's Resource Manual* was created to provide instructors or CLIA-waived lab supervisors with a wealth of material needed to run a successful class or clinical laboratory. All the material has been "field-tested" to help ensure the accuracy and quality of material. This valuable tool is available on-line in Word document format, so that instructors have the ability to edit and update the files to suit their own needs. The *TEACH Instructor's Resource Manual* on Evolve contains:

- TEACH lesson plans to help you prepare for class and make full use of the rich array of ancillaries and resources that come with your textbook. They are organized into easily understandable sections—Instructor Preparation, Student Preparation, the 50-Minute Lesson Plan, an Assessment Plan, and a Laboratory Activities Plan.
- In TEACH, the content covered in each textbook chapter is divided across several lesson plans, each designed to occupy 50 minutes of class time. The consistent time for each lesson plan allows you to re-sequence them in any order to fit your class calendar. And if you are using TEACH lesson plans from multiple Elsevier textbooks their "building block" timing and design make it especially easy to combine them, even within the same class period.
- Information on how to set up course schedules, grading, record keeping, and so forth.
- Field-tested tips and supplies needed for each chapter.
- Structured notes for students that follow the chapter lecture outlines and include fill-in-the-blank answers.
- Comprehensive PowerPoint lecture slides that include the procedures covered in each chapter and provide the answers to the students' structured notes. (NOTE: The PowerPoint lectures are also available in the student resources.)

- An Image library of all the images found in the text organized by chapter. NOTE: The procedure images are located at the end of all the text pictures in each chapter.
- Answer keys to student workbook exercises.
- Interactive electronic skill check-off sheets that will provide a numerical outcome result.
- Test Bank in ExamView format.

Evolve Course Management System for *Laboratory and Diagnostic Testing in Ambulatory Care:* http://evolve.elsevier.com/Garrels/laboratory

Evolve is an interactive learning environment that works in conjunction with *Laboratory and Diagnostic Testing in Ambulatory Care: A Guide for Health Care Professionals,* providing Internet-based course content that reinforces and expands on the concepts that instructors deliver in class. In addition to the resources available to students, instructors are able to access all of the components of the *TEACH Instructor's Resource Manual* previously listed.

Instructors may also use Evolve to:

- Publish class syllabi, outlines, and lecture notes.
- Set up "virtual office hours" and email communication.
- Share important dates and information through the on-line class *Calendar.*
- Encourage student participation through *Chat Rooms* and *Discussions Boards.*

Online Learning

The wealth of materials provided with this product suite (textbook, Workbook, and Evolve resources for both the student and instructor) also lends itself to being used in an online learning environment. In an online atmosphere, students can read the textbook, fill in the structured notes (from the PowerPoint slides on Evolve), and complete their workbook exercises, all at home (and all at their own pace) prior to arriving on campus for their hands-on lab session. Using this method, the face-to-face student-instructor time could be fully devoted to reinforcing the text material, demonstrating the lab skills, and checking out the students in the lab.

Acknowledgments

I would like to acknowledge the valuable input of all the reviewers, medical assisting educators, and students who have helped to make this third edition even better than the previous editions.

I am grateful to all the Elsevier publishers, editors, reviewers, and staff who have personally supported and guided me through this exciting adventure: Adrianne Rippinger, Rae Robertson, Katherine Judge, Elizabeth Tinsley, Michael Ledbetter, Susan Cole, Jennifer Bertucci, Jennifer Hermes, David Stein, Jeanne Genz, Kristen Mandava, and Jayashree Balasubramaniam. I am thankful to have had the opportunity to work with Carol Oatis, co-author of the first edition.

It has been a pleasure to see the wonderful talents of my son-in-law and daughter, Zack and Gala Bent, who have graciously provided us with almost 200 of the high-quality, up-to-date procedure photos and drawings during all three editions. I have also been blessed by the unwavering support from my husband, Mike. Thanks for seeing me through this arduous process!

Marti Garrels, MSA, MT (ASCP), CMA (AAMA)

I would like to thank my family for all of their support during the time that I was involved in the writing of the first edition of this textbook. Also, it has been a great pleasure to work with my co-author, Marti Garrels, who is a tremendous asset to the medical assisting profession.

Carol Oatis, MSEd, MT SM (ASCP), CMA (AAMA)

Contents

Procedures

1 Introduction to the Laboratory and Safety Training

OBJECTIVES   *After completing this chapter you should be able to do the following:*

1. Define and match key terms and abbreviations in this chapter.

Introduction to the Clinical Laboratory

2. List the reasons why laboratory tests are ordered, and describe how specimens are analyzed.
3. Do the following regarding the types of medical laboratories and their personnel:
   - Describe the organization and function of medical laboratories.
   - Compare the advantages of performing laboratory tests in a physician's office laboratory versus an outside reference laboratory.
   - Identify the educational credentials of various personnel who work in laboratories.
   - Describe the necessary attributes required of the laboratory professional.
4. Identify and use laboratory requisitions and reports with proper documentation and confidentiality.
5. Interpret common metric system values used in laboratory test reporting.

Safety Training

6. Explain the categories of hazards found in medical laboratories.
7. Do the following regarding the CDC's Standard Precautions for infection control:
   - Explain the steps involved in the "chain of infection."
   - Identify and apply the CDC's latest Standard Precautions for infection control and its recommendations regarding proper hand hygiene.
   - Perform a medical hand wash followed by application of PPE and proper removal of PPE.
   - Locate Internet sources for updates on CDC and OSHA recommendations regarding laboratory safety.
8. Do the following regarding OSHA regulations and training:
   - Explain the latest OSHA regulations regarding the Bloodborne Pathogens Standard and the Hazard Communication Standard
   - Identify waste classified as biohazardous, and select appropriate containers for disposal.
   - Describe the proper actions that should be taken after exposure to bloodborne pathogens.
   - Complete a mock exposure incident report in the workbook appendix.
   - List and explain the safety rules that must be observed in the laboratory.
   - Identify and note the location of safety equipment, apparel, and safety manuals in the classroom laboratory.
   - Successfully complete a posttest on safety training.
   - Locate Internet sources for updates on OSHA regulations regarding laboratory safety.

KEY TERMS

ambulatory setting outpatient facility versus hospital or bedridden setting

analyte the substance being tested, such as glucose or cholesterol in a blood specimen

biohazard danger related to exposure to infectious and bloodborne pathogens

bloodborne pathogens infectious microorganisms that are transmitted by blood or bloody body fluids from an infected host into the blood of a susceptible host

Bloodborne Pathogens Standard (BBPS) rigorous standard of policies and procedures developed by OSHA to protect employees who work in occupations where they are at risk of exposure to blood or other potentially infectious materials (i.e., other body fluids that may contain blood)

CD4 cell a T lymphocytic white blood cell that fights infections

chemical hazard danger related to exposure to toxic, unstable, explosive, or flammable substances

chronic disorders long-lasting, debilitating conditions

CLIA-waived tests tests that provide simple, unvarying results and require a minimum amount of judgment and interpretation

clinical laboratory a facility or an area within a medical setting in which materials or specimens from the human body are examined or analyzed

coagulation clotting ability of blood

contaminated an area that has been in contact with infectious materials or surfaces where infectious organisms may reside

C-reactive protein (CRP) protein associated with myocardial infarctions (heart attacks)

critical value a test result far from the reference range indicating a threat to a patient's health (also referred to as "panic value")

cross-contamination transmitting a pathogen from one individual to another

diabetes mellitus disease caused by the lack of insulin or the inability to regulate blood sugar (glucose) levels

don to put on

engineering controls efforts and research toward isolating or removing bloodborne pathogens from the workplace (i.e., biohazard disposal containers, safety devices on needles, and sharps containers)

ergonomic practices proper movements and conditions that make a worker less prone to work-related injuries

exposure control plan documented plan provided by a facility to eliminate or minimize occupational exposure to bloodborne pathogens

glucose sugar

Hazard Communication Standard federal law protecting employees' "right to know" about the dangers of all the hazardous chemicals to which they may be exposed under normal working conditions

hepatitis A virus (HAV) highly contagious virus that enters the body through the gastrointestinal tract and attacks the liver

hepatitis B virus (HBV) most prevalent bloodborne virus that attacks the liver: an individual can build a protective resistance against this virus by prior immunization or vaccination

hepatitis C virus (HCV) bloodborne virus that attacks the liver and is very likely to reach the chronic stage later in life

homeostasis steady state of internal chemical and physical balance

human immunodeficiency virus (HIV) retrovirus that attacks the immune system by destroying the white blood cells known as CD4+ T lymphocytes

laboratory reports results of laboratory tests that have been ordered

laboratory requisitions laboratory orders indicating the tests that should be performed

medical assistants multiskilled professionals dedicated to assisting in patient care management in medical offices, clinics, and ambulatory care centers

nosocomial infection disease spread within a health care facility (also referred to as HCAIs [health care associated infections])

occupational exposure occurs when blood or other potentially infectious material comes in contact with open skin, eyes, or mucous membranes, or by parenteral exposure (through the skin) in the workplace

opportunistic infections infections that occur because of the body's inability to repel pathogens normally found in the environment

panels/profiles a series of tests associated with a particular organ or disease

parenteral contact when blood enters the body through the skin or mucous membrane by means of a needle stick, bite, cut, or abrasion

pathogen disease-causing microorganism

patient compliance a patient's willingness to follow a treatment plan and take an active role in his or her health care

percutaneous through the skin

physical hazards dangers related to electricity, fire, weather emergencies, bomb threats, and accidental injuries

polydipsia excessive thirst

polyphagia excessive hunger

polyuria excessive urination

portal of entry a body opening or break in the skin through which an infectious agent enters the body

portal of exit the route by which an infectious agent leaves the host's body, such as through the mouth, broken skin, rectum, or body fluids

reference range the numerical range of analyte values with which the general population will consistently show similar results 95% of the time

reservoir host an infected person who is carrying an infectious agent (pathogen)

Standard Precautions CDC recommendations for infection control within health care facilities

susceptible host an individual who is unable to defend herself or himself against a pathogen

thrombosis the formation of internal clots

transient microorganisms organisms from contaminated objects or infectious patients that adhere to the skin and can be transmitted to others

transmission the means by which an infectious agent or pathogen is transported from an infected individual to another person by indirect or direct contact

Universal Precautions assumption that blood or other potentially infectious material from any patient or test kit could be infectious

venipuncture removal of blood from a vein

work practice controls policies that are recorded, monitored, and evaluated to protect employees from exposure to the pathogens in blood or body fluids

ABBREVIATIONS

CDC Centers for Disease Control and Prevention
HCAIs health care associated infections
HHS Health and Human Services
HMIS Hazardous Materials Information System
MSDS material safety data sheets
NFPA National Fire Protective Association
OPIM other potentially infectious material, such as bloody body fluids

OSHA Occupational Safety and Health Administration
PEP postexposure prophylaxis; preventive treatment after exposure to blood or OPIM
POCT point-of-care testing
POL physician's office laboratory
PPE personal protective equipment

To enter the investigative world of medical laboratories, a general understanding of laboratory testing and the various laboratories that perform medical tests on specimens is needed. Then, a solid foundation in laboratory safety issues is required before laboratory procedures can be performed in the **ambulatory setting** (outpatient facility versus hospital or bedridden setting).

Introduction to the Clinical Laboratory

The medical laboratory plays a critical role in patient care. This section provides information on the following:

- Why and how laboratory tests are performed
- Where the tests are performed
- How various medical laboratories are organized
- The people involved in the testing process
- The basic terminology and paperwork used in the laboratory

Purpose of Medical Laboratories

A medical or **clinical laboratory** is defined as a facility or an area within a medical setting in which materials, or specimens, from the human body are examined or analyzed. The results of the various laboratory tests performed on the specimens give the physician a wealth of information regarding the status of the patient or client.

Why Laboratory Tests Are Ordered

Physicians order laboratory tests for one or more of the three following reasons:

To Screen Patients for Possible Disorders

Screening test results are used to determine if a disease or medical condition exists in patients who may not have signs or symptoms of an underlying disease process. These tests are becoming increasingly popular because they can detect potential **chronic disorders** (long-lasting, debilitating conditions) such as coronary heart disease and diabetes well before irreversible damage occurs. Primary care physician offices and community health centers are encouraged by the latest Medicare policies to participate in screening programs. NOTE: The workbook appendix has a health screening report form that includes the various screening tests that will be presented throughout the text and in the laboratory sessions.

To Establish a Diagnosis

Diagnostic test results help the physician identify or confirm a disease or medical condition. These results can significantly affect the medical care and treatment of the patient. Diagnostic tests should be conducted by well-trained individuals and must correlate with other clinical findings (e.g., the patient's medical history and physical examination).

To Monitor the Patient's Condition or Treatment

Monitoring test results helps the physician keep track of the patient's specific medical condition or response to treatment on a periodic basis. The following three medical conditions commonly require routine testing to monitor the effects of medication treatments:

- *Patients at risk of heart disease* who are taking cholesterol-lowering medications are checked periodically for levels of cholesterol and liver enzymes. The medication goal is to bring cholesterol levels to less than 200 mg/dL and to determine whether the medication is harming the liver, which would raise the levels of the blood enzymes alanine aminotransferase (ALT) and aspartate aminotransferase (AST) (this will be covered in Chapter 6). They may also be tested for **C-reactive protein (CRP),** which is associated with myocardial infarction (heart attack) and indicates the health status of the patient's cardiovascular system.
- *Patients at risk of forming internal clots* **(thrombosis)** who are taking anticoagulant medications are checked to see if their blood **coagulation** (clotting) time is too fast or too slow.
- *Patients with diabetes* have their blood sugar levels checked periodically at the office. They also may have their self-monitored blood sugar results interpreted by the physician. In both cases the physician needs to determine if these patients are maintaining blood sugar levels within the recommended **reference range** (the numerical range of analyte values with which the general population will consistently show similar results 95% of the time).

Advances in medical instrumentation have allowed the monitoring of all these patients to take place in an ambulatory setting rather than in a hospital or reference laboratory. This allows the physician to see the results immediately, while the patient waits, and then advise the patient accordingly.

Three General Ways to Analyze Specimens

Medical laboratories analyze specimens in the following three basic ways:

Measuring the Levels of Analytes Compared with Reference Values

The human body is a remarkable organism, capable of maintaining **homeostasis** (a steady state of internal chemical and physical balance). This universal ability is seen when a healthy population is tested for the presence of a particular **analyte** (a substance being tested, such as the level of glucose or cholesterol in a blood specimen). Most of the population will test within a range of similar results. This is referred to as the reference range for that analyte. When disease strikes, a person's homeostatic balance is disrupted, causing the analyte results to fall outside the reference range.

Figure 1-1 is an example of a reference laboratory's comprehensive report for blood tests. Note that the reference range for each analyte tested is listed above the patient's test value. If a test result is far from the reference range, it may be referred to as a **critical value**

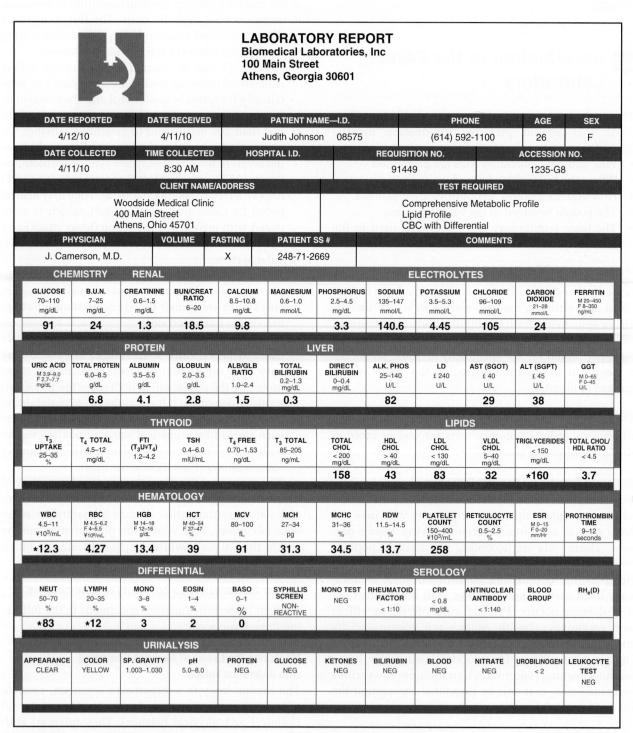

Fig. 1-1 Blood test report showing the levels of a comprehensive panel of analytes. Compare the patient's results with the reference range found above each of the patient's values. Note the four results that fall outside of their reference ranges. In this report the TRIGLYCERIDES, WBC (white blood cells), and NEUT (neutrophils) are high, and the LYMPH (lymphocytes) are low. *(From Bonewit-West K: Clinical procedures for medical assistants, ed 9, St Louis, 2015, Saunders.)*

or *panic value* (indicating a threat to a patient's health). The laboratory report must mark or highlight the critical result requiring immediate attention. In the figure, Judith Johnson does not have any critical values. But she does have a few values outside of the reference range as indicated with an asterisk (*). A variety of **laboratory reports** are shown and discussed throughout this text.

Here is an example of a critical value that may be obtained by monitoring the level of a patient's **glucose** (sugar) analyte and comparing it to its established population's reference range. A physician obtained a variety of abnormal clinical signs and symptoms when examining a female patient—rapid weight loss, lack of energy, **polyphagia** (excessive hunger), **polydipsia** (excessive thirst), and **polyuria** (excessive urination). These symptoms caused the physician to suspect the disease **diabetes mellitus** (a disease caused by the lack of insulin or the inability to regulate blood sugar levels). The physician then ordered a blood glucose test and received a result of 300 mg/dL (milligrams per deciliter). The population's reference range for blood glucose levels was 70 to 110 mg/dL. The patient's extremely high (critical) glucose result, along with all the other signs and symptoms, indicated that her pancreas was unable to produce the insulin necessary to regulate glucose levels in a homeostatic way. A repeat fasting blood glucose test showed the same high result that confirmed the diagnosis of diabetes. The physician then prescribed a course of treatment and continued to monitor the blood glucose levels until the patient's test results returned to the proper reference range.

Observing and Detecting Abnormal Cells under the Microscope

Another way to analyze a specimen is to search for abnormal cells or **pathogens** (disease-causing microorganisms) under the microscope. In the ambulatory

Fig. 1-2 Microscopic analysis of a urine specimen, with a red blood cell on the left and a budding yeast cell on the right. *(From Stepp CA, Woods M: Laboratory procedures for medical office personnel, Philadelphia, 1998, Saunders.)*

setting this form of testing is generally limited to basic identification of abnormal cells and microorganisms found in urine, blood, or samples taken from infected tissues. Figure 1-2 shows the abnormal presence of red blood cells and yeast cells in a urine specimen.

This book discusses some of the normal and abnormal microscopic findings in urine, blood, and microbiology specimens to highlight their significance. Additional training beyond this text is required to identify and report microscopic findings.

Detecting the Presence or Absence of an Infection

The third way to analyze specimens is to test for the presence of pathogens causing an infection. In the ambulatory setting increasing numbers of rapid screening tests are available to help the physician identify the presence of common pathogens. Figure 1-3 shows the Rapid Strep test results from two throat-swabbed

Fig. 1-3 Analyzing the presence of group A strep. **A** is negative and **B** is positive for strep throat infection. *(From Mahon CR, Manuselis G: Textbook of diagnostic microbiology, ed 5, St Louis, 2015, Saunders. Courtesy Becton Dickinson.)*

specimens. The test result shown on the left is negative for streptococcus A, and the test on the right is positive for streptococcus A. For example, test *kits* (all components of a test packaged together) are available that can detect the presence of bacteria that cause strep throat, peptic ulcers, and Lyme disease as well as the viruses that cause influenza, mononucleosis, and acquired immunodeficiency syndrome (AIDS).

Further microscopic, chemical, and growth analysis of the pathogen, along with analysis of the pathogen's sensitivity to antibiotics, is performed by sending the infected swabbed specimen to a microbiology laboratory.

Types of Medical Laboratories and Personnel

The types of medical laboratories range from large, departmentalized institutions to small designated laboratory counters within an ambulatory setting. Personnel in the ambulatory setting interact with staff from all the other types of laboratories and need a basic understanding of how the various laboratories are organized and what types of health care professionals work in each setting.

Reference (or Referral) Laboratories

Reference, or referral, laboratories tend to be the largest laboratories, with specialized departments and extensive state-of-the-art equipment. Figure 1-4 is a sample organizational chart showing the departments typically found in a reference laboratory facility: Specimen Collection and Processing, Hematology, Chemistry, Immunology/Immunohematology, Microbiology, Pathology, and Toxicology.

Reference Laboratory Professionals

- **Pathologists** are physicians with doctorate degrees who have specialized in test methodology and the diagnosis of diseases.
- **Clinical laboratory scientists** and **medical technologists** have master's and bachelor's degrees, are specialists in laboratory testing, and have received one of the following nationally recognized credentials: MT (ASCP), MT (AMT), CLS (NCA), RMT (ISCLT), or CLT.
- **Medical technicians** have 2-year associate degrees in laboratory training and have received one of the following nationally recognized credentials: MLT (ASCP), MLT (AMT), CLT (NCA), or RLT (ISCLT).
- **Phlebotomists** have received one of the following nationally recognized credentials: PBT (ASCP), RPT (AMT), CPT (ASPT), CPT (NHA), and others.

These teams of laboratory professionals collect, process, and evaluate volumes of tests daily and are heavily regulated by the government to ensure that they produce accurate and reliable test results. It is interesting to note that 80% of final definitive diagnoses come from the results of laboratory tests. The testing methods in each department require extensive training in instrument maintenance, problem-solving, test interpretation, and statistical monitoring of test reliability.

Medical offices, health clinics, and hospitals send either their clients or their clients' specimens along with **laboratory requisitions** (laboratory orders indicating the tests that should be performed) to the reference lab. Some insurance companies require a specific reference laboratory for their clients. The client's specimen and requisition must go to the correct reference laboratory for proper insurance reimbursement.

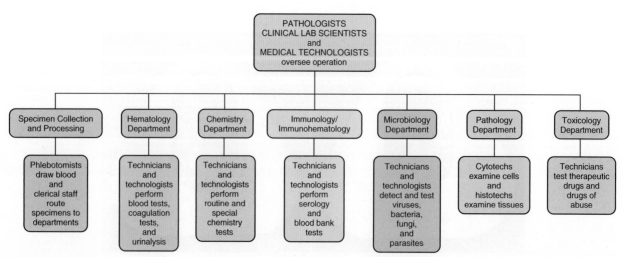

Fig. 1-4 Organizational chart for reference and hospital laboratories showing the departments and individuals involved in testing.

Hospital Laboratories

Hospital laboratories are organized into departments and staffed similarly to reference laboratories. They are involved in diagnostic testing and monitoring the testing of inpatients as well as specimen collection and testing of outpatient specimens from ambulatory settings.

New technology has provided a new approach to patient testing in hospitals called point-of-care testing (**POCT**). Rather than sending specimens to the laboratory, a testing device can be brought directly to the patient's bedside and accurate results can be immediately obtained. These user-friendly portable tests are administered by nurses and other health care professionals (e.g., critical care technicians) when a patient's medical condition, location, or treatment requires immediate results to determine proper medical care. Figure 1-5 shows a patient's blood glucose readout of 71 mg/dL on a point-of-care glucometer.

Another popular point-of-care instrument is the i-STAT portable clinical analyzer (PCA) seen in Chapter 6. It uses disposable cartridges to determine a variety of analytes in whole blood. The analyzer stores up to 50 patient records and permits on-screen viewing of test results. It is capable of transmitting the results to a data management system by using infrared signals. Nonlaboratory hospital personnel must be trained to perform POCT properly.

Ambulatory Care Settings

Unlike the extensive reference laboratories and hospital laboratories, an ambulatory laboratory generally consists of a small, limited space located within

a designated area of the physician's office. Ambulatory care settings generally perform tests that have been designated by the government as **CLIA-waived tests** (tests that provide simple, unvarying results and require a minimal amount of judgment and interpretation). These government-approved tests provide rapid POCT for screening and monitoring patients in a variety of laboratory areas. The CLIA-waived user-friendly tests most frequently performed in the ambulatory setting that will be presented in this text are the following:

- Routine urinalysis and pregnancy testing
- Basic hematology tests—hemoglobin, hematocrit, sedimentation rate
- Coagulation—prothrombin time and its computed international normalized ratio result
- Chemistry—glucose, hemoglobin A_{1c}, lipid panel, alanine aminotransferase (ALT) and aspartate aminotransferase (AST), electrolytes, blood urea nitrogen (BUN), creatinine, and carbon dioxide (CO_2)
- Immunology/serology—mononucleosis test, *Helicobacter pylori* test, OraQuick test for HIV
- Microbiology—rapid tests for streptococcus A, influenza A/B, rapid urine culture
- Fecal occult blood

The physician's office laboratory (**POL**) has greatly benefited and will continue to benefit from the technical advancements that have improved and simplified so many medical testing methods.

Advantages of POL Testing

Ambulatory patients can now obtain their screening and monitoring test results immediately rather than needing to drive to an external laboratory. Also, the physician's interpretation and therapeutic recommendations can now be given during the same office visit. This has led to better patient care and **patient compliance** (a patient's willingness to follow a treatment plan and take an active role in his or her own health care).

Advantages of Reference and Hospital Laboratories

Advantages are to provide physicians with the results of the more complex tests. Patient specimens must be sent to these laboratories for the critical test results that provide the physician with sufficient information to make definitive diagnoses. Because of the complexity of these diagnostic tests, they must be performed by individuals with extensive laboratory training, education, and credentialing. A complete description of such knowledge and training is beyond the scope of this book.

Physician Office Laboratory (POL) Personnel

POL personnel are physicians, physician assistants, nurse practitioners, medical assistants, and/or phlebotomists. **Medical assistants** are multiskilled

Fig. 1-5 POCT with a glucometer to determine the patient's blood glucose level. The specimen, taken from the patient's finger, registers 71 mg/dL, normal for a fasting glucose level.

professionals who assist in patient care management in medical offices, clinics, and ambulatory care centers. They perform administrative duties and clinical procedures, including performing phlebotomies and the basic CLIA-waived laboratory tests, and diagnostic cardiopulmonary tests. Medical assistants attend a 1- or 2-year program and are nationally credentialed as CMA (AAMA), RMA (AMT), NCMA (NCCT), or CCMA (NHA). There may also be laboratory technicians and technologists working in the larger POLs that service multiple physicians.

Table 1-1 lists all the health care professionals involved in medical laboratory and diagnostic testing. They are organized by educational credentials, from doctorates to associate degrees and technical certificates. (NOTE: Nurses are not listed because laboratory training is not part of their education. They are often trained while working in physicians' offices.)

Attributes of a Laboratory Professional

Everyone performing laboratory tests, regardless of educational background and credentials or place of work, must possess the following personal characteristics to guarantee proper patient care:

- Professional attitude—discreet, respectful, proper attire and personal hygiene
- Strong interpersonal communication skills with patients, co-workers, and supervisors
- Motivation, efficiency, commitment, and dedication to serving others in need
- Good organizational skills when setting up a series of tests—ability to manage time and multitask

Table 1-1   Personnel Involved in Laboratory Testing

Title	Credential	Years of College Training and Degree	Laboratory Setting
Board-certified pathologists and specialists	MD or DO	8 or more years: doctorate degree	Reference and hospital laboratories
Primary care physicians and specialists	MD or DO or ND (naturopathic doctor)	6 or more years: doctorate degree	Physician's office laboratory and health clinics
Physician Assistants and Nurse Practitioners	PA, NP	6 or more years: master's degree	Physician's office laboratory and health clinics
Clinical Laboratory Scientist, Medical Technologist, Clinical Laboratory Technologist	CLS (NCA) MT (ASCP) MT (AMT) RMT (ISCLT) CLT (HHS)	4 or more years: bachelor's or master's degrees	Reference and hospital laboratories
Medical Laboratory Technician, Clinical Laboratory Technician, Registered Laboratory Technician	MLT (ASCP)* MLT (AMT)* CLT (NCA)* RLT (ISCLT)*	2 years: associate	Reference and hospital laboratories, and physician's office laboratories
Certified or Registered Medical Assistant	CMA (AAMA)* RMA (AMT)* NCMA (NCCT)* CCMA (NHA)*	1-2 years: technical certificate or associate degree	Physician's office laboratory and ambulatory setting laboratories
Clinical Laboratory Assistant, Medical Laboratory Assistant, Physician Office Laboratory Technician	CLA* MLA* POLT*	1-or less years: technical certificate	Physician's office laboratory and ambulatory setting laboratories
Certified and Registered Phlebotomist	PBT (ASCP)*, RPT (AMT)* CPT (ASPT)* CPT (NHA)* and others*	1 or less years: technical certificate	All laboratories needing blood specimen collection

*This book is designed to provide these professionals with the necessary information to perform specimen collection and CLIA-waived tests in ambulatory settings with confidence, accuracy, and precision.

- Focus, good power of observation, ability to pay attention to details during entire process
- Ability to solve problems if test results are unexpected
- Honesty, integrity, ability to admit when unsure of procedure or results
- Manual dexterity, using both hands to accomplish the task
- Ability to perform precise calculations and measurements and neatly document all findings
- Good eyesight and normal color vision for reading color changes on test strips

Laboratory Documentation

Everyone involved in medical laboratory testing and specimen processing must understand and complete the paperwork and the electronic data accurately and completely. The documentation begins with the physician's laboratory test order being entered onto a requisition form and ends with the laboratory report being evaluated and filed in the patient's chart.

Laboratory Requisitions

When ordering tests from outside reference and hospital labs, the laboratory professionals must understand all forms of written and electronic communication between their office and the laboratory. Communication begins when the physician orders a particular test or series of tests. The laboratory order is recorded on a requisition form that must be entirely completed. Different laboratories have different requisition forms, but most will require all the following areas to be completed, as seen in Figure 1-6.

Fig. 1-6 Bar code requisition and labels for matching specimens with their laboratory order. Note the bar code and its number at the top *(a)* as well as its corresponding peel-off labels with the same requisition number and space for the patient's name *(b)*. The reference laboratory may also have the patient sign the requisition and initial the labels to confirm identity.

1. Demographics on the patient: name, zip code, date of birth, and gender. These are used to identify the patient when collecting specimens.
2. Insurance and billing information for the patient
3. Specimen collection information: date, time, and if the patient is fasting
4. Priority status of specimen and where and how to send the reported results
5. Additional physicians needing the results
6. A listing of laboratory tests to be ordered. NOTE: Each test ordered has a procedure code on the left-hand side. (These codes are found in the latest CPT coding reference book.) Each test must also have a diagnostic code written on the requisition for insurance purposes. Figure 1-6 has a line to the right of each test to add the ICD-9 codes. NOTE: The ICD-9 diagnostic reference code will be replaced by an ICD-10 updated coding reference, which will be a new alpha-numeric coding system.
7. Also notice in Figure 1-6 that the *(a)* **bar code** in the top left and the corresponding *(b)* **labels** on the left are removed and placed on the specimen before sending it to the laboratory

Electronic bar codes on requisitions are becoming more common, along with adhesive labels for the specimens, in an effort to eliminate specimen identification errors and maintain confidentiality. When these convenient labels are used, confirmation of the patient's identity with at least three identifiers is crucial (e.g., patient's name spelled out, birth date, phone number, or picture identification). As an additional safeguard, the patient should write his or her name on the bar code label placed on the requisition and on the specimen labels.

Figure 1-7 is another example of a laboratory requisition with a detailed organization of laboratory tests divided into the following categories:

- **Panels/profiles**—a series of tests associated with a particular organ or disease
- Hematology/coagulation tests—focus on the numbers and quality of blood cells and coagulation
- Chemistry tests—measure the levels of various chemicals, enzymes, and hormones
- Serology/immunology tests—analyze blood serum for evidence of infection or disease by evaluating antigen-antibody reactions in the laboratory
- Microbiology tests—identify the pathogen that is causing the disease
- Toxicology tests—measure the therapeutic levels and abuse of toxic drugs
- Urinalysis tests—indicate the health status of the urinary tract and the liver and the presence of diabetes

Notice how each test item has its five-digit procedure code on the left that is used for insurance billing. Each test item also has a collection container abbreviation on the right that tells the office which color-coded blood collection tube to use or which type of microbiology or urine specimen container to use. The codes are explained at the bottom of the requisition.

When the requisition is entirely completed, it goes to the laboratory with the patient or with the patient's specimen (e.g., blood, urine).

Laboratory Reports

After the specimen has been tested, the laboratory calls in or sends the results on a laboratory report (refer back to the results of laboratory tests as was seen in Figure 1-1). Another type of report is a computer printout, which shows the results of a chemistry panel of tests (Figure 1-8).

New health care laws also allow laboratory results to be sent to patients if they request.

All laboratory reports must be reviewed by the physician as soon as possible. The physician must sign and date the report. Depending on the results of the test, the physician may need to see or contact the patient. Each office has a specific protocol regarding how the patient is notified. Be sure to follow the protocol, and then file the report in the patient's file folder after charting any additional information. Understanding the process and making sure all parties are informed in a timely manner are crucial.

Laboratory Measurements

Medical laboratories must communicate their test results in a universal way. Therefore all laboratories report their results with international metric units for weight, volume, and length. Tables 1-2, 1-3, and 1-4 show the most common metric units used in medical laboratory reports.

Analytes measured in a liquid such as blood or urine are frequently expressed on laboratory reports in milligrams per deciliter (mg/dL). This is an expression of concentration, which is the *weight* of the analyte per *volume* of the specimen. If the analyte is very small, it is expressed in micrograms (mcg), where 1 mcg is 1/1,000,000 of a gram. NOTE: Use of "mcg" is preferred over the lower case Greek letter "μ" because of possible lab errors caused by misinterpretation: the Institute for Safe Medication Practices (ISMP, 2004) has published a list of error-prone abbreviations and strongly recommends that the use of "μg" be discontinued.

Many tests are temperature sensitive and must either be stored at room temperature or be refrigerated. The Centigrade temperature for refrigeration is usually 4° to 8° C (Figure 1-9), and room temperature is 15° to 30° C. (The workbook appendix for Chapter 1 contains a daily temperature monitoring chart that must be filled out daily if test kits or supplies are refrigerated and/or stored at room temperature.)

LABORATORY REQUISITION
Biomedical Laboratories, Inc.
100 Main Street
Athens, Georgia 45760

☐ Fax Send additional copy of report to:
☐ Call Client Number/Physician's Name ( ) Phone/Fax number
☐ Mail Physician's Address City, State, Zip

Patient's Name (Last)	(First)	(MI)	Sex	Date of Birth MO DAY YEAR	Collection Time : AM PM	Fasting YES NO	Collection Date MO DAY YEAR

NPI/UPIN	Physician's ID #	Patient's SS #	Patient's ID #	Urine hrs/vol hrs___ vol___

PATIENT

Physician's Name (Last, First)	Physician's Signature	Patient's Address	Phone
Medicare # (Include prefix/suffix)	☐ Primary ☐ Secondary	City	State ZIP
Medicaid # State	Physician's Provider #	Name of Responsible Party (if different from patient)	
Diagnosis/Signs/Symptoms in ICD-9 Format (Highest Specificity) REQUIRED		Address of Responsible Party (if different from patient) APT #	

RESP. PARTY
City State ZIP

INSURANCE

Patient's Relationship to Responsible Party ☐ 1–Self ☐ 2–Spouse ☐ 3–Child ☐ 4–Other

Insurance Company Name	Plan	Carrier Code
Subscriber/Member #	Location	Group #
Insurance Address	Physician's Provider #	
City	State	ZIP
Employer's Name or Number	Insured SS # (If not patient)	Worker's Comp ☐ Yes ☐ No

Performance Lab ☐ Carrier Group # Employee # Mem

I hereby authorize the release of medical information related to the service subscribed herein and authorize payment directed to LabCorp.
X _____ Patient's Signature _____ Date

MEDICARE ADVANCE BENEFICIARY NOTICE
I have read the ABN on the reverse. If Medicare denies payment, I agree to pay for the identified test(s).
X _____ Patient's Signature _____ Date

NOTE: WHEN ORDERING TESTS FOR WHICH MEDICARE OR MEDICAID REIMBURSEMENT WILL BE SOUGHT, PHYSICIANS SHOULD ONLY ORDER TESTS THAT ARE MEDICALLY NECESSARY FOR THE DIAGNOSIS OR TREATMENT OF THE PATIENT. COMPONENTS OF THE ORGAN OR DISEASE PANELS/COMBINATIONS PRINTED BELOW ARE SHOWN ON THE REVERSE SIDE AND MAY ALSO BE ORDERED INDIVIDUALLY BELOW. COMPONENTS MAY BE BILLED SEPARATELY PER CARRIER POLICY.

PROFILES (See reverse for components)

80049	Basic Metabolic Profile	SST
80054	Comp Metabolic Profile	SST
80051	Electrolyte Profile	SST
80058	Hepatic Profile	SST
80059	Hepatitis Profile	SST
80061	Lipid Profile	SST
80091	Thyroid Profile	SST
80055	Prenatal Profile	RED LAV
80072	Rheumatoid Profile	SST

HEMATOLOGY/COAGULATION

85025	CBC w Diff	LAV
85027	CBC w/o Diff	LAV
85014	Hematocrit	LAV
85018	Hemoglobin	LAV
85595	Platelet Count	LAV
85041	RBC Count	LAV
85048	WBC Count	LAV
85007	WBC Differential	LAV
89190	Nasal Smear, Eosin	Nasal Smear
85060	Pathologist Consult– Peripheral Smear	LAV
85651	Sed Rate	LAV
85610	Prothrombin Time (PT)	BLU
86900 86901	PT and PTT Activated	BLU
85730	PTT Activated	BLU

CHEMISTRY

82040	Albumin	SST
84075	Alkaline Phosphatase	SST
84460	ALT (SGPT)	SST
82150	Amylase, Serum	SST
84450	AST (SGOT)	SST

ALPHABETICAL TESTS CON'T

82607 82746	B₁₂ and Folate	SST
82250	Bilirubin, Total	SST
84520	BUN	SST
82310	Calcium	SST
82378	CEA	SST
82465	Cholesterol, Total	SST
82565	Creatinine	SST
82670	Estradiol	SST
82728	Ferritin, Serum	SST
82985	Fructosamine	SST
83001	FSH	SST
83001 83002	FSH and LH	SST
82977	GGT	SST
82947	Glucose, Plasma	GRY
82947	Glucose, Serum	SST
82950	Glucose, 2-hr. PP	SST
83036	Glycohemoglobin, Total	LAV
84703	hCG, Beta Subunit, Qual	SST
84702	hCG, Beta Subunit, Quant	SST
83718	HDL Cholesterol	SST
83036	Hemoglobin A₁c	LAV

SEROLOGY/IMMUNOLOGY

85610 85730	ABO and Rh	LAV
86038	Antinuclear Antibodies	SST
86677	Helicobacter pylori, IgG	SST
86706	Hep B Surface Antibody	SST
87340	Hep B Surface Antigen	SST
86803	Hep C Antibody	SST
86701	HIV Antibodies Serology	SST

ALPHABETICAL TESTS CON'T

83540	Iron, Total	SST
83540 83550	Iron and IBC	SST
83615	LDH	SST
83002	LH	SST
83690	Lipase	SER
83735	Magnesium, Serum	SST
84132	Potassium	SST
84146	Prolactin, Serum	SST
84153	Prostate-Specific Antigen	SST
84066	Prostatic Acid Phos	SST
84155	Protein, Total	SST
86431	Rheumatoid Arthritis Factor	SST
86592	RPR	SST
86762	Rubella Antibodies, IgG	SST
84295	Sodium	SST
84403	Testosterone	SST
84436	Thyroxine (T₄)	SST
84478	Triglycerides	SST
84480	Triiodothyronine (T₃)	SST
84443	TSH, High Sensitivity	SST
84550	Uric Acid	SST

TOXICOLOGY

80156	Carbamazepine (Tegretol®)	SER
80162	Digoxin	SER
80178	Lithium (Eskalith®)	SER
80184	Phenobarbital (Luminal®)	SER
80185	Phenytoin (Dilantin®)	SER
80198	Theophylline Toxicology	SER
80164	Valproic Acid (Depakene®)	SER

URINALYSIS

81003	Urinalysis	Microscopic on Positives	URN
81001	Urinalysis	with Microscopic	URN

MICROBIOLOGY See Reverse Side
☐ ENDOCERVICAL ☐ THROAT ☐ URINE
☐ STOOL ☐ URETHRAL INDICATE SOURCE

87070	Aerobic Bacterial Culture	Bact Trnspt
87490 87590	Chlamydia/GC DNA Probe w/ Confirmation on Positives	Probe Trnspt
87490 87590	Chlamydia/GC DNA Probe Without Confirmation	Probe Trnspt
87490	Chlamydia DNA Probe	Probe Trnspt
87081	Genital, Beta-Hemolytic Strep Cult, Group B	Bact Trnspt
87070	Genital Culture, Routine	Bact Trnspt
87070	Lower Respiratory Culture	Steril Trnspt
87590	N. gonorrhoeae DNA Probe	Probe Trnspt
87015 87211	Ova and Parasites	O & P Kit
87081 X2 87045	Stool Culture	Fecal Trnspt
87081	Throat, Beta-Hemolytic Strep Cult, Group A	Bact Trnspt
87060	Upper Respiratory Culture, Routine	Bact Trnspt
87086	Urine Culture, Routine	Urn Cul Trnspt

Clinical Information/Comments

OTHER TESTS/INDIVIDUAL COMPONENTS
TEST # TEST NAMES

LAB USE ONLY	STAT ☐998074	VENIPUNCTURE ☐998085	TRAVEL ☐998096	NON LABCORP ☐998239	VERBAL ORDER ☐998250	CHART ORDER ☐998261	HANDWRITTEN ☐998272	24 HR TUV ☐998283	PST/PSC #

CONTAINERS RECEIVED	SST SPUN	USST UNSPUN	SER SERUM TRNSPT	FRZ FRZ TRNS	RED RED	LAV LAVENDER	SLD SLIDE	BLU LT. BLUE	GRY GREY	GRN GREEN	RYB RYL BLU	YEL ACD	PLS PLASMA	URN URINE	24U 24 HR URINE	TA-U TART. ACID	FL FLUID	OT OTHER	BACT TRNSP	O & P KIT	PROBE TRNSP	URN CULT TRNSP	STERIL TRNSP	FECAL TRNSP	VIRAL TRNSP

300-0384

Fig. 1-7 Laboratory requisition. *(From Bonewit-West K: Clinical procedures for medical assistants, ed 9, St Louis, 2015, Saunders.)*

DATE AND TIME RECEIVED	ACCESSION NUMBER
10/20/2014 20:45	
LOCATION	DATE REPORTED
	10/21/2014

PHYSICIAN	PATIENT'S INFORMATION

TEST		RESULTS	REFERENCE RANGE	UNITS
Chemistry 23 - panel B				
Calcium, total, serum	LO	7.4	8.5-10.5	MG/DL
Phosphorus	LO	2.8	3.0-4.6	MG/DL
Uric acid	LO	3.2	3.5-7.2	MG/DL
Cholesterol	LO	123	151-240	MG/DL
Triglyceride		121	58-258	MG/DL
LDH		217	118-242	IU/L
SGOT (AST)	HI	41	10-37	IU/L
SGPT (ALT)	HI	45	10-40	IU/L
GGTP	LO	8	11-51	IU/L
Alkaline phosphatase		63	39-117	IU/L
Bilirubin, total		0.3	0.1-1.5	MG/DL
Albumin	LO	2.4	3.7-5.2	G/DL
Total protein	LO	3.6	6.0-8.5	G/DL
Albumin/globulin ratio		2.0	1.0-2.2	RATIO

Final report		(Summary)	Page 2 of 2	

Fig. 1-8 Blood chemistry laboratory report. Note the patient's results compared with the reference range and the additional column indicating if the result is "HI" or "LO" compared with the reference range. *(From Zakus SM: Mosby's clinical skills for medical assistants, ed 4, St Louis, 2001, Mosby.)*

Table 1-2 Metric Units of Measurement

Measurement	Metric Unit	Abbreviation	Relative Comparison to American Units
Weight	Gram	G, g, or gm	1 g is approximately the weight of a raisin and is used in place of ounces
			1 kg (the weight of 1000 g) is used in place of pounds
Volume	Liter	L or l	1 L is a little more than a quart (used in place of the liquid measurements cup, quart, and gallon)
			1 mL (1/1000 of a liter) is used in place of a liquid ounce or teaspoon
Length	Meter	M or m	A meter is a little longer than a yard
			Centimeters (1/100 of a meter) are used in place of inches
			Kilometers (1000 meters) are used in place of miles
Temperature	Centigrade (Celsius)	°C	0° C = freezing; 100° C = boiling
			(Fahrenheit: 32° F = freezing; 212° F = boiling)
			4°-8° C = refrigerator temperature storage
			15°-30° C = room temperature storage
			37° C = body temperature

Table 1-3 Common Metric System Prefixes Used in Laboratory Reports

Metric Prefix	Abbreviation	Value to Unit	Examples in Laboratory Reports
Deci-	d	1/10 or 0.1	dL or dl = deciliter (one tenth of a liter)
Centi-	c	1/100 or 0.01	cm = centimeter, cc = cubic centimeter (which is the same volume as a milliliter, one thousandth of a liter)
Milli-	m	1/1000 or 0.001	ml or mL = milliliter (one thousandth of a liter, which is the same as a cubic centimeter); mg = milligram (one thousandth of a gram)
Micro-	mc	1/1,000,000	mcg = microgram (one millionth of a gram) (NOTE>: When handwriting, use "mc" for micro, not the Greek letter μ.)

Table 1-4 Greenwich Time and International Military Time

Greenwich Time	Military Hours	Greenwich Time	Military Hours
1:00 AM	0100 hours	1:00 PM	1300 hours
2:00 AM	0200 hours	2:00 PM	1400 hours
3:00 AM	0300 hours	3:00 PM	1500 hours
4:00 AM	0400 hours	4:00 PM	1600 hours
5:00 AM	0500 hours	5:00 PM	1700 hours
6:00 AM	0600 hours	6:00 PM	1800 hours
7:00 AM	0700 hours	7:00 PM	1900 hours
8:00 AM	0800 hours	8:00 PM	2000 hours
9:00 AM	0900 hours	9:00 PM	2100 hours
10:00 AM	1000 hours	10:00 PM	2200 hours
11:00 AM	1100 hours	11:00 PM	2300 hours

Fig. 1-9 Thermometer used to monitor refrigerator temperature. The reading of 6° C, an acceptable refrigerator temperature, would be logged.

When a *liquid* is measured in the laboratory, the most common volume is milliliter (mL or ml), which may also be referred to as a cubic centimeter (cc; the use of cc is discouraged, however, because it is often mistaken as "u," meaning units [ISMP, 2004]).

When the *length* of a test tube or a specimen within a capillary tube is measured, millimeters (mm) are used. There are approximately 25 mm in 1 inch, so 100 mm is approximately 4 inches.

NOTE: When recording whole numbers, *do not place a zero after the decimal* (e.g., the whole number 2 should be written 2, *not* 2.0). When recording a fraction, *a zero must be placed in front of the decimal* (e.g., one half should be written as 0.5, *not* .5).

Safety Training in the Laboratory

Potential hazards are present in the medical laboratory setting. Various government agencies have evaluated the most common laboratory dangers and created regulations and guidelines to help protect and to prevent harm to laboratory employees. These agencies continually monitor potential hazards and periodically update their regulations. Checking their websites and staying current with the latest changes and required dates of implementation are wise practices.

The hazards found in medical laboratories are divided into the following categories:

- **Biohazards**—dangers related to exposure to infectious or **bloodborne pathogens** (infectious microorganisms that are transmitted by the blood or bloody body fluid from an infected host into the blood of another)
- **Chemical hazards**—dangers related to exposure to toxic, unstable, explosive, or flammable materials
- **Physical hazards**—dangers related to electricity, fire, weather emergencies, bomb threats, and accidental injuries

Biohazard Training

Laboratory personnel must also learn how to prevent the spread of disease to themselves and others according to the regulations of two federal agencies: the Centers for Disease Control and Prevention (**CDC**) and the Occupational Safety and Health Administration (**OSHA**).

CDC and Infection Control

The basic means by which diseases are spread must be understood before beginning laboratory work.

Transmission and the Chain of Infection

For a disease to spread, the following conditions must exist as seen in Figure 1-10. A pathogen must be present in a **reservoir host** (an infected person who is carrying an infectious agent). The pathogen must then find a **portal** of exit (a means of leaving the infected host's body, e.g., through the mouth, broken skin, rectum, or body fluids). Next, each pathogen has a particular transportation mode or **transmission** (a means of transporting itself from the infected individual to another person, by direct or indirect contact, e.g., by air, food, hand-to-hand contact, insects, or body fluids). The pathogen must then find a **portal of entry** (a body opening or break in the skin) in another person. Once inside the new person, the pathogen will not cause disease unless the person is a **susceptible host** (an individual who is unable to protect himself or herself against the infectious agent). A susceptible person who becomes infected becomes a reservoir host, and the cycle begins again.

Health care workers must understand the chain of infection and endeavor to break the chain whenever possible to stop the spread of disease. If a disease is spread within a health care facility, it is referred to as a **nosocomial infection** (also referred to as **HCAIs** [health care associated infections]).

Standard Precautions

The CDC has issued a list of **Standard Precautions** for infection control within health care facilities (Figure 1-11). The most important way to stop the transmission of infectious disease, and first on the list, is hand washing. Next on the list is wearing various barriers

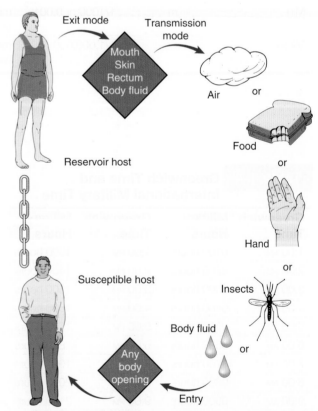

Fig. 1-10 Transmission and chain of infection. *(From Stepp CA, Woods M: Laboratory procedures for medical office personnel, Philadelphia, 1998, Saunders.)*

referred to as personal protective equipment (PPE), which is "specialized clothing or equipment worn by an employee for protection against infectious material." Examples of PPE are gloves, goggles, fluid-impermeable gowns, face shields, and masks. The remainder of the Standard Precautions list consists of recommendations for equipment disinfection, environmental control, linen disposal, bloodborne pathogen guidelines, and patient placement (e.g., in isolation within a hospital setting). The serious occupational hazard of blood-borne pathogens has been further defined and regulated by OSHA and is discussed later in this chapter.

Fig. 1-11 CDC Standard Precautions for infection control. *(From Zakus SM:* Mosby's clinical skills for medical assistants, *ed 4, St Louis, 2001, Mosby.)*

Hand Hygiene

The most common mode of transmission of pathogens is by the hands. The major cause of nosocomial infections (HCAIs) is the transmission of pathogens from health care workers' hands. These infections can also spread bacteria that may become resistant to antibiotics, which makes the treatment and eradication of infections more difficult.

Proper hand hygiene has proved to be the primary factor in infection control. Research has shown, however, that many health care workers do not practice routine hand washing. Their reasons have been as follows:

- Irritation and dryness caused by hand washing agents
- Inconvenient location of sinks
- Lack of soap and paper towels
- Too busy/insufficient time
- Understaffing/overcrowding
- Priority of patient needs
- Misinformation about risk of acquiring infection from patients

In response, new guidelines developed by the CDC and infection-control organizations now recommend that health care workers use an alcohol-based hand rub (gel, rinse, or foam) to routinely clean their hands between patient contacts as long as their hands are not visibly soiled. Alcohol-based hand rubs require less time, are more effective than soap for routine hand washing, are more accessible than sinks, reduce bacterial counts on hands, and improve skin condition. The following three ways to clean the hands are now recommended (Figure 1-12):

1. Washing with plain soap—good for removing microorganisms and dirt
2. Washing with antimicrobial detergent soap—better for removing and killing microorganisms
3. Using an alcohol-based hand rub—best for destroying transient microorganisms obtained from patients, specimens, and objects that are **contaminated,** that is, likely to have been in contact with materials or environmental surfaces where infectious organisms may reside.

Antimicrobial Soap Hand Wash

Laboratory employees' hands should be washed with antimicrobial soap (Figure 1-13) at the beginning and end of work, before eating, after using the rest room, and whenever hands have visible dirt or are visibly contaminated with blood or body fluids. Hand washing with soap and water involves the following process:

1. Remove all hand jewelry.
2. Wet the hands with warm water (avoid hot water).
3. Apply 3 to 5 mL of liquid antiseptic soap to the hands. Use a towel on the pump dispenser to avoid contaminating the dispenser with soiled hands.
4. Rub the hands together for at least 15 seconds, covering all surfaces of the hands and fingers with soap.
5. Clean the fingernails with a brush if necessary.
6. Rinse the hands with water and dry thoroughly.
7. Use a clean, dry paper towel to turn off the water faucet.
8. Apply appropriate hand lotion or cream provided by employer.

Healthy, intact skin acts as a barrier against **cross-contamination** (transmitting a pathogen from one individual to another) and harbors fewer pathogens. When the skin is damaged, **transient microorganisms** (organisms from contaminated objects or from infectious patients that adhere to the skin and can be transmitted to others) are harder to remove. Therefore gloves and alcohol-based hand rubs are also required.

Alcohol-Based Hand Rub

Hand sanitizing with alcohol-based hand rubs should be routinely used between patients and after having direct hand contact with patients, their wounds, broken skin, or body fluids (specimen containers) or after touching equipment used on the patient. Some patients may harbor "colonies" of infectious microorganisms on their skin with no sign of infection. Therefore the Standard Precautions pertaining to the use of gloves and proper hand hygiene apply to *all* patients. Use an alcohol-based hand rub routinely before putting on gloves and after removing gloves.

Fig. 1-12 Effectiveness of hand hygiene preparations in killing bacteria.

Fig. 1-14 Sanitize hands with alcohol-based hand rub before and after using disposable gloves. *(Photo by Zack Bent.)*

Fig. 1-13 Hand washing with antimicrobial soap should be used at the beginning and end of work, after using the rest room, and before eating. Also, apply antimicrobial hand lotion to prevent the skin from drying and cracking. *(Photo by Zack Bent.)*

The following are tips on how to use an alcohol-based hand rub:

1. Apply 1.5 to 3 mL (or manufacturer's recommended amount) of an alcohol gel or foam to the palm of one hand, and then rub the hands together (Figure 1-14).
2. Cover all surfaces of the hands and fingers, including the areas around and under the fingernails.
3. Continue rubbing the hands together until the alcohol dries (15 to 25 seconds).
4. Make sure the hands are completely dry before putting on gloves.
5. Wash the hands with soap and water when a buildup of emollients can be felt on the hands.

Fingernail hygiene consists of maintaining natural nail tips at ¼ inch in length and refraining from using nail polish. Artificial nails should not be worn by employees who have contact with any patients.

NOTE: Access the Evolve site to find videos demonstrating both methods of hand hygiene: aseptic hand wash and alcohol hand rub. (See front of textbook for how to register and access the Evolve site.)

Personal Protective Equipment

Along with hand hygiene recommendations, the CDC also recommends when and how to use PPE. OSHA also specifies and regulates the circumstances in which PPE must be used. (It also requires the employer to provide employees with their needed PPE along with training on how to use it.) These OSHA requirements are discussed next and are demonstrated on the Evolve site and in Procedure 1-1 located at the end of this chapter.

OSHA Biohazard Training in Bloodborne Pathogens Standard

The federal Department of Labor has appointed OSHA to find ways of promoting worker safety and health in every workplace in the United States. On the basis of the history of hazards to health care workers, OSHA has developed a rigorous standard of policies and procedures called the **Bloodborne Pathogens Standard (BBPS)** to protect employees who work in occupations where they are at risk of exposure to blood or other potentially infectious materials **(OPIM)**. **Occupational exposure** is defined as skin, eye, mucous membrane, or parenteral contact with blood or OPIM in the workplace. **Parenteral contact** means the blood entered the body through the skin or mucous membrane by means of a needle, bite, cut, or abrasion. Those who work in a medical laboratory or perform **venipuncture** (removal of blood from a vein) are at an increased risk for occupational exposure to bloodborne pathogens.

OSHA regulations require that an **exposure control plan** be provided by your facility to eliminate or minimize your occupational exposure to bloodborne pathogens. It is a key document developed to assist the employer in implementing and ensuring compliance with the Bloodborne Pathogens Standard, thereby protecting employees. It consists of the following elements:

- Determination of employee risk of exposure
- Implementation of methods of exposure control, including **Universal Precautions** (the assumption that the blood or body fluid containing blood from *any* patient or test kit could be infectious) when dealing with all patients, engineering and work practice controls to improve safety of employees, PPE for employees, and safe housekeeping practices

- Hepatitis B vaccination for employees at risk of bloodborne pathogen exposure
- Postexposure evaluation of patient and employee immediately after an exposure incident
- Evaluation of circumstances surrounding exposure incidents
- Communication of hazards by annual training of employees
- Documentation showing compliance to all the afore-mentioned elements

New employees of a laboratory receive initial training in the Bloodborne Pathogens Standard and subsequent annual training to learn of any changes in the standard. The following OSHA training session is divided into three sections:

1. Education on the causes, symptoms, and transmission of bloodborne pathogen diseases
2. Instruction on preventive measures to minimize exposure
3. Actions and procedures to follow when exposed to blood or OPIM

Diseases Caused by Bloodborne Pathogens

Three main bloodborne pathogens pose a threat to health care workers: human immunodeficiency virus (HIV), hepatitis B, and hepatitis C. A fourth disease, hepatitis A, is not caused by a bloodborne virus but is similar to hepatitis B and hepatitis C in that it is a viral infection of the liver. Table 1-5 summarizes the comparative information on the three bloodborne viruses and the infectious hepatitis A virus (HAV).

The **human immunodeficiency virus (HIV)** is a retrovirus that attacks the immune system by destroying the white blood cells known as CD4+ T lymphocytes. An HIV infection has four stages:

1. An *acute stage* after exposure characterized by flu-like symptoms with swollen glands
2. An *asymptomatic period* in which no symptoms are readily apparent but the person is still infectious
3. A *symptomatic stage* with the appearance of **opportunistic infections** (infections that occur because of the body's inability to repel pathogens normally found in the environment)
4. The *AIDS (acquired immunodeficiency syndrome) stage,* when the immune system is severely weakened and the following conditions start to appear: an extreme decrease in the number of **CD4 cells** (the T lymphocytic white blood cell that fights infection); any combination of the following opportunistic infections that are known to occur when the CD4 cells are no longer defending the body—Kaposi's sarcoma, *Pneumocystis jirovecii* pneumonia, cytomegalovirus infection, herpes simplex 1 and 2 infection, mycobacterial infection (e.g., tuberculosis), candidiasis (yeast infection), cryptosporidiosis, toxoplasmosis, and cryptococcosis

Currently, there is no preventive vaccination for HIV or any cure for the infection of CD4 cells. Management consists of early diagnosis of the HIV infection followed by treatment to reduce the growth rate of the retrovirus and its effect on the CD4 cells.

Hepatitis B virus (HBV) is the most prevalent bloodborne virus. It first infects the liver with acute flulike symptoms and possible jaundice. Most people recover and become immune to the virus, but approximately 2% enter the chronic stage and develop cirrhosis of the liver, cancer, or both. The good news is that a vaccine is available to produce immunity against the virus before an exposure incident. OSHA requires employers to provide the hepatitis B vaccine series free of charge to all health care employees who may be exposed to blood or OPIM. (Some health care employees who work only with medical records would not need the vaccination.)

Hepatitis C virus (HCV) is another bloodborne virus that attacks the liver. It is not as prevalent as HBV, but it is much more likely to reach the chronic stage. In fact, 75% to 85% of infected HCV individuals will reach the chronic phase with cirrhosis of the liver, cancer, and death. Because no vaccine for HCV exists, the health care worker cannot establish an immunity against the disease. Health care workers exposed to HCV are at risk.

Hepatitis A virus (HAV) is not a bloodborne virus; however, similar to HBC and HCV, it does attack the liver. It is highly contagious and is transmitted by direct or indirect contact through the gastrointestinal tract. Patients with HAV are generally placed in isolation during their illness.

Additional Facts Regarding the Bloodborne Viruses

- The average health care professional is more likely to contract HBV or HCV than HIV.
- Although all these diseases have initial flulike symptoms, HIV attacks the immune system, causing swollen glands, whereas HBV and HCV attack the liver, causing jaundice (a yellowing of the skin caused by excess bilirubin levels).
- HCV is becoming a threat because many individuals are chronic carriers and no vaccination is available.

Preventive Measures to Minimize Exposure

Practicing Universal Precautions is the most important way to prevent exposure incidents. The most common exposure to bloodborne pathogens in health care is from accidental puncture wounds with contaminated needles, glass, or other sharp items. All sharp items should be treated with respect.

The **HBV vaccine** should be made available to all health care employees who have the potential of being exposed to blood and OPIM. Employers must

Table 1-5	Three Bloodborne Pathogens and Hepatitis A Virus			
	Human Immunodeficiency Virus (HIV)	**Hepatitis B Virus (HBV)**	**Hepatitis C Virus (HCV)**	**Hepatitis A Virus**
Transmission	Contact with infected blood or blood products, semen, vaginal secretions; perinatal transmission Must get into bloodstream by direct entry into a vein or break in skin or mucous linings	Found in body fluids; spread by blood transfusions, contaminated needles, and sexual contact HBV is most common bloodborne pathogen	Intravenous drug use, body piercing, organ and blood transfusions, contaminated needles Contaminated needles carry a tenfold greater chance of causing HCV than HIV	Not bloodborne Usually spread by contaminated food
Symptoms	Flulike symptoms, fever, diarrhea, swollen glands, and fatigue HIV infection leads to AIDS and an inability to fight infections	Flulike symptoms generally do not appear until 6 months after viral infection; they can include jaundice, fatigue, and abdominal and joint pain	Milder than HBV; symptoms (if appearing) occur generally 1-2 months after exposure; they include jaundice, fatigue, dark urine, abdominal pain	Jaundice, fatigue, abdominal pain, flulike symptoms
Effects	Once infected, HIV is not curable; the majority of infected individuals do not develop AIDS until many years after infection	Most people recover and become immune; death can result in the 2% who become chronically infected	85% of infected individuals acquire chronic form; of those, cirrhosis of the liver develops in 1-15%	Infection results in immunity; symptoms can last 6-9 months
Prevention	No vaccination available; self-testing is now available for early detection and early treatment to prevent the retrovirus from replicating itself	HBV vaccination	No vaccination available	HVA vaccination, good hygiene
Treatment	Postexposure prophylaxis must start in 1-2 hours; antiretrovirals (AVRs) reduce HIV infection, but it is never cured	Postexposure treatment with immunoglobulins should begin as soon as possible—within 24 hours and no later than 7 days	Treated with immunoglobulin, HepatoZYME (inhibits viral synthesis), and alpha interferon	Treatment consists of immunoglobulins and isolated bed rest to prevent spread
Trends	Health care workers are more likely to contract HBV and HCV infections than HIV, although the incidence of HIV infection is rising	10- to 49-year-olds most affected; approximately 1.25 million are chronically infected	2.7 million have chronic form; this number is expected to triple in the next 5-10 years; it is the leading cause of liver disease and liver cancer	

provide a three-vaccination series, and new employees should begin their series within the first 2 weeks of employment. Any employee who does not wish to be vaccinated must sign a Hepatitis B Vaccine Declination form. Health care students should also begin the series if they will be working with blood and blood products.

Many advances have also been made in HIV/AIDS prevention and treatment including rapid self-testing and effective antiretroviral therapies that have reduced the development of HIV opportunistic diseases and early deaths. Early detection of HIV infection is now recognized as a critical component in controlling the spread of HIV infection. Figure 1-15 shows the Ora-Quick self-test kit.

Engineering controls are efforts and research aimed at isolating and removing bloodborne pathogens from the workplace. Some examples of engineering controls involve the use of the following:
- Biohazard bags for blood-contaminated paper and plastic products and biohazard sharps disposal containers made of puncture-resistant material that will safely receive contaminated needles, syringes, and other sharp implements immediately after use
- Safer medical devices to cover contaminated needles immediately after use (Figure 1-16), self-sheathing needles, and needleless systems when performing intravenous (IV) therapy
- Plastic supplies and equipment to replace breakable glass supplies when collecting and processing blood

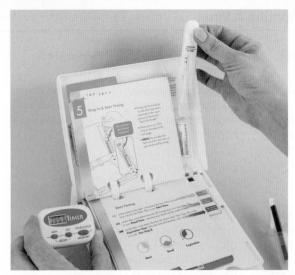

Fig. 1-15 The new OraQuick self-test kit for HIV. This test and the rapid blood test for HIV are presented in Chapter 7: Immunology. *(Photo by Zack Bent.)*

The OSHA standard requires that everyone in the workplace explore new procedures and products regularly to provide greater safety to the health care worker while affording comfort and quality of care to the patient.

Work practice controls are policies that are recorded, monitored, and evaluated to protect employees from exposure to the pathogens in blood or body fluids. Various individuals (both administrators and front-line workers) are assigned the task of identifying, evaluating, and implementing changes in work behavior to reduce the risk of exposure. The implementation and commitment to adhere to work practice controls is required of each individual.

Examples of safe practices in the medical laboratory include the following:

- Do not eat, drink, smoke, or apply makeup or contact lenses in areas with a reasonable likelihood of exposure.
- Sanitize the hands before donning and after removing gloves.
- Bandage cuts and other lesions on the hands before gloving.
- Label all biohazard containers and appliances.
- Place all biohazard waste in appropriately labeled biohazard containers (e.g., sharps versus bag containers).
- If mucous membranes (eyes, mouth, nose) come in contact with blood, flush them with water as soon as possible.
- Do not store food or drink with biohazardous materials.
- Wear and use appropriate protective barriers and closed-toe shoes when working with blood or OPIM.

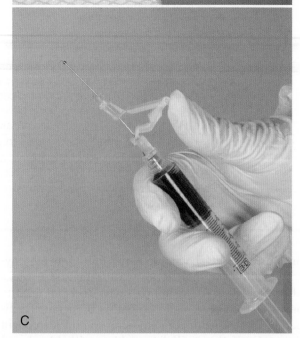

Fig. 1-16 Examples of needle safety devices being activated immediately after drawing blood. **A,** One-hand, thumb-activated device. **B,** One hand using surface to activate device. **C,** One-hand, thumb-activated spring device.

- Use mechanical means to pick up broken contaminated glass.
- Double-package specimens with a biohazard label when sending them to another laboratory.

In the medical laboratory gloves and fluid-impermeable gown barriers are routine requirements when dealing with blood or OPIM. Each procedure should be evaluated to determine if face shields or goggles are also necessary to protect the mucous membranes. This equipment should be used if the procedure is likely to generate splashes or sprays of blood, body fluids, secretions, or excretions.

Housekeeping guidelines in the laboratory consist of several measures:

- Disinfect counters at the beginning and end of each day with an OSHA-approved disinfectant such as freshly diluted 10% bleach solution. Figure 1-17 shows a double-bottle system that dilutes the bleach with water on demand and a CaviWipe container with tissues to thoroughly disinfect contaminated surfaces. NOTE: Always wear protective gloves when working with either of these products.

Fig. 1-17 A bleach/water dispenser automatically delivers a freshly diluted 10% bleach solution and CaviWipes for thorough disinfection of contaminated surfaces. *(Photo by Zack Bent.)*

- When a waste receptacle contains biohazardous material, it must be red or contain the universal symbol for biohazard, or both (Figure 1-18). An understanding of the various waste receptacles and their functions is vital (Figure 1-19).
1. Regular wastebaskets should be used for paper wrappers, paper towels, and other materials that do not have blood or body fluids on them.
2. Biohazard wastebaskets containing red plastic liners and bags with biohazard labels should be used for contaminated gloves, gowns, gauze, and soft plastic supplies.
3. Biohazard sharps containers with biohazard labels should receive only sharp items such as needles and glass that could cut or penetrate a soft biohazard bag. They should be snapped closed when they are approximately three-fourths full.
4. Biohazard-labeled bags and sharps containers are gathered into large cardboard boxes supplied by a regulated waste facility. The boxes are collected and incinerated twice at a cost based on the total weight of the waste. Do not throw unnecessary items in biohazard receptacles.

If a biohazard spill of blood or OPIM occurs, it should be cleaned with a spill kit specifically designed to protect the person during the cleanup process (e.g., gloves and cleanup tools), the area should be decontaminated using the absorbent material and chemicals, and everything should be disposed of properly (biohazard-labeled bag or box) (Figure 1-20; also see the video on the Evolve website).

BIOHAZARD
SYMBOL

Fig. 1-18 Biohazard label. *(From Stepp CA, Woods M: Laboratory procedures for medical office personnel, Philadelphia, 1998, Saunders.)*

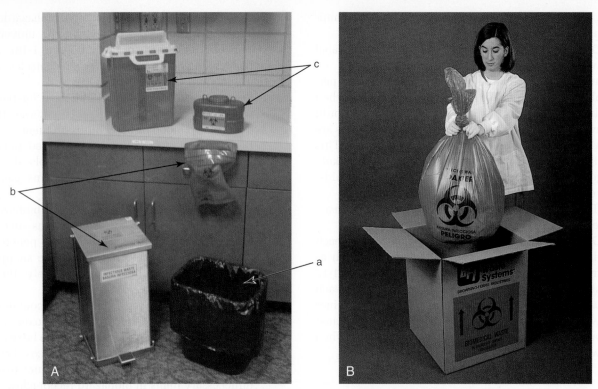

Fig. 1-19 A, Waste containers in the laboratory. *a,* Regular waste receptacle; *b,* nonsharps biohazard waste receptacles; and *c,* biohazard sharps containers. **B,** Biohazard waste is collected in boxes for managed-waste pickup. *(B, from Bonewit-West K:* Clinical procedures for medical assistants, *ed 9, St Louis, 2015, Saunders.)*

Fig. 1-20 Biohazard spill kit and cleaning procedure. *(From Proctor D, Adams A:* Kinn's the medical assistant: an applied learning approach, *ed 12, St Louis, 2014, Saunders.)*

Procedure After Exposure to Blood

If exposed to blood by a **percutaneous** (through the skin) injury or a splash on the mucous membranes of the eyes or mouth, the following postexposure steps must be taken immediately:

1. Flush with water, and wash the exposed area.
2. Report the incident immediately to your supervisor.
3. File an incident report that includes detailed information about how the exposure occurred. (See the Sample Blood and Body Fluid Exposure Report form in the workbook appendix for Chapter 1.)
4. Seek medical attention and permission to determine if the patient was infected with HIV, HBV, or HCV; then determine baseline blood defenses for each of the viral infections. If HIV is suspected, retest at 6, 12, 24, and 52 weeks after exposure to see if any change indicates infection.
5. Because a possibility always exists that the blood contained infectious viruses, postexposure prophylaxis **(PEP)** (preventive treatment after being exposed to blood or OPIM) must begin as soon as possible. The PEP for each of the viral infections is based on the risk evaluation of a qualified health care professional and may consist of the following:
   - Hepatitis B: Passive HBV immune globulin and active HBV vaccine should be administered within 72 hours.
   - Hepatitis C: Immunoglobulin, HepatoZYME, and alpha interferon should be administered as soon as possible.
   - HIV: Antiretrovirals (ARVs) are now proven to reduce HIV infection, although they do not eliminate it. Therefore, it is crucial to begin taking the daily pill as directed by the physician.
6. Counseling and confidentiality are also available and required by OSHA.

Documentation of BBPS Compliance

Compliance with all the steps involved in OSHA's Bloodborne Pathogens Standard must be proven by each facility's documentation of its exposure control plan. The paperwork that must be presented during an OSHA inspection includes the following:

- Written job categories of employees at risk of exposure to blood
- HBV vaccination guidelines and records for each employee at risk
- Record of initial and annual Universal Standards training sessions for bloodborne pathogens and safety training for each employee
- Definition and listing of safe work practices
- Sharps injury log of all work-related needle sticks and cuts from sharp objects contaminated with blood, including date and time of exposure, details of the procedure being performed, the exposure, the exposure source, the exposed person, and postexposure follow-up
- A written plan to maintain the privacy of employees
- Documentation showing the evaluation of new technology by employees and their selection of safety devices based on effectiveness in decreasing injuries, acceptance by users, and ability to not adversely affect patient care

Chemical Hazard Training

Hazardous chemicals in the workplace are also regulated by OSHA in a federal document referred to as the **Hazard Communication Standard.** The document states that employees have the right to know about the dangers of all the hazardous chemicals to which they may be exposed under normal working conditions. As with the Bloodborne Pathogens Standard, the employer must develop a program that consists of taking an inventory of hazardous chemicals in the workplace, labeling the chemical hazards, collecting and maintaining a material safety data sheet **(MSDS)** for each hazardous chemical, properly storing and disposing of hazardous chemicals, and providing employees with information and training. Examples of chemical hazards are dangerous acids, caustics, flammables, and inhalants.

In small medical laboratories, most of the chemicals used are fortunately in small, prepackaged quantities. The most common chemical hazard is the bleach used to disinfect counters. All labels on chemicals such as bleach should be read to understand their hazards. Figure 1-21 shows a bleach label with the following eight container label requirements provided by the manufacturer:

1. Brand name of the chemical
2. Common or chemical name
3. Amount of the contents
4. Signal words such as *danger* (if flammable, corrosive, or highly reactive with other substances), *poison* (if toxic when ingested or inhaled), *warning,* or *caution* (if any other hazardous condition is present)
5. Instructions for the safe use of the chemical (storage, usage, and disposal)
6. Manufacturer information
7. Description of possible hazards such as physical hazards (ability of material to explode, ignite, or react with other chemicals), health hazards (whether material can irritate tissue or cause cancer), toxicity (whether material is toxic if swallowed or inhaled), and safety precautions (whether material requires protective clothing, gloves, or eye protection)
8. First-aid instructions if necessary

Product Label Example

1. **BRITE BLEACH** **Contains No Phosphates**

2. Active Ingredient: Sodium Hypochlorite 5%

3. 64 fl. oz (2 Quarts)

4. **Caution: Keep Out Of The Reach Of Children**

BRITE: Household Uses

5. Use *BRITE* to clean your bathroom and kitchen. *BRITE* is an excellent disinfectant and deodorizer. *BRITE* cleans by removing stubborn stains and eliminating odor-causing germs from surfaces all around the house.
• Toilet Bowls — Pour in 1/2 cup of *BRITE*. Brush entire bowl. Let stand 10 minutes. Do not use with toilet bowl cleaners. See caution statement.
• Kitchen Sinks — Cover stains with water. Pour 1/2 cup of *BRITE* directly into standing water.
• Floor — Clean with a solution of 1 cup of *BRITE* per gallon of sudsy water. Do not use on cork.
• Bathtubs and Showers — Clean with a solution of 1 cup of *BRITE* per gallon warm water.
Laundry
Direction for Use:
For best results, use the proper amount of *BRITE* in your wash water.
• Large top-loading automatic: 1-1/2 cups
• Regular top-loading automatic: 1 cup
• Front-loading automatic: 1/2 cup
• Heavy-soiled laundry: increase 1/2 cup
• Hand laundry: 2 gallons of sudsy water, 1/4 cup *BRITE*

6. WRITE for a free *BRITE* "Guide to Cleaner Laundry" booklet or other information on laundry and house cleaning to the BRITE Co., P.O. Box 12345, Braselton, WA 44150.
For Use On The Following Fabrics: Cotton, linen, synthetics, permanent press and all color-fast fabrics. Do not use *BRITE* on silk, wool, mohair, leather, spandex or non-color fast fabrics.

7./8. **Caution:** *BRITE* may be harmful if swallowed or may cause severe eye irritation if splashed in eyes. If swallowed, feed milk. If splashed in eyes, flood with water. Call Physician. **Skin irritant:** If contact with skin, wash off with water. Do not use *BRITE* with ammonia or products containing acids such as **toilet bowl cleaners, rust removers, or vinegar;** to do so will release **hazardous gases.** Prolonged contact with metal may cause pitting or discoloration. **Do not use this bottle for storage of any other liquid but** *BRITE.*

Fig. 1-21 Product label. Note the eight required elements for labeling a hazardous chemical.

Fig. 1-22 Safety procedure manuals and MSDS manual. *(From Stepp CA, Woods M: Laboratory procedures for medical office personnel, Philadelphia, 1998, Saunders.)*

Along with being properly labeled, each hazardous chemical must be listed on a chemical hazard inventory sheet and have its own MSDS. The sheets are compiled in an inventory notebook available to all employees (Figure 1-22).

On the basis of the information in the MSDS or the manufacturer's label, chemical hazard labels must be placed on all containers holding hazardous chemicals. The National Paint and Coatings Association (NPCA) and the Hazardous Materials Information System **(HMIS)** are two of the most popular systems for labeling hazardous chemicals. The systems use standard labels to communicate hazards through the use of colors, numbers, letters, and symbols (Figure 1-23).

The HMIS is a five-part rectangle that provides identification of the chemical using the information that appears on the MSDS in four categories:
• Blue: health hazards (injuries that may occur if material is inhaled or ingested, skin irritants or carcinogens present in material)
• Red: flammability (volatility of material, ability of material to ignite)
• Yellow: reactivity (stability of the chemical, whether it reacts with other chemicals)
• White: the need for PPE (such as gloves, masks, and gowns)

The numerical ratings range from 0 for no hazard to 4 for extreme hazard. An alphabetical designation is used to denote recommended PPE.

Another way to label hazardous chemicals is the National Fire Protective Association **(NFPA)** coding

HMIS Label

ACETONE	
1	Health
3	Flammability
0	Reactivity
C	Protective Equipment

HAZARD RATING

4 EXTREME	1 SLIGHT
3 SERIOUS	0 MINIMAL
2 MODERATE	

Fig. 1-23 HMIS system showing the labeling of acetone (used in staining procedures).

Fig. 1-24 NFPA coding system showing the color-coded numbering system in four categories. *(From Mahon CR, Manuselis G: Textbook of diagnostic microbiology, ed 3, St Louis, 2006, Saunders.)*

Fig. 1-25 **A** to **C,** Laboratory dispenser bottles with NFPA labels indicating acetone and bleach hazards. Compare the label for acetone with the HMIS label in Figure 1-22, and compare the bleach (sodium hypochlorite) label with the BRITE manufacturer label in Figure 1-21.

system (Figure 1-24). The label uses the same four colors in a diamond pattern and a similar rating system of 0 to 4. Examples of typical NFPA-labeled solutions found in the laboratory are shown in Figure 1-25.

Each facility must use a labeling system that everyone understands. Another way of identifying extremely hazardous chemicals is to use icons representing each chemical hazard: flammable, explosive, corrosive, poisonous, radioactive, compressed gas, and carcinogenic (Figure 1-26).

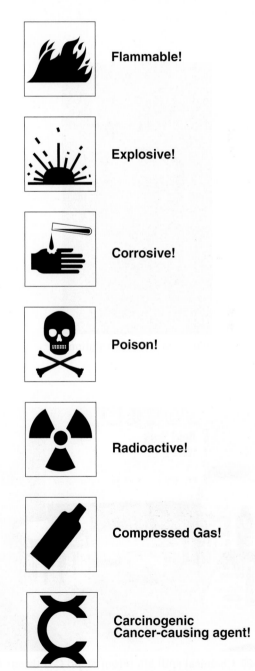

Fig. 1-26 Warning signs for extremely hazardous chemicals.

HIGH VOLTAGE

ELECTRICAL HAZARD

Fig. 1-27 Warning signs for electrical hazards. *(From Stepp CA, Woods M: Laboratory procedures for medical office personnel, Philadelphia, 1998, Saunders.)*

Fig. 1-28 Eye wash station.

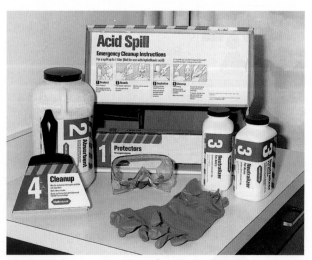

Fig. 1-29 Chemical spill kit. *(From Stepp CA, Woods M: Laboratory procedures for medical office personnel, Philadelphia, 1998, Saunders.)*

Physical Hazard Training

The third area requiring safety awareness involves potential physical hazards. This area relies on common sense and physical hazard orientation in areas such as lifting, weather alerts, bomb threats, and electrical dangers.

- Make sure electrical instruments are grounded and the wires are intact when working with electrical instruments. Never operate electrical equipment with wet hands. Note the electrical hazard icons in Figure 1-27.
- Run periodic drills for physical safety (e.g., fire drills, emergency weather protocol, terrorist attacks).
- Lift with the legs, not the back, and avoid twisting the back when carrying something heavy from one place to another.
- Keep hair shorter than shoulder length, or tie it back to avoid contamination or getting it tangled in moving instruments.
- Never push waste down into a wastebasket with the hands or reach into a biohazard disposal container.
- Learn **ergonomic practices** (proper movements and conditions that make you less prone to work-related injuries) such as proper positioning of seat and computer to prevent carpal tunnel syndrome, leg cramping, and undue stress on back and neck.

Laboratory Safety Evaluation

Laboratory safety training is completed by performing the following:

1. Complete the Chapter 1 Review Questions and the Chapter 1 workbook questions.
2. Complete the following on-line interactive exercises for Chapter 1:
   - Introductory terminology exercises
   - Exercise on ordering laboratory tests
   - Exercise on matching laboratory departments with their functions
   - Evolve on-line videos and training activities found in Chapter 1 student resource
3. Tour the laboratory using the Laboratory Safety Checklist at the end of Chapter 1 in the workbook. Be sure to locate and/or be familiar with how to use the biohazard spill kit (see Figure 1-20), the eye wash station (Figure 1-28), and the chemical spill kit (Figure 1-29).
4. Turn in the OSHA Bloodborne Pathogen Quiz at the end of Chapter 1 in the workbook and a mock exposure incident form in the appendix of the workbook.
5. Observe and perform Proper Use of Personal Protective Equipment found in Procedure 1-1.

✳ PROCEDURE 1-1 Proper Use of Personal Protective Equipment

A, Examples of PPE. *a,* Goggles; *b,* face shield; *c,* fluid-impermeable gown with elastic wrist bands; *d,* box of latex gloves and two pairs of colored nonlatex gloves.

B, A Plexiglass shield provides splash protection in place of goggles and face mask when performing laboratory procedures.

C, Sanitize hands before donning personal protective equipment.

(Continued)

1-1

PROCEDURE 1-1 Proper Use of Personal Protective Equipment—cont'd

D, Order of donning PPE: *(1)* fluid-impermeable coat, *(2)* face protection, *(3)* gloves.

E, Removing gloves correctly. Pull off the glove on the nondominant hand using the dominant hand.

F, Hold the dirty glove in the dominant hand while slipping the nondominant fingers under the cuff.

G, Flip the glove inside out while holding the other glove on the inside.

PROCEDURE 1-1 Proper Use of Personal Protective Equipment—cont'd

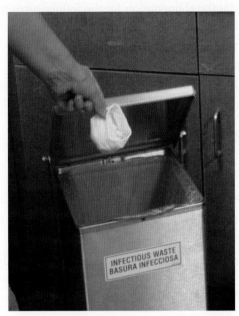

H, Properly dispose of soiled gloves.

PPE used in health care settings is displayed in Figure A. In the laboratory nonpowdered gloves *(D)* and fluid-impenetrable gowns with cuffs at the wrists *(C)* are typically worn to protect the clothes and hands from direct contact with specimens. Latex gloves are not recommended because of potential allergic reactions. Vinyl, nitrile, and other nonlatex gloves are now available in a variety of sizes and colors. A Plexiglass shield can also be placed between you and your work area (Figure B).

Procedure

1. Before **donning** (putting on) PPE, remember to perform either the hand wash or the hand rub appropriately as described in the Hand Hygiene section of the text.
2. Also refer to the Chapter 1 videos on the Evolve website showing proper aseptic hand wash and alcohol-based hand rub methods (see Figure C).

3. If the procedure to be performed has the potential of splashing, eye goggles *(A)* or a face shield *(B)* or both will be required to protect the mucous membranes of the eyes, nose, and mouth.
4. Follow the proper sequence for donning PPE: (1) put on the gown, (2) put on any face protectors, and (3) don disposable nonsterile, nonpowdered, nonlatex, well-fitting gloves. Extend the gloves over the gown cuffs (see Figure D).
5. Keep gloved hands away from the face.
6. Remove gloves if they become torn. (Perform hand hygiene before donning new gloves.)
7. Avoid touching other surfaces and items not involved in the testing process.
8. The outside of the front of the gown is considered contaminated. The clean areas of the gown and gloves are on the inside and the back of the gown.
9. The sequence for removing PPE is to take off (1) the gloves, (2) then the face shield, and (3) then the gown.
10. The proper removal and disposal of gloves is as follows:
    a. Remove one glove by grasping the outside with the other gloved hand and pulling it off (see Figure E).
    b. Wad up the removed glove in the gloved hand. Slip an ungloved finger under the cuff and fold it over until you can grasp the inside area of the second glove (see Figure F).
    c. Pull off the second glove inside out with the first glove still inside (see Figure G).
    d. If the gloves have visible blood or body fluid on them, dispose of them in a biohazard waste receptacle (see Figure H).
11. Next, remove the goggles and then the gown.
12. Close the gown with the clean inside protected before hanging it up. The gown must not leave the lab area.
13. Perform hand hygiene (hand wash or hand rub) immediately after removing PPE.

Photos **A-G** by Zack Bent.

1-1

Review Questions*

1. The head of a hospital laboratory is usually a
   _____.

2. Phlebotomists perform _____.

3. Two nonhospital locations of medical
   laboratories are _____ and
   _____.

4. The educational degree of a pathologist is
   _____.

5. Five qualities important in a laboratory
   professional are:
   _____
   _____
   _____
   _____
   _____

6. Match the prefix on the left with the definition on
   the right.
   _____ milli-   a. one hundredth
   _____ centi-   b. one millionth
   _____ deci-   c. one tenth
   _____ micro-   d. one thousandth

7. Write the abbreviation for the following units:
   milliliter _____
   deciliter _____
   centimeter _____
   micrometer _____
   cubic centimeter _____

8. The three major types of hazards are _____,
   _____, and _____.

9. An example of a physical hazard is _____.

10. An example of a chemical hazard is _____.

11. What is an appropriate surface disinfectant for
    use in the laboratory?

12. Bloodborne pathogen precautions apply only
    to patients who are known to have infectious
    disease.
    True _____ False _____

13. Laboratory apparel includes fluid-impermeable
    laboratory coats and closed-toe shoes.
    True _____ False _____

*Answers to these Review Questions are located in the Appendix.

Websites

HHS information on disease control:
www.hhs.gov/diseases/index.html
OSHA's Bloodborne Pathogens Standard:
www.osha.gov/SLTC/bloodbornepathogens/index.html
FDA website on antiretroviral treatments:
www.fda.gov/ForConsumers/byAudience/ForPatientAdvocates/HIVandAIDSActivities/ucm118915.htm
NIH's website showing the latest research on the hepatitis viruses A thru E:
www.niaid.nih.gov/topics/hepatitis/research/Pages/activities.aspx
The International Health Care Worker Safety Center at the University of Virginia Health System, dedicated to
the prevention of occupational transmission of bloodborne pathogens:
www.healthsystem.virginia.edu/internet/epinet/
Example of bleach MSDS:
www.sciencelab.com/xMSDS-Sodium_Hypochlorite_5_-9925000

2

Regulations, Microscope Setup, and Quality Control

protected health information (PHI) any health information in any form (written, electronic, or oral) that contains patient-identifiable information (e.g., name, Social Security number, telephone number) that must be kept confidential

qualitative test test that simply looks for the presence or absence of a substance

quality assurance (QA) overall process to aid in improving the reliability, efficiency, and quality of laboratory testing in general

quality control (QC) process in which known manufactured samples (controls) are routinely tested to establish the reliability, accuracy, and precision of a specific test system

quantitative test test that produces a numerical value indicating the amount of a substance present

reactive/positive a visible result indicating the presence of a substance a test is designed to detect

reagent substance or ingredient used in a laboratory test to detect, measure, examine, or produce a reaction

reliability when both accuracy and precision are accomplished

semiquantitative test determines the approximate quantity of an analyte (i.e., small, moderate, large)

standard deviation (SD) statistical term describing the amount of variation from the mean in a dataset

wet mount specimens microscope slides that contain cells in water without a stain

ABBREVIATIONS

CLIA	Clinical Laboratory Improvement Amendments
CMS	Centers for Medicare and Medicaid Services
FDA	Food and Drug Administration
HHS	Health and Human Services
HIPAA	Health Insurance Portability and Accountability Act

PPM	provider-performed microscopy
PPMP	provider-performed microscopic procedures certification
certification	

This chapter presents additional government regulations, microscope setup, and quality assurance procedures as they apply to the medical laboratory.

 ## CLIA: Government Regulations

Whenever a specimen is removed from a human body and an analysis occurs that translates to a result, that activity is considered a medical laboratory test. As stated earlier, physicians use test results for the following reasons: (1) to *screen* and detect possible diseases, (2) to confirm a clinical *diagnosis* and make treatment decisions, and (3) to *monitor* the progress of diseases and treatments. If testing is not performed properly, the incorrect results can pose a threat to the patient's overall care and treatment. For example, if a clinical laboratory misreads or misreports a patient's blood sample as having a normal cholesterol level when in fact the patient's cholesterol level is abnormally high, that patient may not receive the necessary treatment to prevent a heart attack. In addition, if the report is misread as high when it is actually normal, the patient may receive unnecessary treatment that could potentially cause harm.

To protect patients from inaccurate test results, Congress passed the Clinical Laboratory Improvement Amendments (**CLIA**) in 1988. CLIA 1988 required that all laboratories examining materials derived from the human body for diagnosis, prevention, or treatment

purposes be certified by the Secretary of Health and Human Services (**HHS**). The Centers for Medicare and Medicaid Services (**CMS**) administers the certification process by requiring all medical laboratories to register and pay a certification fee based on the level of complexity of the tests they perform.

CLIA Levels of Complexity and Their Certification Requirements

There are four complexity levels: high complexity, moderate complexity, provider-performed microscopy (**PPM**; a subset of moderate complexity), and waived testing. The Food and Drug Administration (**FDA**) is involved in determining the level of complexity for all commercial medical laboratory tests on the market.

CLIA Certificate of Waiver

The CLIA **Certificate of Waiver (CoW)** is used predominantly by physician's office laboratories (POLs), ambulatory settings, and institutions with point-of-care testing (POCT).

According to CLIA, CoW laboratories can perform only tests that are determined by the FDA to be so simple that there is little risk of error. Examples of **CLIA-waived tests** with their appropriate procedure codes are listed in Table 2-1.

The number and types of tests waived under CLIA have increased from the 8 originally approved tests in 1992 to now more than 100 tests. The number of waived laboratories has also grown exponentially, from 20% to more than 60% of the total laboratories enrolled in CLIA.

Table 2-1	Tests Granted Waived Status under CLIA 1988	
CPT Codes	**Test Name**	**Use**

Original Eight Tests Approved in 1988

Hematology

83026	Hemoglobin by copper sulfate—nonautomated	Monitors hemoglobin level in blood
85013	Blood count; spun microhematocrit	Screens for anemia
85651	Erythrocyte sedimentation rate—nonautomated	Nonspecific screening test for inflammatory activity, increased for majority of infections and most cases of carcinoma and leukemia

Chemistry

| 82962 | Blood glucose by glucose monitoring devices cleared by FDA for home use | Monitoring of blood glucose levels |

Urine and Feces

81003QW	Dipstick or tablet reagent urinalysis—nonautomated for bilirubin, glucose, hemoglobin, ketones, leukocytes, nitrites, pH, protein, specific gravity, and urobilinogen	Screening of urine to monitor or diagnose various diseases and conditions such as diabetes, the state of the kidney or urinary tract, and urinary tract infections
81025	Urine pregnancy tests by visual color comparison	Diagnosis of pregnancy
84830	Ovulation tests by visual color comparison for human luteinizing hormone	Detection of ovulation (optimal for conception)
82271	Fecal occult blood	Detection of hidden blood in feces from any cause, benign or malignant (colorectal cancer screening)

Examples of More Recently Approved Waived Tests

Hematology (See Tests in Chapter 5)

85014QW	STAT-CRIT/hematocrit	Screen for anemia
85018QW	HemoCue hemoglobin system	Measures hemoglobin level in whole blood
85610QW	ProTime test	Measures time it takes to clot blood and calculates patient's international normalized ratio (INR)

Blood Chemistry (See Tests in Chapter 6)

80061QW	Cholestech LDX	Measures total cholesterol, high-density lipoprotein cholesterol (HDL), triglycerides, and glucose levels in blood
82947QW	HemoCue B—glucose photometer	Measures glucose levels in whole blood
83036QW	Bayer A1CNOW+	Measures percent concentration of hemoglobin A_{1c} in blood, which is used in monitoring long-term care of people with diabetes
80047QW	i-STAT basic metabolic panel	Measures sodium (Na), potassium (K), chloride (Cl), ionized calcium (Ca), total carbon dioxide (TCO_2), creatinine (Crea), glucose (Glu), blood urea nitrogen (BUN), hematocrit (Hct), and hemoglobin (Hgb) in whole blood
82274QW	iFOB fecal occult blood	Immunological detection of hidden blood in feces

Drug Screening (See Chapter 9)

| G0434QW | Multiple drug cup test | Screening test to detect presence of amphetamines, barbiturates, benzodiazepines, tetrahydrocannabinol (THC), cocaine metabolites, methadone, methamphetamines, opiates, oxycodone, and phencyclidine (PCP) in urine |
| K121247 | Alcohol saliva test for ethanol | Measures amount of ethanol in saliva |

(Continued)

Table 2-1	Tests Granted Waived Status under CLIA 1988—cont'd	
CPT Codes	**Test Name**	**Use**
Examples of More Recently Approved Waived Tests, cont'd		
Immunology/Serology (See Chapter 7)		
86308QW	Rapid whole blood mononucleosis tests	Qualitative screening test for presence of heterophile antibodies to aid in diagnosis of infectious mononucleosis
86318QW	Rapid whole blood test for *Helicobacter pylori* antibodies for determining possible cause of peptic ulcers	Immunoassay for rapid, qualitative detection of immunoglobulin G antibodies specific to *H. pylori*
86618QW	Rapid whole blood test for *Borrelia burgdorferi* (causative agent of Lyme disease)	Qualitative detection of immunoglobulin G and M antibodies to *B. burgdorferi*
86701QW	Rapid HIV-1 antibody test with whole blood	Qualitative immunoassay to detect antibodies to HIV-1 in fingerstick and venipuncture whole blood specimens
86703QW	OraQuick rapid HIV-1 and HIV-2 antibody test	Qualitative immunoassay to detect antibodies to HIV-1 in oral liquid specimen
Microbiology (See Chapter 8)		
87804QW	Quick influenza A and B test	Qualitative detection of influenza type A and B antigens in nasal wash and nasopharyngeal swab specimens
87889QW	Quick *Streptococcus* A test	Rapidly detects *Streptococcus* A antigen from throat swabs as an aid in diagnosis of strep throat, tonsillitis, and scarlet fever
Urinalysis (See Chapter 3)		
81003QW	Bayer Clinitek 50 urine chemistry analyzer—qualitative dipstick for glucose, bilirubin, ketones, specific gravity, blood, pH, protein, urobilinogen, nitrites, leukocytes (automated)	Screening of urine to monitor or diagnose various diseases and conditions such as diabetes, the state of kidney or urinary tract, and urinary tract infections
82044QW	Bayer Clinitek 50 urine chemistry analyzer—microalbumin, creatinine	Semiquantitative measurement of microalbumin and creatinine in urine for detection of patients at risk for developing kidney damage
84703QW	Bayer Clinitek 50 urine chemistry analyzer— pregnancy test using cartridge in analyzer	Qualitative test for HCG hormone in urine to detect pregnancy
Semen		
89321QW	Fertell male fertility test	Measures concentration of motile sperm
83900Q	SpermCheck vasectomy	Detects presence of sperm

To become a CLIA-waived laboratory, the physician or facility simply needs to enroll in the CLIA-waived program through CMS, pay an applicable certification fee of $150 every 2 years, and follow the manufacturer's instructions for each FDA-approved waived test.

The following are some benefits of becoming a CLIA-waived lab in an ambulatory setting:
- Rapid availability of results while the patient is available for immediate follow-up
- Simple tests have minimal need for training
- Portability of many waived tests allows for easier testing in nontraditional settings

CLIA High and Moderately Complex Laboratories

Hospital and reference laboratories are staffed with highly educated laboratory professionals who have been trained to perform the complex tests in the various laboratory departments, such as hematology, chemistry, microbiology, and blood bank. To be registered and certified by CLIA, professional laboratories must obtain a Certificate of Registration, and then be surveyed to receive a Certificate of Compliance and then a Certificate of Accreditation. They must maintain their accreditation status by being surveyed periodically to validate that they are performing only tests within their level of complexity and that their personnel are qualified and sufficiently trained in the test procedures.

All testing procedures are continuously monitored by the following systems:
1. **Quality assurance (QA)**—the overall process to aid in improving the reliability, efficiency, and quality of all laboratory tests in general. QA has three major phases: preanalytical, analytical, and

postanalytical. Each of these steps must be evaluated regarding the effectiveness of the laboratory's policies and procedures in producing and documenting the test results, the identification of any problems, and the correction of the problems. The policies must ensure the accurate and prompt performance and reporting of tests.

2. **Quality control (QC)**—a part of QA that takes place during the analytical phase. It uses manufactured samples with known values that are tested along with the patient samples to establish the reliability, accuracy, and precision of a specific test system.

3. **Proficiency testing program**—biannual confirmation of laboratory competency by testing specimens from an outside accreditation agency and obtaining the correct results (**proficiency testing**).

Further details concerning high and moderate complexity testing may be found at the government websites for HHS, CMS, CDC, and FDA. The purpose of this text, however, is to explore the lesser regulated CLIA certificates most commonly used in physicians' offices, ambulatory care, and point-of-care settings, specifically the CLIA-waived tests and the PPM tests.

CLIA: Provider-Performed Microscopy Procedures Certificate

The PPM procedures (**PPMP**) certificate allows qualified health care providers to conduct waived testing and basic microscopic examinations during the patient's visit. The microscopic tests are performed on specimens that are not easily transportable. To receive PPMP certification, the physician or medical facility must enroll in the CMS program for PPMP certification, pay applicable certificate fees of $200 every 2 years, and maintain certain quality assurance (QA) and administrative requirements such as the following:

- Proficiency testing by an outside agency to evaluate microscopic accuracy twice a year
- Documentation of microscope/centrifuge maintenance
- Confirmation that competent personnel are interpreting the microscopic findings

Some of the microscopic tests that require proper preparation before being interpreted are presented in this text. The preparations for these microscopic tests include the following:

- Urine sediment preparation as part of a complete urinalysis
- Direct wet mount preparations for the identification of bacteria, fungi, parasites, and abnormal human cellular elements
- Potassium hydroxide preparations for identifying fungi
- Cellulose tape preparations for identifying pinworms

The actual reading and reporting of the microscopic findings must be done by the physician or a laboratory professional trained and certified to interpret the particular test. Table 2-2 lists the approved PPM tests and their numerical Current Procedural Terminology (CPT) codes.

Table 2-2   CLIA-Approved Provider-Performed Microscopy Tests

Q0111	Wet mounts, including preparations of vaginal, cervical, or skin specimens to view organisms in living state
Q0112	All potassium hydroxide preparations to detect fungal infections
Q0113	Pinworm examinations to detect *Enterobius vermicularis*
Q0114	Fern test (to detect leakage of amniotic fluid caused by ruptured membranes)
Q0115	Postcoital direct, qualitative examinations of vaginal or cervical mucus to detect presence and motility of sperm after sex regarding infertility
81015	Urinalysis, microscopic only to examine, count, and categorize solid structures in urine
81000	Urinalysis, by dipstick or tablet reagent for bilirubin, glucose, hemoglobin, ketones, leukocytes, nitrite, pH, protein, specific gravity, urobilinogen, and any number of these constituents; nonautomated, with microscopy
81001	Urinalysis, by dipstick or tablet reagent for bilirubin, glucose, hemoglobin, ketones, leukocytes, nitrite, pH, protein, specific gravity, urobilinogen, and any number of these constituents; automated, with microscopy. (NOTE: This may be used only when the laboratory is using an automated dipstick urinalysis instrument approved as waived.)
81020	Urinalysis; two- or three-glass test: to determine the location of an infection in the male urinary system
89055	Fecal leukocyte examination to count and categorize white blood cells in a fecal specimen
G0027	Semen analysis; presence and motility of sperm, excluding Huhner test to detect the presence and motility of sperm
89190	Nasal smears for eosinophils to identify and count eosinophils to assess allergic reactions

Microscope Procedure

If the physician chooses to register and perform basic microscopic examinations of specimens, his or her employees will need to learn how to set up a microscope slide for observation. They will also need to focus and maintain the microscope for optimal performance. The microscopic structures and procedure for using a clinical microscope are described in the following section. Procedure 2-1: Using a Microscope skill checklist is found at the end of Chapter 2 in the workbook.

Identifying the Parts and Functions of a Microscope

The microscope can be divided into the following three basic functional areas:

1. *The foundational structures*—consisting of the base, arm, stage, and mechanical slide holder and its controls
2. *The illuminating structures*—consisting of the light source and condenser, with the condenser containing both a control knob and an iris diaphragm lever to open and close the diaphragm
3. *The magnifying structures*—consisting of the objectives lenses that are attached to the nosepiece, the ocular lenses, and the coarse and fine focus adjustment knobs. As you look at the picture of the microscope in Figure 2-1, note the name of each lettered structure in the text as it is described in the three subsequent categories.

Foundational Structures and Their Functions

First, always carry the microscope with two hands—one under the *(a) base* and the other holding the *(b) arm.* The slide with the specimen is placed on the *(c) stage* and clipped into place with the *(d) mechanical holder,* which can then precisely move the slide back and forth and side to side when the operator turns the *(e) mechanical controls* located under the stage.

Illuminating Structures and Their Functions

The slide is illuminated by the *(f) light source* in the base of the microscope. The light flows up into the *(g) condenser,* where it becomes highly concentrated. The condenser can be raised or lowered to a position just under the slide by using the *(h) condenser adjustment* when viewing densely stained specimens. The condenser can be lowered for more transparent **wet mount specimens** (slides that contain cells in water without a stain). The condenser

also contains the *(i) iris diaphragm lever,* which opens the iris for dense slides and closes the iris, thus reducing the amount of light, for more transparent slides (similar to the way the iris of the eye opens and closes the pupil).

Magnifying Structures and Their Functions

After the light flows up through the condenser and through the slide on the stage, it enters one of three or four *(j) objectives lenses.* These lenses are usually color coded, with tubes of different lengths marked with the magnification power. The shortest tubes are the low power objectives and are usually marked with 4× and/or 10× magnification, meaning they make the image 4 and 10 times larger, respectively. The middle-length tube contains the high power objective and usually magnifies 43×. The longest tube objective usually magnifies 100×. This extremely high power objective contains the only lens that requires oil to be placed between it and the slide to prevent air from bending (refracting) the light out of focus. Thus it is called the *oil immersion objective.* The *(k) revolving nosepiece* is used to move from one objective to another. (NOTE: Do not turn the objectives by pushing on the objective tubes.)

After passing through the objectives, the lighted image strikes a mirror that sends the image through the *(l) ocular lenses* (eyepieces), where the operator can see the result. The ocular lenses enlarge the image an additional 10 times, which is multiplied by the objective magnification to determine total magnification.

Objective Magnification (×) Times	Ocular Magnification (×) =	Total Magnification
Low power 4×	10×	40×
Low power 10×	10×	100×
High power 43×	10×	430×
Oil immersion 100×	10×	1000×

The ocular lenses can also be adjusted to focus each eye individually and can move closer together or apart to become aligned with the operator's eye span. The specimen is brought into focus by starting with the low power objective and then turning the *(m) coarse adjustment* knob followed by moving the hand to the *(n) fine adjustment* knob to focus the objects more clearly.

After all the names and locations of the parts of the microscope have been mastered, the first microscope laboratory procedure can be undertaken as seen in Procedure 2-1 and in the workbook.

Fig. 2-1 Microscope. *a*, Base; *b*, arm; *c*, stage; *d*, slide holder; *e*, mechanical slide controls; *f*, light source; *g*, condenser; *h*, condenser adjustment; *i*, iris diaphragm lever; *j*, low power objective; *k*, nosepiece; *l*, ocular lens; *m*, coarse focus adjustment; *n*, fine focus adjustment.

✳ PROCEDURE 2-1 Using a Microscope

A, Clean with lens paper.

B, Move the objectives by rotating the nosepiece to where the low power objective is pointing down toward the slide.

C, Adjust the condenser height control on the left, and the diaphragm control on the right.

D, Place the slide on stage into the mechanical holder.

E, Use the mechanical stage controls to move the slide sideways or forward and back to place the slide above the light source.

F, After finding the image with the large coarse knob, use the small fine focus knob with one hand while moving the slide slightly using the mechanical stage control with the other hand.

PROCEDURE 2-1 Using a Microscope—cont'd

G, Adjust the oculars to the width of your two eyes and then adjust each of the oculars to your eyes' vision.

Equipment and Supplies

Microscope; lens paper; a stained slide; immersion oil; soft, lint-free tissue

Set Up the Microscope and Slide (See Figure 2-1)

1. Always carry the microscope with one hand under the base (a) and the other grasping the arm (b) of the scope.
2. Clean the ocular (l) and objective (j) lenses with lens paper (clean the oil immersion lens last). Note that in Figure A the soft part of the finger is used to clean the lens. Use a different part of the lens paper for each lens, and always clean the oil immersion lens last to keep from spreading the oil to the other lenses.
3. Turn the nosepiece (k) until the low power objective is directly above the stage (Figure B). Do not push the objective tubes.
4. Turn the coarse adjustment (m) until the stage (c) and the low power objective (j) are farthest apart.
5. Turn on the light source (f), and turn the condenser adjustment (h) until the condenser (g) is at its highest level for viewing stained slides. With the other hand, completely open the iris with the diaphragm lever (i) to adjust for the maximum amount of light (Figure C).
6. Place the slide in the slide holder (d) (Figure D) and use the mechanical controls (e) to move the stained portion of the slide directly above the light source (Figure E).
7. Adjust the ocular lens (l) to align with your eyes.

H, After cleaning the lenses and stage, always store the microscope with its protective cover.

Low Power Focus

8. Always start with the low power objective in place, and initially focus using the coarse adjustment. While looking through the oculars, turn the coarse adjustment (m) until color starts to appear, and then turn very slowly, bringing the image into coarse focus (Figure F). *Tip:* Moving the mechanical slide knob slightly back and forth with your right hand while finding the focus position with your left hand helps realize movement for ease in focusing.
9. Next, move the focusing hand to the fine focus adjustment (n) and turn it one way and then the other until the image becomes clear. Both eyes should see a clear image. If not, adjust the oculars by turning their individual focus controls. In Figure G the left hand is adjusting the ocular focus while the right hand is pulling the ocular lenses apart to align with the operator's eyes.
10. Once the image is in focus, move the slide so that the object of interest is in the center of the visual field. Then turn the nosepiece to high power.

(Continued)

2-1

PROCEDURE 2-1 Using a Microscope—cont'd

High Power Focus

11. Refocus the image by turning the fine adjustment one way and then the other until you see color and then the clear image. (NOTE: Do not use the coarse adjustment because it will make too drastic a change and possibly break the slide and/or damage the objective. If you are unable to focus with the fine adjustment, go back to low power and start again with the coarse and fine focus adjustments.) Move the slide so that the desired object is once again in the middle of the visual field.

Oil Immersion Preparation and Focus

12. You are now ready to use the oil immersion lens for maximum magnification. Turn the nosepiece halfway between high power and the oil immersion objective.
13. Place a drop of oil directly on the slide where the condenser light is shining through the slide.
14. Carefully turn the nosepiece until the oil immersion lens dips into the oil and snaps into place.

15. Now, while looking into the oculars, move the small fine focus adjustment back and forth until the image pops into view. The slide can be moved and refocused by using the mechanical stage controls with one hand, while the other hand is turning the fine focus to continuously make adjustments while moving to different areas of the slide. The instructor or supervisor will verify the successful focused result.

Cleanup and Microscope Maintenance

16. When you are finished observing the slide, turn off the light and turn the nosepiece back to the low power objective. By using the large coarse focus knob, maximize the distance between the lens and the stage. Remove the slide, and clean the stage with soft, lint-free tissue. Clean the oil off the slide with tissue or xylene.
17. With a new piece of lens paper, clean the ocular lenses, and then the objective lenses. Always clean the oil immersion lens last.
18. Cover the microscope with a dust-proof cover (Figure H), and store it in a clean, protected area.

Keys to Proper Condenser and Objective Lens Settings Based on Three Common Slides

A. (From Stepp CA, Woods M: Laboratory procedures for medical office personnel, *Philadelphia, 1998, Saunders;* Zakus SM: Mosby's clinical skills for medical assistants, ed 4, St Louis, 2001, Mosby.)

B. (From Rodak BF: Hematology: clinical principles and applications, *ed 4, St Louis, 2012, Saunders.)*

C. (From   Proctor   D, Adams A: Kinn's the medical assistant: an applied learning approach, *ed 12, St Louis, 2014, Saunders.)*

	Liquid Urine	Stained Blood Slide	Stained Microbiology
Condenser setting	Down with diaphragm almost closed	All the way up against the bottom of the slide with the diaphragm open	All the way up against the bottom of the slide with the diaphragm open
Objective lens setting	Low and then high "dry" lenses only— no oil immersion (10× and 43×)	Start on low, then high, then oil immersion for identification	Start on low, then high, then oil immersion for identification

Good Laboratory Practices

The CLIA CoW is the least regulated category of laboratory testing. Waived tests can be performed by individuals with little or no previous experience in laboratory testing, and they do not require the rigorous QC or QA documentation, periodic surveys, and proficiency testing of the other CLIA categories. These facts, along with the ever-increasing number of approved waived tests, have raised the following question: Are the waived test results accurate and reliable? The HHS, CMS, FDA, CDC, laboratory professionals, and test manufacturers are all looking for ways to better educate the personnel performing waived tests. Anyone performing a test on a specimen must know how to achieve accurate and reliable results to ultimately improve the quality of health care.

Quality Assurance

How can the patient be assured that the results were obtained in a reliable, efficient, and well-monitored way? This is where quality assurance (QA) becomes a factor. Remember, QA is an overall process to aid in improving the reliability, efficiency, and quality of the laboratory as a whole. Also remember that QA has three major phases: preanalytical, analytical, and postanalytical.

Table 2-3 describes the QA that must be assessed and documented during the three phases of laboratory testing. Table 2-4 lists the problems or variables that may occur within each phase causing inaccurate results. These tables are a good review of the concepts presented in this chapter. Everyone involved in the laboratory process must take personal responsibility for his or her part in providing safe, high-quality patient care.

Eight quality assurance questions should always be asked when testing specimens:

1. Are the patients and specimens properly identified?
2. Are the patients' charts up to date, with the proper patient test information?
3. Was the quality control performed and documented?
4. Did the laboratory get the right answers for the QC?
5. Do the waived test results correlate with the patient's history or symptoms?
6. Are there any complaints about the laboratory testing?
7. Are the testing personnel trained before performing laboratory testing?
8. Are there periodic discussions about laboratory concerns?

Table 2-3 Quality Assurance and the Three Stages of Laboratory Testing

Preanalytical Phase	Analytical Phase	Postanalytical Phase

1. Physician examines patient and **orders the tests** that need to be performed to:
  a. screen for possible disorders
  b. confirm tentative diagnosis
  c. monitor existing disorder
2. A **requisition** is completed, and patient is instructed in any preparatory procedure, such as fasting (no eating) before some blood tests or first morning urine specimen (for some urine tests).
3. Appropriate **specimen is collected** in proper container:
  a. urine
  b. blood in proper tubes
  c. specimen from infected site
  d. fecal specimen
4. The **specimen is processed:**
  a. labeled
  b. stored at proper temperature
  c. preservatives or additives added if needed
5. The **specimen is transported** to:
  a. laboratory area in office
  b. reference laboratory
  c. hospital laboratory
	6. If tested in the physician's office laboratory, **quality control** is run and logged before patient testing:
	  a. Instrument is calibrated daily and results are logged.
	  b. Controls provided by manufacturer are run and results are logged.
	  c. Proficiency test is successfully run on sample from outside source twice annually and results are logged.
	7. If all the preceding are verified, the **patient specimen is tested.**
	8. A **laboratory report** is produced showing the results of the tests:
	  a. In-office results are recorded directly on the patient's chart with reference ranges and on a patient log.
	  b. Reference laboratory reports are sent to the office by mail, phone, fax, or electronically. They are logged when received.
		9. **Specimen is properly disposed** in biohazard container and sent to a managed waste company.
		10. **Quality control results are analyzed** to determine if test method is "in control" based on precision, accuracy, reliability, shifts, trends, and random errors.
		11. Patient reports are interpreted and signed by:
		  a. the ordering physician
		  b. laboratory pathologists
		  c. additional consulting physicians
		12. **Patient is notified** in the proper confidential manner. Communication is documented in the patient record.
		13. The **final signed report is filed** in the patient record.

Table 2-4	Variables That Can Negatively Affect the Quality of Laboratory Results
Preanalytical Phase	**Analytical Phase**	**Postanalytical Phase**

• Improper patient identification
• Improper patient instruction or compliance (e.g., did not fast, did not collect first morning urine specimen)
• Improper collection of specimen (e.g., wrong time, wrong container, wrong volume, wrong site)
• Improper labeling of specimen
• Improper processing of specimen (e.g., spun versus unspun blood)
• Improper storage of specimen (e.g., refrigerator or room temperature)
• Improper transportation of specimen (e.g., timing, temperature, light exposure)
• Contamination
	• Instrument not functioning correctly
	• Instrument not calibrated
	• Not running and observing controls before patient test
	• Reagents or test kit expired
	• Reagents or test kit not stored at proper temperature
	• Reagents from one kit used with another kit
	• Poor testing technique of operator
	• Not following manufacturer's instructions regarding
	  1. amount of specimen
	  2. amount of reagents
	  3. steps involving time
	  4. proper temperature for testing (e.g., refrigerated test kit must first come to room temperature before testing)
		• Incorrectly recording in-office results on patient log or patient record
		• Not identifying when controls are out of their range and problem-solve reasons for this
		• Not providing physician with reference range along with patient's results to aid in interpretation
		• Not notifying physician when results have arrived from outside reference laboratory
		• Not notifying patient in proper confidential manner regarding results of test
		• Results lost in mail or fax machine
		• Report filed in wrong patient chart

Quality Control

A major concern facing all medical laboratories is how to ensure that the test kit or test instrument is producing the correct results consistently. As mentioned earlier, if the patient's test result is *not* right, it can have a harmful effect on the patient's future course of diagnosis and treatment. The answer to the problem during the analytical phase is to implement QC for each test. This is done by testing a control sample (a manufactured specimen that already has a known value) before testing the patient specimen. If the control sample's test result is within the acceptable range of its known value, then the values from patients' specimens are surmised to also be reliable. When all the QC sample results are recorded on a dated log sheet, the overall performance of the test system can also be monitored over time.

In CLIA-waived laboratories, two different types of tests require QC: qualitative and quantitative.

Quality Control Monitoring of Qualitative Waived Tests

The method of simply testing for the presence or absence of an analyte (the substance being tested in the specimen) is considered a qualitative test. Most qualitative test kits are designed to show three possible test results expressed as the following:

• Reactive/positive—a result that indicates the presence of the substance a test is designed to detect
• Nonreactive/negative—a result that indicates the absence of the substance a test is designed to detect

• Invalid test—when the internal control area on a qualitative test shows no reaction during the testing process

Figure 2-2 shows three qualitative pregnancy test kits. These individual testing devices usually have a built-in positive control *("C")* that produces a colored band to prove the device is operational. If the built-in internal control does not show a color reaction, the test would need to be repeated. If the repeated test also fails, the test system would be considered invalid and corrective action must be taken by checking for the following possible causes:

1. Were the directions followed?
2. Were the reagents (substances used in a test to detect, measure, examine, or produce a reaction) added in the correct order and at the correct time?
3. Were the reagents outdated or stored at the wrong temperature (e.g., room temperature, in the refrigerator)?
4. If everything seems accurate and problems still exist, contact the manufacturer and use a new kit.

Many manufacturers also supply and recommend external controls (liquid positive and negative controls that are tested the same way as the patient's liquid specimen to check the reliability of the instrument and the testing). These manufactured external controls must be run daily, weekly, or monthly as recommended by the manufacturer to further check the reliability of the test system. The dated results of these external controls must also be logged and evaluated.

Fig. 2-2 Qualitative pregnancy tests. *a,* Test kit before adding urine specimen; *b,* a positive reaction in the test area *(T)* indicates that the pregnancy hormone human chorionic gonadotropin (HCG) is present; *c,* a negative reaction (nonreaction) in the test area indicates that no pregnancy HCG is present. NOTE: In both tests *b* and *c,* the internal control area *(C)* indicates the results are valid.

You will be using the qualitative log sheets in your workbook when testing for occult blood, immunology tests, and microbiology tests.

Quality Control Monitoring of Semiquantitative Waived Tests

It is also possible to semiquantify the amount of an analyte by its color reaction with a particular reagent, as seen when testing urine specimens (see Chapter 3). A urine test strip contains reagent pads that react specifically with each analyte, causing a variety of color changes. The more a particular analyte is present in urine, the darker the color will be on the reagent pad. This is referred to as **semiquantitative testing**. A *qualitative* test indicates if a particular analyte is present, whereas *semiquantitative* testing determines the approximate quantity of an analyte. Urine reagent strips provide both qualitative and semiquantitative measurements, with results recorded as negative and/or positive, or in ranges such as trace, 1+, 2+, or 3+; small, moderate, or large.

QC monitoring consists of running two manufactured liquid controls, one with normal results and a second with abnormal results. The manufacturer will provide the semiquantitative predicted results of its control to be compared with the results obtained when running the liquid control. If the results do not match, the same four questions listed in the preceding section should be addressed and the necessary corrections made.

Quality Control Monitoring of Quantitative Waived Tests

Quantitative test results have a numerical value indicating the amount of a substance present (e.g., the glucose monitor in Chapter 1, Figure 1-5, showed a numerical readout of 71 mg/dL). The quantitative result is compared with a population's reference range. A typical reference range for fasting glucose level in the general population might be 70 to 100 mg/dL. If the patient's results are drastically less than or greater than the reference range, it may be clinically significant. For example, if the glucose level in a patient with diabetes is drastically low, the patient could transition into insulin shock. If the glucose level is drastically high, the patient could present with a diabetic coma.

Optics

Monitors that measure the quantity of a substance often send a light through the specimen or reflect off the specimen to determine how much of the analyte is present. With this method of testing, an **optics check** (process of confirming that the light source and light sensor in optical analyzers are working properly) must be performed daily with the results documented on a log sheet. The manufacturer may refer to this process as *calibrating the instrument.* **Calibration** is the process of setting the instrument's optics to the test reagents or test devices that will be used. **Coding** the instrument may also be necessary after receiving a new set of testing supplies in order to reset the instrument's optics. Be sure to read the manufacturer's directions to determine if and when optic checks and/or coding are necessary.

External Controls

Quantitative tests produce numerical results that indicate whether the analyte value is high, normal, or low compared to its reference range. Therefore, it is often necessary to run two or three levels of manufactured control samples on the instrument to ensure that all levels are being accurately detected (i.e., high, low, and normal controls). These QC samples are generally manufactured liquids that are tested in the same way as the patient's specimen. They, too, must be documented on log sheets at specific intervals (daily, weekly, or monthly), dated, and evaluated over time.

External controls can be further evaluated by statistical means. For example, if a control specimen was tested 10 times, the results could be added and then divided by 10 to determine a **mean** (average test result). Each result could then be compared with the mean, and a mathematical calculation could be made to determine how much each control result varied from the mean. Another mathematical calculation could then be made to determine the **standard deviation (SD)** (a statistical term describing the amount of variation from the mean in a dataset). Once these figures are determined, a graph can be created showing the value of the mean and the value of one and two SDs above and below the mean (abbreviated as +1 SD, +2 SD, –1 SD, and –2 SD). When manufactured controls are being run, the goal is to make sure the results fall within ±2 SDs of the manufacturer's mean (referred to as the control's range). In Figure 2-3 the mean for a glucose normal standard control is 100 mg/dL. If 1 SD is calculated to be 5 mg/dL, then ±1 SD would be 105 and 95 mg/dL. Two SDs would be equal to 10 mg/dL, and their values above and below the mean would be 110 and 90 mg/dL, respectively. In this example, 6 days of control results have been plotted and all the results fall within ±2 SDs. This indicates the test method is "in control." NOTE: CLIA-waived test controls have been statistically measured by the manufacturers and will be packaged with the control "range" already determined.

The graph in Figure 2-3 is called a **Levey-Jennings chart**, which is used to plot the ongoing results of test control samples. If a control test result falls higher or lower than 2 SDs or outside the manufacturer's given range, it is considered "out of control" and corrective action must be taken before testing and reporting patient samples.

By plotting quantitative results on a Levey-Jennings chart over time, the laboratory professional can identify possible problems and correct them before running patient samples. Examine each of the graphs in Figures 2-4 to 2-6, and note the possible causes for each of the patterns. In all these cases, the control may be within 2 SDs, but reason for concern still exists.

The following are some patterns seen in weekly control graphs and examples of ways they may be corrected:

Excessive scatter (see Figure 2-4): Values scatter widely above and below the mean. Possible cause: operator variability (e.g., days 2 and 5 were logged by technician A, and days 1, 3, 4, and 6 by technician B). Correction: Observe each technician's technique to see how he or she is performing the test and interpreting the results.

Trends (see Figure 2-5): Values move up or down incrementally in the same direction on each subsequent day. Possible cause: Reagents are outdated or instrument is losing its calibration. Correction: Use a new set of reagents, and run a calibration check.

Shift (see Figure 2-6): Values shift from a consistent set of results to another set of results. Possible cause: new reagents, new person testing, or sudden deterioration of reagents. Check lot numbers and expiration dates on reagents, and observe new technician's performance.

Additional statistical terms must be understood when analyzing control results. **Accuracy (correctness)** occurs when control results consistently fall within 1 SD of the mean. **Precision (reproducibility)** is the ability to produce the same test result each time a test is performed. **Reliability** is the result when both accuracy and precision are accomplished. Reliability is the goal that must be achieved before testing patient specimens.

A way to visualize these three terms is to take the mean of a control and place it in the middle, or bull's-eye, of a target (Figure 2-7). The two circles around the mean represent 1 SD and 2 SDs. The arrows in "A" are inaccurate because they all incorrectly miss the center of the target, and they are not precise because they are scattered around the central area. The arrows in "B" are precise because they are clustered together (reproducible) but none of them are accurate because they all incorrectly miss the inner circle. The goal for a *reliable* test system is seen as the arrows in "C" that show all the values *accurate* (in the center of the target) and *precise* (all showing a similar value). NOTE: These same terms apply when observing CLIA-waived control results. The controls should fall close to the manufacturer's stated mean (the bull's-eye), and they

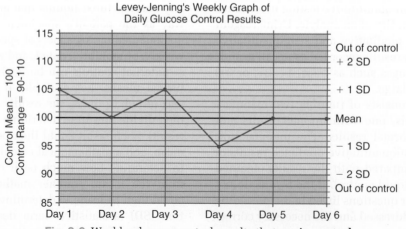

Fig. 2-3 Weekly glucose control results that are **in control**.

Fig. 2-4 Weekly glucose control results showing **excessive scatter.**

Fig. 2-5 Weekly glucose control results showing a **trend.**

Fig. 2-6 Weekly glucose control results showing a **shift.**

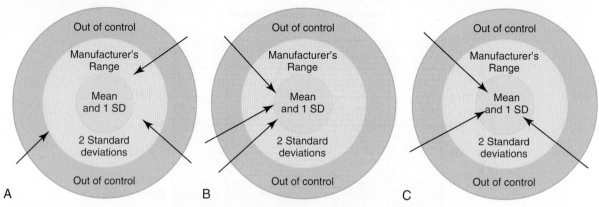

Fig. 2-7 Visual examples of quality control test results using a target to facilitate understanding of terms. **A,** Results are not *accurate* (not within required standard deviations, or the bull's-eye) and are not *precise* (not consistently reproducible, or hitting the same area). **B,** Results are precise but not accurate. **C,** Results are both precise and accurate and are therefore *reliable.*

should also be within the manufacturer's stated range (the circle around the bull's-eye).

See Figure 2-8 for an example of the manufacturer's liquid control ranges for a glucose meter.

A **proficiency testing program** requires a lab to enroll in an accreditation organization that sends the lab unknown samples to test twice a year. The received samples must be run in exactly the same manner as patient specimens. The results are then sent back to the accreditation agency so it can confirm that the results agree with their known values. This method of QC is *required* for CLIA complex tests (including physician-provided microscopy) and is *recommended* for CLIA-waived testing.

Quality Assurance and Quality Control Checklist

This text is designed to follow the latest booklet and its check sheet provided by the CDC (Centers for Disease Control and Prevention) entitled "Ready? Set? Test!" (Figure 2-9).

HIPAA Privacy Rule

Another area of concern that has generated governmental intervention in the medical community is that of patient confidentiality. On April 14, 2003, the Health Insurance Portability and Accountability Act (**HIPAA**) Privacy Rule went into effect. HIPAA is a federal law consisting of several components, one of which contains provisions to protect a patient's privacy. The privacy rule provides patients with more control over the use and disclosure of their health information. During the three phases of laboratory testing, many individuals handle what is referred to as **protected health information (PHI)**, which is any health information in any form (written, electronic, or oral) that contains patient-identifiable information, such as name, Social Security number, and telephone number. This information must be kept confidential. Because of this new approach to medical records and medical information, employees are trained regarding how their specific office uses, stores, maintains, and transmits laboratory testing information. No test result should be given to a patient or family member without the physician's permission. If a patient asks for his or her results or those of another person, you should explain that you are not authorized to disclose that information and that the physician will interpret and explain the results to the patient or family member

Fig. 2-8 Example of *(a)* glucose *meter* with its *(b)* test strip that calibrates the instrument when inserted and "draws in" the specimen or liquid control. *(c) External liquid control* used to check whether its results fall in the normal range, and *(d)* the test strip container with the *LOT #, expiration date,* and *manufacturer's normal control range of 96 to 133 mg/dL (the mean would be 114 mg/dL).*

Tips, Reminders, and Resources

Ready?

- [ ] Clean work surfaces before and after testing.
- [ ] Perform testing in a well lit area.
- [ ] Check and record temperatures of the testing and reagent storage areas.
- [ ] Check inventory regularly to ensure you will have enough reagents and supplies on hand for testing.
- [ ] Check and record expiration dates of reagents/kits, and discard any reagents or tests that have expired.
- [ ] Check that all kit reagents came from the same kit lot. Do not mix reagents.
- [ ] Inspect reagents for damage, discoloration, or contamination, and discard if found.
- [ ] Prepare reagents according to manufacturer's instructions.
- [ ] Allow time for refrigerated reagents/samples to come to room temperature prior to testing.
- [ ] Inspect equipment and electrical connections to be sure they are working.
- [ ] Perform calibration checks, as needed, following the manufacturer's instructions.
- [ ] File the old manufacturer's instructions and replace with the new copy if there are changes.
- [ ] Communicate all changes in the manufacturer's instructions to other testing personnel and to the person who directs or supervises testing.
- [ ] Treat and test quality control (QC) samples the same as patient samples.
- [ ] Perform QC as recommended in the manufacturer's instructions.

Set?

- [ ] Check patient identification and test orders.
- [ ] Discuss pretest instructions and counseling needs with the patient.
- [ ] Wear appropriate personal protective equipment (PPE) such as gloves.
- [ ] Collect and label a good sample for testing.
- [ ] Clean hands and change gloves between patients.
- [ ] Use the proper biohazard containers to dispose of waste and sharps.

Test!

- [ ] Do not test samples that are improperly collected or handled.
- [ ] Have the manufacturer's instructions or a quick reference guide at the work station.
- [ ] Follow the manufacturer's instructions in the exact order.
- [ ] Follow required timing for testing.
- [ ] Identify and correct problems before reporting test results.
- [ ] Identify and report critical values in a timely manner.
- [ ] Perform or refer confirmatory or additional testing, if needed.
- [ ] Make sure patient reports are legible and reported in a timely manner.
- [ ] Make sure reports are standardized and easily distinguishable from referral laboratory test reports.
- [ ] Report patient test results only to authorized persons.
- [ ] Document verbal reports, followed by a written test report.
- [ ] Report public health diseases.
- [ ] Dispose of biohazardous waste safely.
- [ ] Participate in proficiency testing (PT).

Fig. 2-9 Ready? Set? Test! *(From Centers for Disease Control and Prevention, Division of Laboratory Science and Standards,* To Test or Not to Test? *Booklet, available at http://www.cdc.gov/dls/waivedtests/ReadySetTestBooklet.pdf.)*

based on the full medical findings and knowledge of the patient. It is also important to guard the patient's test results from being seen or heard by others.

Risk Management

Medical office risk management is a term that refers to both the physical and the procedural risks that may bring about an injury or legal action against a practice. In the laboratory and office, the best defense against legal accusations is proper documentation. The following documentation recommendations contribute to sound risk management practices in the laboratory:

- Provide written office procedures that inform patients how to prepare for tests (e.g., how to collect home specimens, fasting requirements, or special diets) and document in the patient's record when this occurred.
- Be accurate and consistent when charting and documenting test and control results on the lab logs.
- Use appropriate abbreviations and legible writing on the patient chart and logs.
- Chart corrections made in the legally required manner (line through error; correction, date, and initials of person correcting error).
- Document immediately when diagnostic tests have been received, reviewed, filed, and communicated to the patient

Electronic Medical Records and Bar Coding

As the demand for more laboratory and safety documentation increases, technological advancements in the area of electronic communications to ease this burden are increasing as well. These advancements will also make the process of test documentation more accurate. For example, electronic medical records are replacing patients' physical charts. These records will be accessible at each phase of the testing process by laptop computers or desktop computers located in the reception area, examination rooms, laboratory area, and reference laboratories. In most of the large reference laboratories and hospitals, the various departments are directly linked to a central computerized health information system. This system takes the test results directly from the laboratory's instruments to the patient's electronic medical record, and then immediately alerts the physician about the results.

Another electronic aid to the laboratory is the use of bar code labels on all requisitions and specimens. Bar coding was introduced to the health care industry in the mid-1970s, when blood banks and blood collection centers began using the technology for error-free tracking, tracing, and positive patient identification (Figure 2-10). Today bar coding is used in virtually every hospital department to help improve accuracy

Fig. 2-10 Blood bank bar code label.

and timely information management. Statistics show that the error rate for manual data entry is 1 in 300 characters compared with 1 in 3 million characters for bar code scanning.

So what exactly is a bar code? Without getting too technical, **bar codes** are a pattern of narrow and wide bars and spaces. Each pattern is encoded with its own particular meaning, just like words in a language are made up of letters and symbols. When a beam of light scans the bar code, the light reflects differences between the dark bar areas and the space areas. These differences are transformed into electrical impulses that are measured, decoded, and entered into a computer.

The single most important use of bar codes in the medical laboratory is for positive patient and specimen identification throughout the entire testing process. An understanding of an office's or reference laboratory's labeling system is important. A typical system consists of a specific bar code printer that prints the bar code labels on the basis of typed input from a computer. As the operator enters the patient's name and the test ordered, a series of bar code labels are generated and then attached to the laboratory requisition and the collected patient specimens. Before the labels can be applied to the specimens, patients must be identified by at least two of the following patient identifiers, depending on specific office protocol:

1. Always ask the patient to give his or her name. Do *not* say, "Are you Mrs. Smith?"
2. Have the patient state his or her Social Security number, *or*
3. Ask the patient's birth date, *or*
4. Ask the patient's telephone number

Once positive identification is made that agrees with the requisition and the bar code labels, have the patient print his or her name on the label that will be affixed to the requisition. The smaller bar code labels are then affixed to the tubes of blood after they have been filled.

Review Questions*

1. What is the purpose of CLIA 1988?

2. What is the purpose of proficiency testing?

3. A slide is initially brought into focus by using the _____ power objective.

4. Ocular lenses have a magnification of _____.

5. The _____ directs and concentrates light through the slide and into the objective lens.

6. The revolving _____ contains the objectives.

7. The _____ objective usually has a magnification of 100×.

8. The total magnification is calculated by multiplying the 10× ocular lens by the magnification of the _____ lens.

9. Match each term on the left with its definition on the right.
   _____ standard deviation   a. uninterrupted rise or decline from the mean
   _____ trend   b. average value of a set of control tests
   _____ mean   c. variability from the mean in a dataset

_____

*Answers to Review Questions are located in the Appendix.

Websites

CDC site with educational information on CLIA-waived testing including an excellent brochure and on-line course: "Ready? Set? Test!":
wwwn.cdc.gov/dls/waivedtests/
CPT codes for CLIA-waived tests:
www.doh.wa.gov/portals/1/Documents/Pubs/681018.pdf
Tests granted waived status under CLIA with CPT codes:
www.cms.gov/Regulations-and-Guidance/Legislation/CLIA/Downloads/waivetbl.pdf
FDA listing of CLIA-waived tests since 2000:
www.accessdata.fda.gov/scripts/cdrh/cfdocs/cfClia/testswaived.cfm

3 Urinalysis

OBJECTIVES — *After completing this chapter you should be able to do the following:*

1. Define and match key terms in this chapter.

Fundamental Concepts

2. Demonstrate an understanding of the urinary system by:
   - Describing the structures and functions of the organs, the formation of urine, the significance of renal threshold, the flow of urine, and the composition of urine.
   - Defining medical terms related to the urinary system and urinalysis.
3. Instruct the patient in the proper method of urine collection for voided urine, clean-catch midstream urine for bacterial studies, and timed urine specimens.

CLIA-Waived Tests

4. Describe the three parts of urinalysis: physical, chemical, and microscopic.
5. State the tests involved in physical urinalysis and recognize the diseases that cause abnormal results.
6. State the 10 dipstick tests involved in manual chemical urinalysis and recognize the diseases that cause abnormal results.

7. Describe the automated method for performing chemical urinalysis, including microalbumin testing.
8. Perform physical and chemical assessments of urine samples demonstrating the following criteria:
   - Perform the stated task, conditions, and standards listed in the Procedure Sheets in the student workbook.
   - Apply the correct quality control.
   - Follow the most current OSHA safety guidelines.

Advanced Concepts

9. Describe the standardized urine microscopic method (e.g., Kova), and perform a microscopic urinalysis setup according to the conditions required while following the most current OSHA safety guidelines.
10. Recognize the pictures of various elements in normal and abnormal urine microscopic sediment.
11. Correlate abnormal microscopic results with certain pathological conditions and correlate the results with the physical and chemical urinalysis results.

KEY TERMS

anuria no flow of urine

Bence Jones protein protein found in the urine of patients with multiple myeloma

bilirubin waste product from the breakdown of hemoglobin

casts elements excreted in the urine in the shape of the renal tubules and ducts

diuresis increase in the volume of urine output from the kidney

dysuria painful urination

electrolyte element or compound that forms positively or negatively charged ions when dissolved and can conduct electricity

glomerular (Bowman's) capsule cup-shaped structure surrounding the glomerulus that collects the glomerular filtrate

glomerulus structure in the renal corpuscle made up of tangled blood capillaries in which the hydrostatic pressure in the capillaries pushes substances through the capillary pores

glycosuria sugars (especially glucose) in the urine

hematuria intact red blood cells in the urine

hemolysis red cells breaking open and releasing hemoglobin

iatrogenic adverse effect or complication caused by treatment or diagnostic procedures

ketonuria ketones in the urine

lyse to break open and be destroyed

micturition expelling of urine from the body, also referred to as voiding and urination

nephron functional unit of the kidney

nocturia voluntarily getting up frequently during the night to urinate

oliguria decrease in the flow and volume of urine

pH scale that measures the level of acidity or alkalinity of a solution

polyuria frequent urinary flow producing abnormally large amounts of urine

porphyrin intermediate substance in the formation of heme (part of hemoglobin)

proteinuria proteins in the urine

pyuria white blood cells in the urine

reducing substance substance that easily loses electrons

renal corpuscle part of the nephron that contains the glomerulus and glomerular capsule

renal threshold level blood reabsorption limit of a substance and the point at which the substance is then excreted in the urine

renal tubules parts of the nephron composed of proximal convoluted tubules, the nephron loop (loop of Henle), and distal convoluted tubules

retroperitoneal located behind the peritoneal cavity

sediment the solid material at the bottom of the centrifuged tube of urine

specific gravity in urinalysis, the weight of urine compared with the weight of an equal volume of water; measures the amount of dissolved substances in urine

supernatant the liquid portion of urine on top of the spun sediment

ureters slender, muscular tubes 10 to 12 inches long that carry the urine formed in the kidneys to the urinary bladder

urethra tube that carries urine to the outside of the body

urethral meatus urethral opening through which urine is expelled from the body

urinary bladder hollow muscular organ that holds urine until it is expelled

Fundamental Concepts and Collection Procedures

Anatomy of the Urinary System

Before the results of urine testing can be interpreted, the overall anatomy and function of the urinary system must be understood.

Function of the Urinary System

The urinary system has the following functions:

- It removes unwanted waste substances.
- It stabilizes blood volume, acidity, and electrolytes.
- It regulates extracellular fluids of the body and the absorption of calcium ions by activating vitamin D.
- It secretes the hormone erythropoietin, which controls the rate of red blood cell (RBC) formation, and the hormone renin, which regulates blood pressure.

Structures of the Urinary System

The urinary system consists of the kidneys, ureters, urinary bladder, and urethra (Figure 3-1).

Kidneys

Each person normally has two kidneys, which are reddish-brown, bean-shaped organs. The kidneys are 4 to 5 inches long and are located in the **retroperitoneal** space (behind the peritoneal cavity) slightly above the waistline in the posterior wall of the abdominal cavity. The kidney is composed of three main sections: the cortex, which is the outer part; the medulla, which is the middle area; and the renal pelvis, which is the hollow inner area (Figure 3-2, *A*).

The functional unit of the kidney is the microscopic **nephron** located within the cortex and medulla of the kidney. Approximately 1 million nephrons are in each kidney. The nephrons filter waste substances from the blood and simultaneously maintain the essential water and electrolyte balance of the body (Figure 3-2, *B*). The structural components of the nephron are the renal corpuscle and renal tubules (Figure 3-3).

The **renal corpuscle** consists of two structures: the **glomerulus** and the **glomerular (Bowman's) capsule**. The glomerulus is made up of tangled blood capillaries in which the hydrostatic pressure in the capillaries pushes substances through the capillary pores. The filtered substance is called the glomerular filtrate, and it is collected in the glomerular (Bowman's) capsule, a cup-shaped structure surrounding the glomerulus.

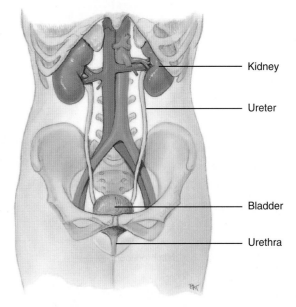

Fig. 3-1 The urinary system. *(From Applegate EJ: The anatomy and physiology learning system, ed 4, St. Louis, 2011, Saunders.)*

Fig. 3-2 **A,** Sections of the kidney. **B,** Enlarged view of renal corpuscle consisting of the glomerulus and glomerular (Bowman's) capsule. *(From Chabner D:* The language of medicine, *ed 10, St. Louis, 2014, Saunders.)*

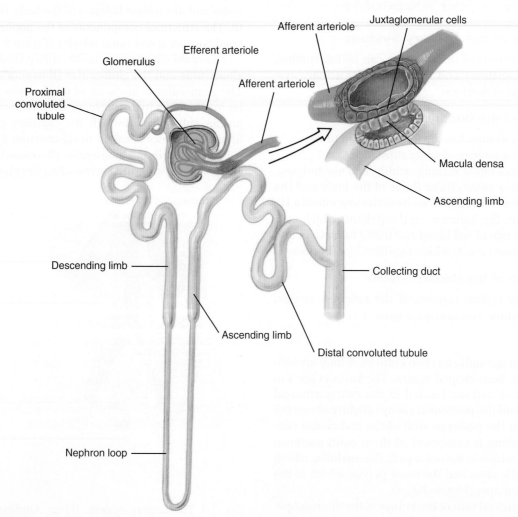

Fig. 3-3 Components of the nephron. *(From Applegate EJ:* The anatomy and physiology learning system, *ed 4, St. Louis, 2011, Saunders.)*

Renal tubules are composed of proximal convoluted tubules, the nephron loop (loop of Henle), and distal convoluted tubules. The glomerular filtrate fluid flows through these tubules and undergoes changes in composition. This process is discussed later in this chapter.

Also in the medulla of the kidney are collecting tubules and ducts that empty into the renal pelvis.

Ureters

The two **ureters** are slender, muscular tubes 10 to 12 inches long. They carry the urine formed in the kidneys to the urinary bladder.

Urinary Bladder

The **urinary bladder** is a hollow muscular organ that holds the urine until it is expelled by a process called **micturition** (also referred to as *voiding* and *urination*).

Urethra

The **urethra** is a tube that carries urine to the outside of the body. The length of a woman's urethra is approximately 1.5 inches. A man's urethra is longer, approximately 8 inches. The opening at the end of the urethra, where the urine is expelled, is called the **urethral meatus**.

Formation and Flow of Urine

Urine is formed in the nephron by three mechanisms: filtration, reabsorption, and secretion.

Filtration

Filtration is the process by which fluids and dissolved substances in the blood are forced through the pores of the glomerulus into the glomerular capsule by hydrostatic pressure. Substances such as water, salts, sugar, and nitrogen waste products (urea, creatinine, and uric acid) can pass through the pores. Substances such as red blood cells (RBCs) and proteins are too large and therefore remain in the blood.

Reabsorption

In the process of reabsorption, some of the substances that flow through the renal tubules that are needed by the body cross back into the blood by the peritubular capillaries surrounding the tubules. Examples of reabsorbed substances are glucose, water, and **electrolytes** (elements or compounds that form positively or negatively charged ions that, when dissolved, can conduct electricity).

When blood levels of a substance such as glucose reach a point at which no more can be reabsorbed, the substance is excreted in the urine. This is the **renal threshold level** for that particular substance. For example, the renal threshold level for glucose is 160 to 180 mg/dL.

Secretion

The final process in the formation of urine is called *secretion,* in which substances are transported from the peritubular blood capillaries into the renal tubules. Metabolized drugs, potassium, and hydrogen ions are examples of substances that are secreted into the urine.

Flow of Blood and Urine Through the Urinary System

Blood is carried into the kidney by the renal artery, which eventually branches into the afferent arterioles. The afferent arterioles carry blood into the capillaries of the glomerulus, and the efferent arterioles carry the blood out of the glomerulus. The glomerular filtrate is collected in the glomerular capsule (Bowman's) and flows through the proximal convoluted tubules to the nephron loop; then to the distal convoluted loop, the collecting tubule, and the collection duct; and finally to the calyces of the renal pelvis. The filtrate then flows into the hollow renal pelvis and at this point is called *urine.* The urine then passes through the ureters to the urinary bladder, where it is stored until released by the process of urination or voiding. The main structures involved in the formation and excretion of urine, in sequence, are the following:

1. Bloodstream—blood enters the kidney via the renal afferent arterioles
2. Glomerulus
3. Glomerular (Bowman's) capsule
4. Renal tubules
5. Collecting ducts
6. Renal pelvis
7. Ureter
8. Urinary bladder
9. Urethra
10. Urinary meatus—urine is expelled from the body

NOTE: The Evolve site for this text has animated pictures showing the formation of urine as it is filtered from the arterioles and then processed through the nephron.

Composition of Urine

Water makes up 95% of urine. Urine also contains nitrogen waste products such as urea, uric acid, ammonia, and creatinine. Urea, uric acid, and ammonia are derived from the breakdown of protein, and creatinine is a waste product of muscle metabolism. Other waste products found in urine include chloride, sodium, potassium, calcium, magnesium, phosphate, and sulfate.

Approximately 1200 mL of blood passes into the renal arteries per minute, with a daily output of 1200 to 1500 mL of urine per day. This amount varies depending on the amount of fluid intake and the amount of fluid lost from perspiration, feces, and water vapor from the lungs.

The following terms are related to urination:

1. **Diuresis**—increase in the volume of urine output from the kidney, which can be caused by the following:
   - Intake of excessive amounts of fluids, especially those that contain caffeine
   - Some drugs, such as diuretics
   - Some types of diseases, such as diabetes mellitus, diabetes insipidus, and renal diseases that prevent the kidney from concentrating the urine
2. **Anuria**—no flow of urine
3. **Dysuria**—painful urination
4. **Nocturia**—voluntarily getting up at night frequently to urinate
5. **Oliguria**—decrease in the flow and volume of urine that can occur in the following situations:
   - Decreased fluid intake
   - Vomiting
   - Profuse sweating
   - Diarrhea
   - Kidney disease
6. **Polyuria**—frequent urinary flow producing abnormally large amounts of urine

Urine Specimen Collection

The urine sample is usually easily obtained, but all types of urine collection methods have the following general requirements:

- The volume needed is usually between 25 and 50 mL.
- The outside of the filled container should be cleaned with a disinfectant.
- The outside of the specimen container must be correctly labeled with the patient's name, the collection date and time, and the type of specimen (e.g., random specimen, first morning specimen, clean-catch midstream, or catheterized). Do not label the lid of the container because it may become separated from the specimen.

Use the correct urine containers (Figure 3-4). The physician's office should provide the patient with a urine container. Containers from the patient's home, such as glass jars, should not be used because their previous contents can affect the accuracy of the tests. The most common types of containers are disposable, nonsterile plastic cups with lids. For infants and children who are not toilet trained, special pliable

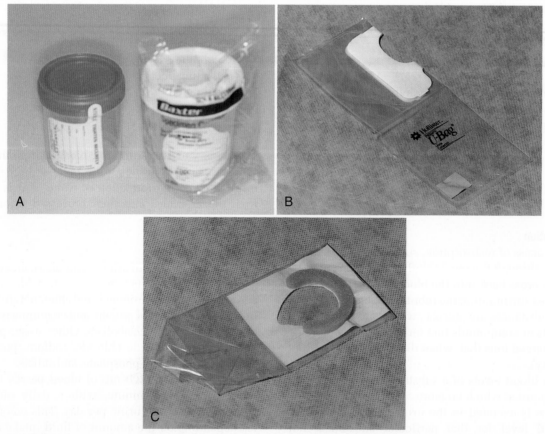

A
B
C

Fig. 3-4 A, Adult urine specimen container. **B** and **C,** Pediatric urine specimen containers. *(From Stepp CA, Woods M: Laboratory procedures for medical office personnel, Philadelphia, 1998, Saunders.)*

polyethylene bags called pediatric urine containers (PUCs) are available that contain an adhesive section to adhere to the skin. If urine is being collected for microbiological studies, a sterile urine container must be used.

- If a woman is having a menstrual period, collection of a urine sample should be postponed. If this is not possible and a urine specimen must be collected immediately, the requisition must note that the patient is menstruating. This will indicate the cause of a false-positive result for blood.
- The urine should be tested as soon as possible after collection. If it is going to sit for more than 1 hour, it must be refrigerated or preservatives must be added.

The method of collection for urine specimens is dictated by the type of test being ordered. For example, special collection procedures are performed if the urine will be cultured for bacteria or if a 24-hour test is ordered. Documentation of the method used to collect the specimen should be noted on the specimen container, the requisition form, and the patient's chart.

Random Specimen

A random specimen is usually collected in the medical office. The patient should collect the midstream portion of urine when voiding. The patient is instructed to void a small amount of urine into the toilet to flush away the normal bacteria in the area around the urinary opening and to get a steady midstream flow. The second portion is collected in the container to a volume of at least 25 mL. Once the specimen has been collected, the remaining urine in the bladder can be emptied into the toilet. A specimen collected this way is more representative of the contents of the bladder. The lid should be tightly placed on the container, and the outside of the container should be disinfected. The sample container (not the lid) should be appropriately labeled.

First Morning Specimen

The first morning specimen is usually the specimen of choice because it is the most concentrated and has the greatest amount of dissolved substances. Provided the patient has not voided during the night, the first morning urine specimen has formed over an approximately 8-hour period. Because this urine is more concentrated, the probability of detecting abnormalities increases and the microscopic elements remain intact for a longer period.

The patient must collect the first morning specimen soon after rising and preserve it by refrigeration until it is brought into the physician's office. The collection procedure is the same as that described for the random specimen.

Clean-Catch Midstream Urine Specimen

The urethra and urinary meatus normally harbor many microorganisms. Therefore, when a urine specimen is collected for culture to determine the source of a urinary tract infection (UTI), only the organisms causing the infection should be cultured. To avoid contamination, the midstream clean-catch method of collection is used. This method consists of having the patient clean the urinary opening first using antiseptic wipes, as seen in Figure 3-5. The patient then urinates into the sterile container by using the midstream method. See (Procedure 3-1 Instructing Patients How to Collect a Clean-Catch Urine Specimen) located at the end of this fundamental section.

NOTE: If the medical assistant does not know if the urine specimen will be needed for culture, collect a clean-catch midstream just in case.

When the urine requires further evaluation, it may be necessary to send it to an outside lab in a sterile tube with preservative to keep the organisms alive during transportation. This transferring of the clean-catch midstream urine specimen to a sterile vacuum tube will be covered in the microbiology chapter (Chapter 8).

Other options for collecting urine specimens for culturing are bladder catheterization and suprapubic aspiration. In catheterization, a sterile tube called a *catheter* is passed through the urethra into the bladder to remove urine. With suprapubic aspiration urine is removed by passing a needle through the abdominal wall into the bladder.

Fig. 3-5 Supplies for collecting a midstream clean-catch specimen. *(From Stepp CA, Woods M: Laboratory procedures for medical office personnel, Philadelphia, 1998, Saunders.)*

Timed Urine Specimen

Some tests require that a urine specimen be collected at a certain time. One example is a 24-hour urine specimen. Collecting all the urine produced over a 24-hour period allows greater accuracy of measurement for urinary components. Substances produced in the urine are affected over time by body metabolism, exercise, and hydration. Substances measured in a 24-hour specimen include calcium, creatinine, lead, potassium, protein, and urea nitrogen. In addition, this type of specimen is used in the diagnosis of the cause, control, and prevention of kidney stones.

24-Hour Collection Procedure

Urine containers for 24-hour collection (Figure 3-6) are quite large, holding approximately 3000 mL. They are dark in color to screen out ultraviolet light and avoid decomposition of substances.

The following guidelines should be given to the patient:
- The specimen should be kept refrigerated.
- Some containers may contain a preservative. Patients should be instructed about the possible hazards associated with these preservatives. NOTE: The proper preservative must be selected to avoid interference with the analyte being tested.
- The patient should be provided with verbal and written directions.
- The patient should be instructed to moderately limit the intake of fluids during the collection process. Also, the patient should not consume alcohol 24 hours before and during the collection procedure.
- The physician should determine whether medication should be discontinued during the procedure because some medications, such as thiazides, phosphorus-binding antacids, allopurinol, and vitamin C, could alter the results. See (Procedure 3-2 Instructing Patients How to Collect a 24-hour Urine Specimen) at the end of this fundamental section.

Fig. 3-6 A 24-hour urine container. (From Stepp CA, Woods M: Laboratory procedures for medical office personnel, Philadelphia, 1998, Saunders.)

✴ PROCEDURE 3-1 Instructing Patients How to Collect a Clean-Catch Urine Specimen

A to C, Procedure for female midstream clean-catch urine collection. **A,** Clean labia from front to back with antiseptic. **B,** Urinate the first part into the toilet. **C,** Next, collect middle of specimen into cup, and then urinate the last part into the toilet.

Equipment and Supplies

Sterile urine collection container, label, antiseptic towelettes

Procedure

For a Female Patient

1. Wash your hands, and gather the equipment.
2. Greet and identify the patient, and provide her with the clean-catch urine supplies.
3. Instruct the patient to sanitize her hands and remove her underwear.
4. Instruct the patient to spread apart her labia with one hand to expose the urinary meatus (Figure A). Tell her to keep this area spread apart with her nondominant hand during the entire cleaning procedure.
5. Instruct the patient to take one antiseptic towelette and clean one side of the urinary meatus from front to back on one side. She should clean from front to back so that microorganisms in the anal region are not spread into the urinary meatus area.
6. Instruct the patient to repeat the same procedure with another antiseptic towelette, wiping from front to back on the other side of the urinary meatus.
7. Instruct the patient to use a third antiseptic towelette to wipe from front to back directly across the urinary meatus.

8. Instruct the patient to continue to keep the labia spread apart and to void a small amount of urine into the toilet to flush away microorganisms that may be around the urinary meatus (Figure B). Tell her to be careful not to touch the inside of the sterile container at any time during the procedure.
9. Instruct the patient to collect the second part of the urine in the container (Figure C). This is the midstream flow of urine.
10. Instruct the patient to urinate the last amount of urine into the toilet. This will ensure that the first and last sections of the urine flow are not in the container, only the midstream section.
11. Instruct the patient to dry the area with a tissue and wash her hands.
12. Instruct the patient to carefully cap the specimen container and put it in a specified place if collected in the office or refrigerate it if collected at home.
13. Gloves should be worn when receiving the specimen from the patient. The sample container (not the lid) should be labeled correctly, and a requisition should be completed if required.
14. The person receiving the sample should remove the gloves and sanitize his or her hands after the urine has been placed in the testing area.
15. The procedure should be charted correctly. The charting should document that midstream clean-catch urine collection instructions were given and that the specimen was received from the patient.

Figures A through C courtesy Gala Bent.

(Continued)

3-1

PROCEDURE 3-1 Instructing Patients How to Collect a Clean-Catch Urine Specimen—cont'd

D to F, **D,** Clean area around penis opening and across the opening. **E,** Void a small amount into the urinal or toilet. **F,** Collect the second part of urine in the container and then void the last part in the urinal. Procedure for male midstream clean-catch urine collection. *(From Stepp CA, Woods M:* Laboratory procedures for medical office personnel, *Philadelphia, 1998, Saunders.)*

For a Male Patient

1. Wash your hands, and gather the equipment.
2. Greet and identify your patient, and provide him with the clean-catch urine supplies.
3. Instruct the patient to sanitize his hands and remove his underwear.
4. If the patient is uncircumcised, instruct him to retract the foreskin, holding it back during the entire procedure.
5. Instruct the patient to clean the area around the penis opening (glans penis) by starting at the tip of the penis and cleaning downward (Figure D), using a separate antiseptic towelette for each side.
6. Instruct the patient to use a third antiseptic towelette to clean directly across the meatus.
7. Instruct the patient to void a small amount of the urine into the toilet to flush away microorganisms that may surround the urinary meatus (Figure E).
8. Instruct the patient to collect the second part of the urine in the container, being careful not to touch the inside of the container (Figure F).

9. Instruct the patient to void the last amount of urine into the toilet so that only the midstream section is collected.
10. Instruct the patient to dry the area with a tissue if needed.
11. Instruct the patient to carefully cap the specimen container and place it in a specified place if collected in the office or refrigerate it if collected at home.
12. Gloves should be worn when receiving the specimen from the patient. The sample container (not the lid) should be labeled correctly, and a requisition should be completed if required.
13. The person receiving the sample should remove the gloves and sanitize his or her hands after the urine has been placed in the testing area.
14. The procedure should be charted correctly. The charting should document that midstream clean-catch urine collection instructions were given and that the specimen was received from the patient.

3-1

PROCEDURE 3-2 Instructing Patients How to Collect a 24-Hour Urine Specimen

Procedure

Sanitize your hands and assemble and label the correct specimen collection equipment. Determine that you are instructing the correct patient by having the patient state his or her name. Provide the patient with the required equipment and written instructions.

1. Wash your hands, and gather the equipment.
2. Greet and identify your patient.
3. Instruct the patient to empty the bladder into the toilet after arising on the first day of the 24-hour procedure. Inform the patient not to save this specimen but to record the exact time the bladder was emptied. The concept is to start the 24-hour period with an empty bladder and then start saving/measuring the urine formed by the kidneys after that time for 24 hours.
4. Instruct the patient that each time he or she urinates for the next 24 hours, the urine must be voided directly into the collection container, including any urine expelled during the night. It might be necessary to give female patients a large sterile container that has a wide opening in which they can void; afterwards, they can pour the contents into the 24-hour jug.
5. Tell the patient to be sure to screw the lid on tightly each time and keep the container refrigerated. If at any time during the procedure some urine is not collected, the test must be started again. Examples include the patient forgetting to collect some urine; spilling some urine; and, if the patient is a child, wetting the bed with urine.
6. Instruct the patient that on the following morning, he or she must collect the last specimen at the same time he or she emptied the bladder on the first day. Therefore the first morning specimen on the second day is kept and it ends the 24-hour collection procedure.
7. Instruct the patient that on the day the procedure is completed, the container must be returned to the physician's office or to the laboratory.
8. After the patient has completed the procedure and returned the container, check the label for completeness and ask the patient whether any problems occurred during the collection procedure.
9. A requisition form must be completed and the 24-hour urine container transported to the laboratory that will perform the test.
10. Document in the patient's chart the instructions and equipment that were supplied to the patient. Also document that the specimen was sent to an outside laboratory. Include the type of specimen that was sent, the date, the time, the name of the laboratory to which it was sent, and the test that was ordered.

3-2

CLIA-Waived Tests

Urinalysis

Urinalysis is the description and measurement of the substances found in urine. It is the most common test performed in the medical office. The specimen is easily obtained, and the testing is not difficult to perform. Urinalysis can be used for screening in a physical exam, to assist the physician in the diagnosis of pathological conditions, and to determine the effectiveness of a treatment. A routine urinalysis consists of three parts: physical analysis, chemical analysis, and microscopic analysis. Figure 3-7 is an example of a urinalysis requisition/report form containing the test results for routine, microscopic, and quantitative analyses. NOTE: The quantitative tests in the right-hand column of the requisition are not CLIA waived and are generally performed on a 24-hour collected specimen in which the total volume of the urine has been measured and recorded.

Fresh or preserved urine can be used when performing a routine urinalysis. Preservatives are usually used for specimens being sent to a lab a long distance away and requiring prolonged storage. Nonpreserved, fresh urine is preferred because some preservatives can interfere with the chemicals used in the testing. Urine should be tested within 1 hour of voiding, but if this is not possible, the urine should be refrigerated. Before testing, the urine must be brought to room temperature and be well mixed.

Urine that stands at room temperature for more than 1 hour may undergo the following changes:

- Bacteria will multiply, causing the urine to be cloudy. Some bacteria can break down urea to ammonia, which will change the **pH** (scale that measures acidity or alkalinity) of the urine to alkaline.
- Glucose that could be present in the urine decreases as it is metabolized by microorganisms.
- Cells in the urine will **lyse** (break open).

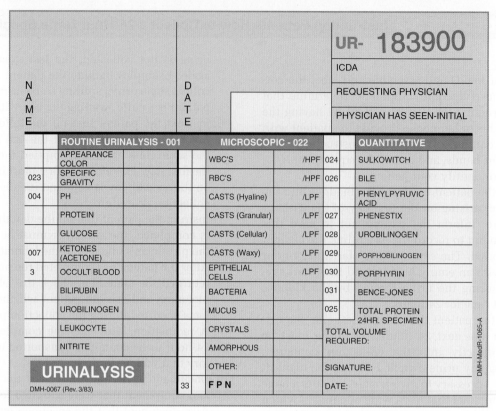

ROUTINE URINALYSIS - 001				MICROSCOPIC - 022				QUANTITATIVE	
	APPEARANCE COLOR			WBC'S	/HPF	024		SULKOWITCH	
023	SPECIFIC GRAVITY			RBC'S	/HPF	026		BILE	
004	PH			CASTS (Hyaline)	/LPF			PHENYLPYRUVIC ACID	
	PROTEIN			CASTS (Granular)	/LPF	027		PHENESTIX	
	GLUCOSE			CASTS (Cellular)	/LPF	028		UROBILINOGEN	
007	KETONES (ACETONE)			CASTS (Waxy)	/LPF	029		PORPHOBILINOGEN	
3	OCCULT BLOOD			EPITHELIAL CELLS	/LPF	030		PORPHYRIN	
	BILIRUBIN			BACTERIA		031		BENCE-JONES	
	UROBILINOGEN			MUCUS		025		TOTAL PROTEIN 24HR. SPECIMEN	
	LEUKOCYTE			CRYSTALS				TOTAL VOLUME REQUIRED:	
	NITRITE			AMORPHOUS					
URINALYSIS				OTHER:				SIGNATURE:	
DMH-0067 (Rev. 3/83)			33	**F P N**				DATE:	

UR- 183900
ICDA
REQUESTING PHYSICIAN
PHYSICIAN HAS SEEN-INITIAL

DMH-MedR-1065-A

Fig. 3-7 Urinalysis laboratory form. *(From Bonewit-West K:* Clinical procedures for medical assistants, *ed 9, St Louis, 2015, Saunders.)*

- **Casts** (elements excreted in the urine in the shape of the renal tubules and ducts) dissolve and disappear, and crystals may dissolve if the pH changes.
- **Bilirubin** (a waste product from the breakdown of hemoglobin that is metabolized by the liver), if present, will be oxidized with exposure to light.

If substances, originally present in the urine, are dissolved, eliminated, or lysed, then the microscopic testing for such analytes will result in false-negative reports.

Physical Routine Urinalysis

The physical part of a urinalysis consists of observing the color, odor, and appearance (transparency) of a urine specimen. To determine the color and appearance, the urine must be viewed through a clear container. NOTE: In the past, the urine would also be tested for pH and specific gravity during the physical analysis. These two tests are now included in the chemical analysis of urine because they are measured using the same test strips as the chemical analytes.

Color

The color of normal urine (Figure 3-8) is typically described as *straw colored (light yellow),* to *yellow,* to *amber (dark yellow).* Varying amounts of a normal

pigment called *urochrome* give the urine its characteristic shades of yellow. Concentrated urine with less water and more substances is dark yellow to amber, whereas more diluted urine is a lighter yellow or straw color. The first morning specimen is most concentrated (dark yellow); the urine becomes more dilute (lighter in color) as the day progresses and more fluid is consumed.

Fig. 3-8 Normal colors of urine with their various descriptions. *(From Bonewit-West K:* Clinical procedures for medical assistants, *ed 9, St Louis, 2015, Saunders.)*

Sometimes additional substances may cause a change in the color of urine, but this is not necessarily associated with disease. Such color changes may be caused by food dyes, some medications, and vitamins.

The colors in the following list, however, may be indications of a pathological condition. The following are abnormal urine colors and their possible causes:

- Yellow-brown—caused by bilirubin resulting from excessive RBC destruction or bile duct obstruction
- Orange-yellow—caused by bilirubin or urobilinogen resulting from a reduction in the functioning of liver cells or excessive RBC destruction
- Green—caused by biliverdin resulting from the oxidation of bilirubin
- Dark red—caused by erythrocytes (red blood cells) resulting from the bleeding of urinary structures, the occurrence of the menstrual cycle, or the presence of hemoglobin from the breakdown of erythrocytes
- Red-brown—caused by erythrocytes and hemoglobin or myoglobin (from skeletal or cardiac muscle breakdown)
- Clear red—caused by hemoglobin and **porphyrin** products
- Cloudy red—caused by intact erythrocytes

Odor

A fresh urine specimen has a slight aroma. Odor is not normally recorded in a urinalysis, but some characteristic odors may indicate certain conditions.

- An *ammonia odor* may indicate bacteria in the urine. Also, if urine is left standing, urea converts to ammonia.
- A *sweet* or *fruity odor* may be an indication of the presence of ketones. Ketones are an intermediate product of fat metabolism found in patients with uncontrolled diabetes and patients consuming low-carbohydrate diets.
- A *foul odor* is characteristic of a UTI. The longer the urine stands, the worse the odor becomes. The decomposition of leukocytes (white blood cells) causes the foul odor.
- A *musty or mousy odor* can be caused by certain foods, such as asparagus, or by an inherited metabolic condition, phenylketonuria (PKU), that occurs in newborns.

Appearance

The appearance part of a physical urinalysis evaluates the transparency of the urine. This can be performed accurately only if the urine is in a clear container; it is usually done at the same time the color is evaluated. The terms used to describe the appearance of urine are *clear, hazy (slightly cloudy), cloudy,* and *turbid (very cloudy)* (Figure 3-9).

Some of the substances that may cause a freshly voided urine specimen to appear cloudy are bacteria,

Fig. 3-9 Appearance of urine showing clear to turbid (very cloudy) characteristics. *(From Bonewit-West K: Clinical procedures for medical assistants, ed 9, St Louis, 2015, Saunders.)*

yeast, blood cells, casts, mucous threads, and sperm. These substances could be clinically important and are evaluated further in the chemical and microscopic parts of the urinalysis. Urine that is clear when voided may become cloudy as it is allowed to stand. Dissolved substances crystallize as urine cools, causing the cloudy appearance.

Chemical Urinalysis

The second part of a urinalysis is the chemical testing, which helps diagnose pathological conditions. A reagent strip is a thin plastic strip containing pads impregnated with chemical reagents that test for specific substances. When each reagent pad reacts with its specific analyte, a color change occurs. The greater the amount of a particular analyte that is present in urine, the darker the color will be on the reagent pad. This is referred to as *semiquantitative testing*. A *qualitative* test indicates whether a particular analyte is present, whereas *semiquantitative* testing determines the approximate quantity of an analyte. *Quantitative* testing measures the exact amount of a substance and usually requires more complex equipment and procedures that are not usually available in a physician's office. Reagent strips provide both qualitative and semiquantitative measurements, with results recorded in ranges such as trace, 1+, 2+, and 3+; small, moderate, and large; and negative and positive.

Reagent strips are also time dependent, which means that each test on a strip must be read at a particular time. The tests on the strips are referred to as *screening tests*. If a result is abnormal, then additional testing may be performed to confirm the presence of the abnormal analyte. Some of these confirmatory tests will be reviewed when individual analytes are discussed.

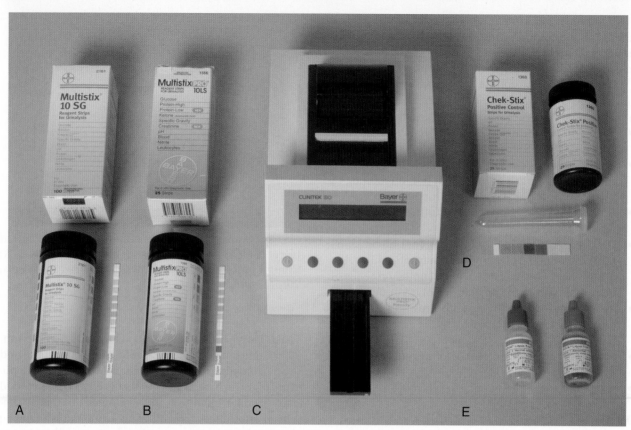

Fig. 3-10 Urinalysis chemistry supplies. *A,* Multistix 10 SG urinalysis chemistry reagent strips; *B,* Multistix Pro10LS urinalysis chemistry reagent strips that also test for microalbumin; *C,* Clinitek instrument; *D,* Chex-Stix positive control strips; *E,* Kova normal and abnormal controls.

Urinalysis chemistry strips (Figure 3-10, *A* and *B)* have multiple reagent pads on each strip. The most commonly used testing strip consists of reagent pads for specific gravity, pH, glucose, ketones, bilirubin, urobilinogen, blood, protein, nitrite, and leukocytes. Some physician offices may use a test strip with fewer test pads more appropriate for their medical practice. For example, an obstetrician may use a two-pad test strip to monitor pregnant patients for only glucose and protein levels.

The color comparisons provided by the manufacturer may indicate more than one set of units for reporting positive results for specific analytes. The physician will indicate to the medical assistant which set of reporting units is to be used. For example, positive glucose results could be reported as *0.25% to 2% or more,* or as *100 to 2000 mg/dL or more.*

Chemical Urinalysis—Quality Assurance

The following guidelines help ensure high-quality results when performing urinalysis testing with a reagent strip:

- The reagent strip bottle must be kept tightly closed when not in use because moisture from air, light, and aerosols can affect the accuracy of the testing.

- The pads on the strip should not be touched or placed on any surface.
- Keep the strips in a cool, dry place but do not refrigerate them.
- Do not use an expired bottle (the expiration date is displayed on the bottle).
- Any bottle that has been open longer than 2 months should not be used. Repeated exposure to air can change the accuracy of the strips. Be sure to note the written date on the label indicating when the bottle was opened.
- Do not combine strips from different bottles.
- Follow all directions from the manufacturer.
- Mix the urine specimen well, and bring it to room temperature before testing.
- Make sure that all pads are covered with the specimen.
- Do not leave the strip in the urine too long because this can cause the chemical in the pads to leach (wash out) into the urine.
- When taking the strip out of the urine, remove excess urine by pulling the back side of the strip against the edge of the container and then briefly blot the side of the strip against absorbent paper.

- Hold the strip horizontally to keep the colors on one pad from running into another while you are comparing the colors to the reference testing chart. Do not touch the bottle with the strip while comparing (see Procedure 3-3). NOTE: There are plastic charts available from the manufacturer that can be cleaned and disinfected should they become contaminated.
- Record observed results for each analyte on the lab log and requisition/report.

Reagent Strip Quality Control

To ensure the accuracy of results, quality control procedures must be followed when performing chemical tests on urine. Quality control determines whether the reagent strips are working properly and whether the test is being correctly performed and accurately interpreted.

Several reagent control methods can be used (see Figure 3-10, *D* and *E*). One method is to use a control strip containing synthetic ingredients *(D)*. The strip is placed in water to dissolve the ingredients, and this solution is then tested as a urine specimen. Another method is to use a dehydrated urine control, which can be purchased from the manufacturer in normal and abnormal levels *(E)*. The controls are rehydrated according to the manufacturer's directions, and then a chemical examination is performed in the same way a patient's urine sample would be examined.

With any quality control method, the results obtained must be compared with the manufacturer's ranges that accompany the controls and the results must be logged in quality control record books. If the results do not fall within the quality control ranges, then appropriate steps must be taken to determine the cause. No patient testing should be performed until the quality control results fall within the acceptable ranges.

Proficiency checklists (also referred to as *procedure sheets*) for any new laboratory test must be documented for each person performing the test. In this case, each person would run the test using the urinalysis controls, write the results on the laboratory log, and then check to see if the results fall within the manufacturer's control range before testing patients. The procedure sheets for urinalysis along with the log sheets for both control results and patient results are available in the workbook and the on-line website.

Automated Clinitek Method

Urine analyzers are available that automatically read the chemistry strips (Figure 3-11). The Clinitek analyzer, for example, runs the chemical analysis according to the principle of reflectance photometry. A microprocessor in the machine controls the movement of the strip into the reflectometer, where a light

Fig. 3-11 Clinitek urine analyzer with tray for measuring reagent strips. *(Photo by Zack Bent.)*

of specific wavelengths is beamed onto the strip. The light that is reflected is measured, converted into a digital reading, and printed.

In the automated method, the timing and color interpretation are consistent and do not vary among individual readers as the visual interpretation of color does. A disadvantage of this method is that if the urine contains a large amount of pigment, the machine cannot recognize this and will give false results based on the pigment rather than the presence of analytes.

Urine Test Strips

The routine tests included in a chemical examination of urine are specific gravity, pH, glucose, ketones, bilirubin, urobilinogen, blood, protein, nitrites, and leukocytes. These tests can provide the physician with information about the status of the patient's acid-base balance, carbohydrate metabolism, liver and kidney functions, and possible UTIs.

Specific Gravity

To measure the **specific gravity** of urine, the weight of the urine is compared with the weight of an equal volume of water, which has a standardized specific gravity of 1.000. Specific gravity measures the amount of particles that are dissolved in the urine, which indicates the ability of the kidneys to concentrate the urine.

Pathological conditions that *increase* urine concentration and raise specific gravity include adrenal insufficiency, congestive heart failure, hepatic disease, and **glycosuria** (sugars in the urine) seen both in diabetes mellitus and in dehydration caused by fever, vomiting, and diarrhea.

Pathological conditions that *decrease* urine concentration include chronic renal insufficiency, diabetes insipidus, and malignant hypertension.

The normal range for urine specific gravity is 1.003 to 1.030, but the range is usually between 1.010 and 1.025. The first morning urine is more concentrated and therefore has a higher specific gravity. Urine becomes more dilute as fluids are consumed throughout the day, so subsequent urine samples have a lower specific gravity.

pH. The pH of a substance measures its level of acidity or alkalinity (Figure 3-12). A pH of 7 is neutral, 0 to 6 is acidic, and 8 to 14 is alkaline. The lungs and kidneys are responsible for maintaining the body's acid-alkaline balance in the blood. The blood pH must be in a range of 7.35 to 7.45. If the blood pH is less than 7.35, acidosis occurs, and if the pH is greater than 7.45, alkalosis occurs. Both acidosis and alkalosis in the blood are critical conditions.

Normal urine pH has a variable range of 5.0 to 8.0. The average is 6.0, slightly acidic. The pH of urine is determined by measuring the amount of hydrogen ions present. The pH should be measured by testing a freshly voided specimen because urea is converted to ammonia by bacteria in urine that has been standing at room temperature. This conversion causes the urine to become alkaline. Freshly voided urine that is alkaline, however, may indicate a bacterial UTI.

Glucose. Glucose is not normally found in urine. In the glomerulus of the nephron, glucose is filtered into a glomerular filtrate, and in the renal tubules this substance is reabsorbed into the blood. However, if a large amount of glucose is present in the blood, glucose in the tubules cannot be reabsorbed because the renal threshold level has been reached. For glucose, the renal threshold level is between 160 and 180 mg/dL.

When sugars are found in the urine (glycosuria), glucose is the most likely to be present (glucosuria). Other sugars that can be found are lactose, fructose, galactose, and pentose. The reagent strip method of testing is an enzymatic reaction using the enzyme glucose oxidase that is specific for glucose. The presence of glucose in the urine may indicate diabetes mellitus, but it may also occur after vigorous exercise or during acute emotional stress. False-positive results can also be obtained in the presence of large quantities of aspirin, ascorbic acid (vitamin C), and any medication containing levodopa.

The Clinitest (Bayer Corp.) is a confirmatory test to determine if other sugars or **reducing substances** (substances that easily lose electrons) in addition to glucose are present in urine.

Galactosemia is a rare metabolic condition in which the body is not able to convert galactose to glucose, resulting in the excretion of galactose in the urine. In infants this condition results in the failure to thrive because of anorexia, vomiting, and diarrhea. In addition, enlargement of the liver and spleen; cirrhosis; cataracts; mental retardation; and, in extreme cases, permanent brain damage or even death can occur. A positive Clinitest and a negative glucose strip test in a pediatric urine analysis could indicate galactose in the urine.

Lactose may be found in the urine of pregnant women, and in rare instances fructose and pentose can be found in urine because of high consumption of honey or fruit (see Procedure 3-5).

Ketones. Ketones are products of fat metabolism that are then oxidized by the muscles. The body normally uses carbohydrates for energy, but if the body is deficient in carbohydrates, it metabolizes fats. Excessive fat metabolism can lead to the production of large amounts of ketones that the muscles cannot oxidize. The excess ketones accumulate in tissues and blood and subsequently in the urine, a condition called **ketonuria**.

Fig. 3-12 The pH scale. *(From Stepp CA, Woods M: Laboratory procedures for medical office personnel, Philadelphia, 1998, Saunders.)*

Ketones and glucose in the urine may be associated with uncontrolled diabetes mellitus. The glucose levels in the blood and urine of a diabetic person are high because insulin is either absent or not working correctly and the glucose cannot be metabolized for energy. Fats are then metabolized for energy, and ketone blood levels increase, causing ketones to spill over into urine. In addition, ketones are acid compounds; therefore ketonuria is correlated with a low pH (acid) urine. If glucose, ketones, and acidity are all present in the urine, this may indicate a condition known as *ketoacidosis,* which may lead to diabetic coma.

Other conditions that may lead to ketonuria are fevers, starvation, anorexia, prolonged vomiting, and diets high in fat and low in carbohydrates. NOTE: These conditions generally do not have glucose present.

Ketones evaporate at room temperature; therefore the urine specimen must be tested immediately or capped tightly and refrigerated. If the reagent strip is positive for ketones, the confirmatory test Acetest (Bayer Corp.) can be performed to confirm the presence of ketones.

Bilirubin. The life span of a RBC is 120 days, after which the red cell lyses and releases hemoglobin. Heme, a product of hemoglobin decomposition, subsequently breaks down to form bilirubin. Bilirubin is an intensely yellow (yellow-orange) pigmented substance that is not soluble in water and must attach to a protein, usually albumin, to be transported through blood. Attached to protein, bilirubin does not pass through the glomerulus because of its large size. Instead, it enters the liver. In the liver it becomes water soluble, enters the gallbladder, and is excreted into the intestines, where it becomes a substance called *urobilinogen.* (See Figure 5-8 for a graphic representation of this process.)

Bilirubin is normally not found in urine. Bilirubin levels are elevated if conditions such as hepatitis, excessive **hemolysis** (red cells breaking open and releasing hemoglobin), liver damage, and obstruction of the bile duct are present. The yellow-orange color is called *jaundice* when it is found in the skin, mucous membranes, sclera of the eye, plasma, and urine. The color of urine containing bilirubin can be yellow-orange to yellow-brown. A yellow foam forms when it is shaken. If the reagent strip is positive for bilirubin, an Ictotest (Bayer Corp.) can be performed to confirm the presence of bilirubin.

Urobilinogen. Urobilinogen results from the breakdown of bilirubin in the intestines by bacteria. The circulatory system reabsorbs approximately half of the urobilinogen that forms in the intestines, and the remaining half then travels to the liver, where it is sent to the intestines and excreted in the feces. It either remains in this form or is further oxidized to urobilin by intestinal flora. Feces derive their color from urobilin, a pigmented substance. Small amounts of urobilinogen may be present in the urine (approximately 1%), but most is excreted in the feces.

Urine urobilinogen levels may be increased in conditions such as excessive hemolysis of RBCs, cirrhosis, infectious mononucleosis, and congestive heart failure.

Blood. Three types of blood components give a positive reagent strip reaction for blood: intact RBCs (nonhemolyzed), hemoglobin (from lysed RBCs), and myoglobin. The presence of intact RBCs in urine is called **hematuria** and usually occurs in UTIs associated with bleeding, such as cystitis and urethritis. Kidney stones, tumors, and lesions may also cause bleeding.

If a female patient is having a menstrual period, a clean-catch, midstream urine specimen is recommended and her menstrual status should be noted on the requisition. In general, if small amounts of blood and protein are detected on the urine dipstick, it may be necessary to repeat the urinalysis in 1 or more weeks, after the menstrual cycle is complete, to rule out possible infection.

Hemoglobin in the urine, *hemoglobinuria,* is caused by blood transfusion reactions, malaria, drug reactions, snakebites, and severe burns. Because it is the result of hemolyzed RBCs that are no longer visible, it is referred to as "occult (hidden) blood." Myoglobin, an oxygen-storing pigment of muscle tissue, can be found in urine after massive muscle injury, physical trauma, or electrical injury.

Protein. Protein molecules are normally too large to pass though the glomerulus. One of the first signs of renal disease is **proteinuria**, the presence of large amounts of protein in the urine. Sometimes protein is temporarily found in the urine and may not be pathogenic—for example, during fever, exposure to heat or cold, excessive exercise, and emotional stress. However, large amounts of protein repeatedly excreted in the urine over a period of time indicate renal disease. In pathological conditions, albumin is the protein found in urine. The types of protein that can be found in urine are listed in Table 3-1. Proteinuria may occur because of damage to the glomerulus or an imperfection in the reabsorption ability of the renal tubules.

In addition, pregnant women are routinely checked for protein in the urine because it may be a sign of preeclampsia. Correlating protein level with specific gravity is important because urine with a low specific gravity (very dilute) showing a trace or small amount of protein may be a significant abnormal result.

A microalbumin test determines if small amounts of albumin are excreted, 30 to 300 mg a day, and is performed if the routine strip is negative for protein

Table 3-1　Proteins Found in Urine

Protein	Associated Causes/Conditions
Albumin	Strenuous physical exercise
	Emotional stress
	Pregnancy
	Infection
	Glomerulonephritis
	Neonates (first week)
Globulins	Glomerulonephritis
	Renal tubular dysfunction
Hemoglobin	Hematuria
	Hemoglobinuria
Fibrinogen	Severe renal disease
Nucleoprotein	White blood cells in urine
	Epithelial cells in urine
Bence Jones	Multiple myeloma
	Leukemia

From Stepp CA, Woods M: *Laboratory procedures for medical office personnel,* Philadelphia, 1998, Saunders.

or shows trace amounts. Annual screening for micro-albuminuria helps identify patients with nephropathy at an early stage. Because urine concentration is so variable, it is recommended that the urine be standardized by performing a ratio of microalbumin to the creatinine concentration, which is excreted at a constant rate. Less than 3.4 mg/mmol (millimole) is considered negative, and levels between 3.4 and 33.9 mg/mmol indicate microalbuminuria. Bayer Corp. has developed microalbumin/creatinine ratio test strips that can be visually read or measured on the Clinitek instrument. The Multistix Pro10LS is a urinalysis strip that measures a protein/creatinine ratio (see Figure 3-10, *B*).

Microalbumin screening is critical for the following conditions:
- Diabetes mellitus
- Hypertension
- Heart attack
- Stroke
- Pregnancy

Bence Jones protein is another protein found in the urine of patients with multiple myeloma, a malignant cancer of the bone marrow. Bence Jones protein coagulates at temperatures between 45° and 55° C and then redissolves when boiled.

Nitrites. Some urinary tract bacteria can convert nitrate, which is found normally in the urine, to nitrite. The first morning specimen is recommended for this test because the urine must stay in the bladder for at least 4 to 6 hours to allow any bacteria that may be present sufficient time to convert nitrates to nitrites. Urine should not be left standing because bacterial contamination may convert nitrate to nitrite and give a false-positive reaction. A negative nitrite test does not necessarily mean that no bacterial infection is present. Some bacteria cannot convert nitrates to nitrites, or possibly the urine did not stay in the bladder for 4 to 6 hours. A positive nitrite test is correlated with a positive leukocyte test and then confirmed with a bacterial culture to determine the quantity and identification of the organisms. The most common organism that causes UTIs, *Escherichia coli,* does convert nitrates to nitrites.

Leukocytes. Another test on the reagent strip determines the presence of leukocytes, or white blood cells (WBCs). The strip tests for esterase, which is produced by lysed granulocytic WBCs (cells broken open). The presence of WBCs usually indicates a UTI and should be correlated with a nitrite test.

Becoming Proficient at Urinalysis Physical and Chemical Testing

Now that you have learned how to describe the physical characteristics of urine and how to measure the specific gravity, pH, and various urine analytes, you are ready to perform a urinalysis and record your results on a form such as that shown in Figure 3-13. NOTE: The physician or laboratory technician will complete the microscopic results on the right side of the report form. The proficiency check-off sheets, report forms, and logs are located in your workbook.

The following are additional ways to increase your knowledge:
1. Answer the questions at the end of this chapter and in the workbook (Chapter 3).
2. View the on-line videos on Evolve to see demonstrations of the skills.
3. Perform the on-line "activities and lessons" designed to reinforce your terminology and reagent strip performance.
4. Study Procedure 3-3: Manual Chemical Reagent Strip Procedure in the text and workbook before your laboratory class.
5. Also study Procedure 3-4: Clinitek Analyzer Method for Chemical Reagent Strip and Procedure 3-5: Clinitest Procedure for Reducing Substances Such as Sugars in the Urine before class.

Patient:						Date/Time Spec. Collected:					
Doctor:			DOB:			Date/Time Spec. Completed:					
☐ VOID	TEST	REFERENCE	RESULT	TEST	REFERENCE	RESULT		TEST	REFERENCE	RESULT	TEST	REFERENCE	RESULT

☐ VOID	TEST	REFERENCE	RESULT	TEST	REFERENCE	RESULT		TEST	REFERENCE	RESULT	TEST	REFERENCE	RESULT
☐ CC	Color	Yellow		Blood	Neg			WBC	0-5 HPF		Bact.	0-5	
☐ CATH	Char.	Clear		pH	5.0-8.0			RBC	0-3 HPF		Mucus	0	
	Glucose	Neg		Protein	Neg		MICRO	Epith.	D		Casts	0	
☐ TURBID	Bilirubin	Neg		Urobili	0.2-1.0 EU			Cryst.	0-3 HPF				
☐ HAZY	Ketone	Neg		Nitrite	Neg		OTHER:						
☐ CLEAR	Sp. Gr	1,000-1,030		Leuk	Neg								

Fig. 3-13 Example of a urinalysis form to be completed and inserted into the patient record. NOTE: The physician or laboratory technician will fill out the microscopic results on the right side of the report form.

✳ PROCEDURE 3-3 Manual Chemical Reagent Strip Procedure

A, Urinalysis chemistry procedure. Dip the reagent strip in the urine, making sure all the reagent pads are wet. *(From Bonewit-West K: Clinical procedures for medical assistants, ed 9, St Louis, 2015, Saunders.)*

B, Slide the back of the reagent strip on the urine cup as it is removed to eliminate excess fluid, and then blot the side of the strip against absorbent paper. *(From Bonewit-West K: Clinical procedures for medical assistants, ed 9, St Louis, 2015, Saunders.)*

C, Compare each color pad on the strip to the reference chart starting with the first pad (glucose) and its corresponding row on the bottom of the chart. *(From Bonewit-West K: Clinical procedures for medical assistants, ed 9, St Louis, 2015, Saunders.)*

(Continued)

PROCEDURE 3-3 Manual Chemical Reagent Strip Procedure—cont'd

D, Multistix 10 SG chart showing each analyte's row with its reading time and possible reactions, beginning on the left with "normal" results and moving to the right as the amount of analyte being tested increases. *(Courtesy Bayer Corp.)*

Purpose

Testing for chemical substances in a urine specimen

Equipment and Supplies

Gloves, reagent strips, timing device, reference chart, patient's requisition

Procedure

1. Sanitize and glove your hands, and assemble the equipment. Check the expiration date and the date the reagent bottle was first opened located on the reagent strip bottle. Do not use them if expired.
2. Have the patient produce freshly voided urine in the appropriate container. The sample must come to room temperature, if necessary. Be sure to mix the urine sample before testing. (NOTE: Urine is usually poured into a conical tube to make it easier to determine the color and appearance. This type of tube is used for centrifugation in the microscopic part of the urinalysis and also keeps the original container sterile if a urine culture is necessary.)
3. NOTE: Perform quality control testing using manufacturer's controls *before* testing patients. Record and compare the control results to ensure accuracy by checking the results against the manufacturer's control values.

PROCEDURE 3-3 Manual Chemical Reagent Strip Procedure—cont'd

4. After you remove the strip from the bottle, close it immediately. Do not touch the pads.
5. Make sure the pads are completely covered with urine, but do not immerse the strip for more than a few seconds (Figure A).
6. Pull the nonpad side of the strip along the edge of the container (Figure B), and then briefly blot the side of the strip against absorbent paper.
7. Hold the strip parallel to the color chart (in a horizontal position) so that the reagents in the pads do not interact (Figure C). To keep from contaminating the chart, do not place the strip on it.
8. The reagents in the pads are time dependent, so read each test on the strip at its particular time and compare it to the reference chart (Figure D). Start with the pad that corresponds with the bottom row of the color chart. The 10 tests on Multistix 10 SG reagent strips and their reading times are as follows:
   - Glucose: 30 seconds
   - Bilirubin: 30 seconds
   - Ketones: 40 seconds
   - Specific gravity: 45 seconds

- Blood: 60 seconds
- pH: 60 seconds
- Protein: 60 seconds
- Urobilinogen: 60 seconds
- Nitrite: 60 seconds
- Leukocytes: 2 minutes

9. After you have read all the pads, discard the strip in a biohazard bag.
10. Remove the gloves, and sanitize your hands.
11. Document the procedure, indicating the results, the brand name of the test strip used, the date, the time, and the name of the person testing in the patient's chart (or record results on the preprinted patient's requisition/report).
12. Pour the remaining urine down the sink, and place the container in the biohazard waste container. Be sure to have a stream of water started before pouring the urine down the sink to keep from splattering the sample. NOTE: If the results of a urine test are abnormal, do not discard the specimen until the physician approves since he or she may want to order additional tests on the specimen.

✳ PROCEDURE 3-4 Clinitek Analyzer Method for Chemical Reagent Strip

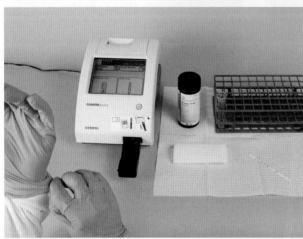

A, Prepare the following: gloves, Clinitek analyzer, absorbent paper, Multistix 10 SG reagent strips or Multistix Pro10LS strips, patient's urine, and/or control specimen.

B, Follow the prompts on the instrument monitor and/or the manufacturer's flow sheet. IMPORTANT NOTE: Before pressing the "start" command, have your test strip ready to dip into the urine.

(Continued)

PROCEDURE 3-4 **Clinitek Analyzer Method for Chemical Reagent Strip—cont'd**

C, Immediately after pressing "start," you have 8 seconds to dip the strip in the urine, remove excess urine from the back of the strip, turn the strip sideways, and blot on the paper.

D, Place the strip in the proper position on the tray (within the 8 seconds). NOTE: This strip still needs to be straightened.

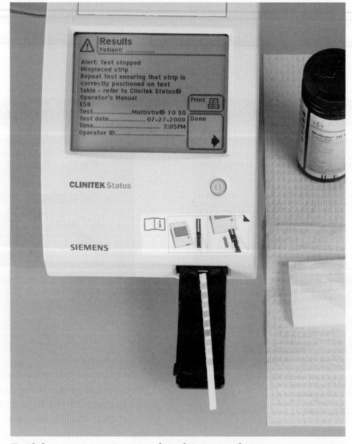

E, If the reagent strip was placed incorrectly, an error message will appear and the tray will push the sample out. You will need to start the test again with a new strip.

PROCEDURE 3-4 Clinitek Analyzer Method for Chemical Reagent Strip—cont'd

Equipment and Supplies

Gloves, Multistix 10 SG reagent strips or Multistix Pro10LS strips, absorbent paper, Clinitek analyzer (Figure A).

Procedure

1. Assemble the equipment. Sanitize and glove your hands. Check the expiration date on the reagent strip bottle. Do not use if expired.
2. Be sure to mix the room temperature urine sample, and pour it into a conical tube before testing.
3. NOTE: Perform quality control using a manufacturer's liquid control. Record the results and check for accuracy.
4. After you remove the strip from the bottle, close it immediately. Do not touch the reagent pads.
5. Follow the instructions on the instrument monitor or the manufacturer's flow sheet.
   - Enter technician identification.
   - Enter patient information.
   - Before pressing the "start" command, have your test strip ready to dip into the urine (Figure B).
6. After pressing start, you will have 8 seconds to do the following:
   - Dip the strip into the urine, making sure all the pads are completely covered with urine, but do not immerse the strip for more than a few seconds.
   - Remove excess urine from the strip by pulling the nonpad side of the strip along the edge of the container.
   - Blot the side of the strip against absorbent paper briefly (Figure C).
   - Place the strip in the Clinitek tray, making sure it is placed correctly (Figure D).
7. When the instrument completes its 8-second countdown, it will pull the specimen into the analyzer. NOTE: If the reagent strip was placed incorrectly, an error message will appear and the tray will push the sample out (Figure E). The reagent strip must be discarded, the instrument will need to be reset, and a new reagent strip must be used to run the test again.
8. While the instrument is measuring each of the timed reagent pads, you will be prompted to record the color and transparency of the urine specimen.
9. When the test is complete, the analyzer will eject the sample tray and print the date, the time, the patient's name, the name of the person performing the test, the results of the 10 tests, and the color and transparency of the specimen.
10. Discard the strip in the appropriate biohazard waste container. Gently wipe off the tray with gauze or paper towel. Pour the remaining urine down the sink, if no additional tests will be ordered, and place the container in the biohazard waste container. Be sure to have a stream of water started before pouring the urine down the sink to keep from splattering the sample.

Photos A through E by Zack Bent.

PROCEDURE 3-5 Clinitest Procedure for Reducing Substances Such as Sugars in the Urine

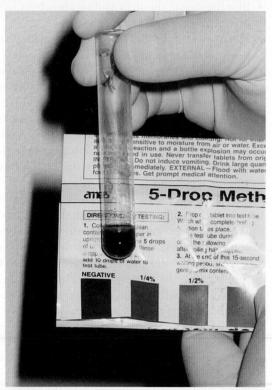

A, Comparison chart for measuring the color results of the Clinitest sugar test. The specimen result is blue, which would be negative for sugar. *(From Proctor D, Adams A: Kinn's the medical assistant: an applied learning approach, ed 12, St Louis, 2014, Saunders.)*

Equipment and Supplies

Bottle of Clinitest tablets, Clinitest glass tube, tube of water with pipette, urine sample with pipette, Clinitest reference chart

Procedure

1. Gather equipment, sanitize your hands, and put on gloves.

2. Add 5 drops of urine to 10 drops of water in a Clinitest tube.

3. Place the tube in a rack. Put a Clinitest tablet into the lid of the bottle so that you do not touch it; the tablet could become caustic if it becomes moist. Tap the tablet into the tube.

4. The boiling reaction that occurs is very hot. Observe it for any color change. Observe for the "pass-through effect" that results, with color changes occurring during the reaction and appearing negative when the reaction is completed and results are determined. The pass-through effect occurs as a result of very high concentrations of reducing substances in the urine. If this does occur, results should be recorded as greater than 2% if using the 5-drop method or as greater than 5% if using the 2-drop method. The final color of either method should not be compared with the color chart when the pass-through effect takes place.

5. Mix the tube 15 seconds after the boiling has stopped to blend the contents.

6. Compare the color of the reaction with the Clinitest chart (Figure A) for the 5-drop method, and record the results. If the rapid pass-through effect has occurred and you briefly see an orange color, the test must be reported as positive.

7. Discard the equipment in the appropriate biohazard waste container. The remaining urine should be rinsed down the sink, and the container should be placed in a biohazard waste container. Be sure to have a stream of water started before pouring the urine down the sink to keep from splattering the sample.

8. Disinfect the work area.

9. Remove gloves, and sanitize your hands.

10. Correctly document the results in the patient's chart.

Advanced Concepts

Microscopic Urinalysis

A microscopic examination of urine consists of examining, counting, and categorizing the solid material seen under the microscope. A standardized method called the *Kova System* is used to prepare the microscopic slide. It consists of centrifuging a standard amount of urine for a specific time with a specific centrifugal force. After centrifugation the urine separates into **sediment**, the material at the bottom of the centrifuged tube of urine, and **supernatant**, the liquid portion of urine on top of the spun sediment. The supernatant is poured off, and the sediment is stained and poured onto a slide or transferred into a Kova slide chamber. The slide is then placed under the microscope and focused in preparation for the analysis by the physician or trained professional (see Procedure 3-6 at the end of this section).

Medical assistants prepare the urine microscopic slide, and either medical technologists or physicians interpret the results. The medical assistant should be familiar with the terminology of the microscopic findings and the basic shapes of the elements found in the urinary sediment in order to understand the complete urinalysis report. The sediment is examined under the microscope for the presence of cells, casts, crystals, and other substances. First, the presence of casts is viewed using the low power objective of the microscope; then all other substances are observed on high power. NOTE: See the "urinalysis videos" on-line showing actual microscopic views of cells, casts and some of the crystals, parasites, and fungi.

Cells (See Atlas)

The following cells may be found and reported during a microscopic examination.

Red Blood Cells

Hematuria is the abnormal presence of RBCs in the urine (Figure 3-14). RBCs are round, biconcave, non-nucleated, colorless disks. They are highly refractile in unstained urine and can be difficult to differentiate from other structures, such as yeasts and oil droplets. Yeast usually shows budding, whereas RBCs do not. RBCs shrink in concentrated urine and are referred to as *crenated.* RBCs will swell and hemolyze in diluted urine. If the RBCs have been hemolyzed (broken open), they will not be seen on the microscopic examination, but the hemoglobin will be detected on the blood pad of the chemical strip test. A few RBCs, 1 to 2 per high power field (hpf), can be normal. Bleeding, damage to the glomerulus (e.g., inflammation of the glomerulus, or glomerulonephritis), and vascular injury are associated with the presence of RBCs in the urine.

White Blood Cells

The condition **pyuria**, or WBCs in the urine, usually indicates the presence of an infection in the genitourinary system (Figure 3-15, *B*). WBCs are larger than RBCs, approximately 12 micrometers in diameter. The most common WBC found in the urine is the neutrophil, which possesses a multilobed nucleus and granules. A urine microscopic examination normally contains 0 to 5 WBCs/hpf. Pyuria can be temporary or caused by fevers or strenuous exercise, but the presence of WBCs can be a factor in pyelonephritis, cystitis, prostatitis, and urethritis.

Epithelial Cells

Another type of cell that can be found in the urine is the epithelial cell. Several types exist.

Squamous epithelial cells (see Figure 3-15, *A*) are the most frequently seen and least significant of the epithelial cells found in urine. They are derived from the lining of the vagina and the lower portion of the male and female urethras. These cells are large and have abundant, irregular cytoplasm with a central nucleus the size of an RBC.

Transitional or *caudate epithelial cells* (Figure 3-16) come from the lining of the renal pelvis, bladder, and upper urethra. They are spherical, polyhedral, or caudate (having a tail), with a central nucleus, and are smaller than squamous epithelial cells. They can be found in pairs and small clumps after catheterizations. The presence of large numbers of transitional epithelial cells may indicate a pathological condition.

Renal tubular epithelial cells (RTEs) (Figure 3-17) are the most significant of the epithelial cells. The presence of increased amounts (more than 2/hpf) indicates tubular necrosis. The size and shape of these cells vary depending on their origin. These cells are round to oval, sometimes rectangular to columnar, and slightly larger than WBCs, and they can be distinguished from leukocytes by the presence of a single round, eccentric nucleus. Renal tubule cells are present in microscopic urine in conditions such as pyelonephritis, toxic reaction, viral infections, allograft rejection, and secondary effects attributable to glomerulonephritis.

Casts (See Atlas)

Casts are formed primarily within the lumen of the distal convoluted tubules and the collecting ducts. They provide a microscopic view of conditions within the nephron. Their shapes usually contain parallel sides and rounded ends. The main component of a cast is a gel-like protein. Four factors can lead to cast formation: decreased urine flow, increased acidity (low pH), increased concentration (high specific gravity), and increased plasma protein. When these factors are present, a cast is formed in the following manner:

1. Protein aggregates into individual protein fibrils that attach to renal tubule cells.
2. The protein fibrils interweave, forming a loose fibril network that becomes a solid structure.
3. Urinary components, such as RBCs or epithelial cells, may attach to the solid structure.
4. The protein fibril structure detaches from the epithelial cells lining the renal tubules and is excreted as a cast.

Casts are observed and counted on low power, but they are identified on high power. They tend to migrate to the edges of the slide, so this area must be examined. Fresh urine should be examined because casts dissolve in alkaline urine that has been standing.

Hyaline Casts

The hyaline cast (Figure 3-18) is the most frequently seen cast. It consists almost entirely of protein and appears colorless in unstained urine. Because the hyaline cast has a refractive index very similar to that of urine, it must be examined with the light subdued. This cast can normally be found in the urine (0 to 2/hpf). Conditions such as strenuous exercise, dehydration, heat exposure, and emotional stress can cause hyaline casts to be present in the urine. These casts can also be found in pathological conditions such as acute glomerulonephritis, pyelonephritis, chronic renal disease, and congestive heart failure.

Red Blood Cell Casts

An RBC cast (Figure 3-19) contains RBCs, is refractile, and is yellow-orange to orange-red in color. RBC casts are primarily associated with glomerulonephritis. As they age, the RBCs lyse and the cast becomes a hemoglobin cast. A hemoglobin cast has the same color as an RBC cast but without visible intact cells.

White Blood Cell Casts

WBC casts (Figure 3-20) most frequently contain neutrophils, one type of WBC, that are refractile because of the presence of granules and multilobed nuclei. They indicate infection or inflammation within the nephron, mostly seen in pyelonephritis.

Renal Epithelial Cell Casts

Renal epithelial cell casts (Figure 3-21) contain renal tubule epithelial cells and can be very difficult to differentiate from WBC casts. They are found in conditions such as heavy metal and chemical- or drug-induced toxicity, viral infection, and allograft rejection.

Granular Casts

Granular casts (Figure 3-22) contain granules throughout the matrix. They can appear as coarse or finely granular, but distinguishing between the two is not necessary. When urinary flow diminishes, a granular cast may form as a result of the disintegration of cellular casts and tubule cells or protein aggregates filtered by the glomerulus. Granular casts result from stress and strenuous exercise but can also be found in conditions such as nephrotic syndrome, orthostatic proteinuria, and congestive heart failure.

Waxy Casts

Waxy casts (Figure 3-23) are very refractile and are homogeneously smooth, with ends that are blunt and cracked. These casts appear dark pink, if stained, and represent extreme urine stasis (stoppage of urine), signifying chronic renal failure.

Crystals (See Atlas)

Crystals are formed by the precipitation of urine salts when changes in pH, temperature (crystals form readily at low temperatures), or concentration occur. The most important aid in the identification of urine crystals is based on the urine pH. Although most crystals are normal when found in acidic and alkaline urine, the few abnormal crystals cited next may represent disorders such as liver disease, inborn errors of metabolism, or renal damage caused by the crystallization of **iatrogenic** compounds (caused by treatment or diagnostic procedures) and must be detected and reported. Crystals are counted and identified under high power and reported as few, moderate, and many.

Crystals in Acidic Urine

The most common crystals normally seen in acid urine are uric acid crystals, amorphous urates, acid urates, and calcium oxalate.

Uric acid crystals (Figure 3-24) are typically four-sided and flat yellow to reddish brown. They can be seen in a variety of shapes, such as rhombic, wedge, and rosette. Although these crystals are usually normal, they can be seen in patients with leukemia who are receiving chemotherapy and sometimes in patients with gout.

Amorphous urates (Figure 3-25) are yellow-brown granules often found in clumps that give the urine a macroscopic (i.e., sufficiently large to see with the eyes) pink "brick dust" color.

Acid urates are found in urine at pH levels below 7 and are frequently seen in urine that has been refrigerated.

Calcium oxalates (Figure 3-26) are frequently found in acid urine but can also be found in neutral and rarely in alkaline urine. They are commonly seen as colorless octahedron crystals that resemble envelopes (they have the appearance of an × on them). The presence of calcium oxalate crystals in fresh urine may indicate the formation of renal calculi (kidney stones). They are also associated with foods high in oxalic acid, such as tomatoes and asparagus, and ascorbic acid (oxalic acid is an end product of ascorbic acid).

Crystals in Alkaline Urine

The majority of normal crystals seen in alkaline urine are phosphates and include triple phosphate, and amorphous phosphate.

Triple phosphate crystals (Figure 3-27) resemble coffin lids and have no clinical significance. They are found in very alkaline urine that contains urea-splitting bacteria.

Amorphous phosphate crystals (Figure 3-28) are found in urine with a pH greater than 7. They are yellow-brown granules with no distinctive shape. These crystals, which form when urine cools to room temperature, have a macroscopic appearance of white turbidity.

Abnormal Crystals

Most abnormal crystals are found in acid urine and only rarely in neutral urine.

Cystine crystals (acid pH) appear as colorless, refractile, hexagonal plates and can be confused with uric acid crystals. Differentiation can be made by the fact that uric acid crystals are very birefringent under a polarized microscope. However, only thick cystine crystals have polarizing abilities. Positive identification can be made with a cyanide-nitroprusside test.

Leucine crystals (acid or neutral pH) are oily-appearing spheres with radial and concentric striations. These crystals are often found with tyrosine crystals in patients who have severe liver disease.

Tyrosine crystals (acid or neutral pH) resemble fine needles in sheaves or rosettes and are found in conjunction with leucine. They may occur in patients with inherited disorders of amino acid metabolism.

Bilirubin crystals are seen in hepatic disorders and appear as clumped needles or granules with the characteristic yellow color of bilirubin.

Cholesterol crystals (acid pH) are rarely seen because lipids do not usually crystallize, but they can be found in urine that has been refrigerated. They appear as rectangular plates with a notch in one or more corners (Figure 3-29). Along with fatty casts and oval fat bodies (discussed later in this chapter), cholesterol crystals are characteristic of disorders such as nephrotic syndrome.

Sulfonamide (Figure 3-30) and *ampicillin crystals* are formed after inadequate hydration in patients being treated with these antibiotics.

Other Substances (See Atlas)

Bacteria

Because bacteria (Figure 3-31) are normally not found in the urine, the presence of bacteria could indicate either contamination of the specimen or the presence of a UTI. WBCs present with bacteria could signify a UTI. Because contaminant bacteria reproduce rapidly if the urine is kept at room temperature for a prolonged period, testing and microscopic examination should be performed on fresh urine. Bacteria are very tiny and must be viewed on high power. They appear as either rod shaped (bacilli) or round (cocci) and are reported as few, moderate, or many, or as 1+, 2+, 3+, or 4+.

Yeast

Yeasts (Figure 3-32) are small, oval organisms that may bud. Differentiating them from RBCs is sometimes difficult, but the budding characteristic is helpful. *Candida albicans* is a yeast that may be found in the urine of women who have a vaginal infection (candidiasis), in patients with diabetes mellitus, and in immunocompromised patients. Yeasts are reported in the same way as bacteria.

Parasites

Trichomonas vaginalis (Figure 3-33) is the most frequently seen parasite in urine specimens. It is a pear-shaped flagellate with an undulating membrane and a characteristic rapid darting movement that helps identify it in a wet preparation. *T. vaginalis* is a sexually transmitted parasite that causes vaginal inflammation in women and infection of the urethra and prostate in men. It is reported as rare, few, moderate, or many per high power field.

Sperm

Spermatozoa, or sperm, can be found in both male and female urine after sexual intercourse. They have oval, slightly tapered heads and long, flagella-like tails. Spermatozoa are reported as 1+, 2+, 3+, or 4+.

Mucus

Mucus (Figure 3-34) is a protein whose major constituent is Tamm-Horsfall protein. It is produced by the glands and epithelial cells of the lower genitourinary tract and renal tubular epithelial cells. Microscopically, mucus appears as threadlike structures. To see mucus, the microscope light must be subdued. The presence of mucus in the urine has no clinical significance.

Artifacts

Artifacts that may be found in the urine may include fecal contamination (Figure 3-35), starch granules from gloves, air bubbles, pollen grains, hair (Figure 3-36), and clothing and diaper fibers (Figure 3-37).

Calculating a Microscopic Urinalysis

Although medical assistants do not read microscopic urinalysis results, they must understand how the calculation and interpretation of this test are performed. NOTE: There are excellent videos on-line that show moving examples of the cells, casts, and crystals seen under the microscope. Between 10 and 15 fields are examined under low power for casts. Casts are observed and counted under low power, but they must be identified under high power. Between 10 and 15 fields are then viewed under high power. Each substance that is seen in each of the high power fields is counted. When all the fields have been counted, the results for each substance are averaged and reported. Casts are reported as the average number seen per low power field (lpf), whereas cells are reported by using numerical ranges based on the average per high power field (hpf). Other substances are reported as rare, few, moderate, or many (or 1+, 2+, 3+, 4+) per hpf. Standard counting and reporting systems must be used by everyone in the same laboratory. Table 3-2 shows an example of how a microscopic urinalysis is calculated and reported.

Cells

Fig. 3-14 Red blood cells in urine. *(From Stepp CA, Woods M:* Laboratory procedures for medical office personnel, *Philadelphia, 1998, Saunders; Zakus SM:* Mosby's clinical skills for medical assistants, *St Louis, 1998, Mosby.)*

Fig. 3-15 Squamous epithelial cell **(A)** and white blood cell **(B)**. *(From Stepp CA, Woods M:* Laboratory procedures for medical office personnel, *Philadelphia, 1998, Saunders; Zakus SM:* Mosby's clinical skills for medical assistants, *St Louis, 1998, Mosby.)*

Fig. 3-16 Transitional epithelial cells. *(From Ringsrud KM, Linne JJ:* Urinalysis and body fluids: a color text and atlas, *St Louis, 1995, Mosby; Zakus SM:* Mosby's clinical skills for medical assistants, *St Louis, 1998, Mosby.)*

Fig. 3-17 Renal tubular epithelial cell. *(From Ringsrud KM, Linne JJ:* Urinalysis and body fluids: a color text and atlas, *St Louis, 1995, Mosby; Zakus SM:* Mosby's clinical skills for medical assistants, *St Louis, 1998, Mosby.)*

Casts

Fig. 3-18 Hyaline casts. *(From Ringsrud KM, Linne JJ: Urinalysis and body fluids: a color text and atlas, St Louis, 1995, Mosby; Zakus SM: Mosby's clinical skills for medical assistants, St Louis, 1998, Mosby.)*

Fig. 3-19 Red blood cell casts. *(From Stepp CA, Woods M: Laboratory procedures for medical office personnel, Philadelphia, 1998, Saunders; Zakus SM: Mosby's clinical skills for medical assistants, St Louis, 1998, Mosby.)*

Fig. 3-20 White blood cell casts. *(From Stepp CA, Woods M: Laboratory procedures for medical office personnel, Philadelphia, 1998, Saunders; Zakus SM: Mosby's clinical skills for medical assistants, St Louis, 1998, Mosby.)*

Fig. 3-21 Renal epithelial cast. *(From Ringsrud KM, Linne JJ: Urinalysis and body fluids: a color text and atlas, St Louis, 1995, Mosby; Zakus SM: Mosby's clinical skills for medical assistants, St Louis, 1998, Mosby.)*

Fig. 3-22 Granular casts. *(From Stepp CA, Woods M: Laboratory procedures for medical office personnel, Philadelphia, 1998, Saunders; Zakus SM: Mosby's clinical skills for medical assistants, St Louis, 1998, Mosby.)*

Fig. 3-23 Waxy casts. *(From Stepp CA, Woods M: Laboratory procedures for medical office personnel, Philadelphia, 1998, Saunders.)*

Crystals

| Acidic | Alkaline |

Fig. 3-24 Uric acid crystals. *(From Ringsrud KM, Linne JJ: Urinalysis and body fluids: a color text and atlas, St Louis, 1995, Mosby; Zakus SM: Mosby's clinical skills for medical assistants, St Louis, 1998, Mosby.)*

Fig. 3-27 Triple phosphate crystals. NOTE: Coffin lid shapes. *(From Stepp CA, Woods M: Laboratory procedures for medical office personnel, Philadelphia, 1998, Saunders; Zakus SM: Mosby's clinical skills for medical assistants, St Louis, 1998, Mosby.)*

Fig. 3-25 Amorphous urate crystals. *(From Ringsrud KM, Linne JJ: Urinalysis and body fluids: a color text and atlas, St Louis, 1995, Mosby.)*

Fig. 3-28 Amorphous phosphate crystals. *(From Ringsrud KM, Linne JJ: Urinalysis and body fluids: a color text and atlas, St Louis, 1995, Mosby.)*

Fig. 3-26 Calcium oxalate crystals. NOTE: X's with crystals. *(From Stepp CA, Woods M: Laboratory procedures for medical office personnel, Philadelphia, 1998, Saunders; Zakus SM: Mosby's clinical skills for medical assistants, St Louis, 1998, Mosby.)*

Abnormal Crystals

Fig. 3-29 Cholesterol crystals. *(From Stepp CA, Woods M: Laboratory procedures for medical office personnel, Philadelphia, 1998, Saunders; Zakus SM: Mosby's clinical skills for medical assistants, St Louis, 1998, Mosby.)*

Fig. 3-30 Sulfonamide crystals. *(From Stepp CA, Woods M: Laboratory procedures for medical office personnel, Philadelphia, 1998, Saunders; Zakus SM: Mosby's clinical skills for medical assistants, St Louis, 1998, Mosby.)*

Other Substances

Fig. 3-31 Bacteria in urine. Note the large white blood cells. *(From Ringsrud KM, Linne JJ: Urinalysis and body fluids: a color text and atlas, St Louis, 1995, Mosby.)*

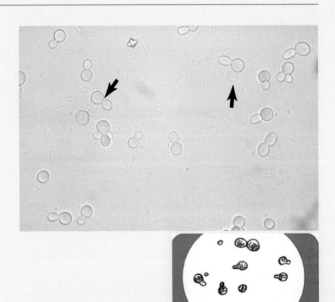

Fig. 3-32 Yeast in urine. Note how they are budding. *(From Stepp CA, Woods M: Laboratory procedures for medical office personnel, Philadelphia, 1998, Saunders; Zakus SM: Mosby's clinical skills for medical assistants, St Louis, 1998, Mosby.)*

Other Substances—cont'd

Fig. 3-34 Mucous threads in urine. *(From Stepp CA, Woods M:* Laboratory procedures for medical office personnel, *Philadelphia, 1998, Saunders.)*

Fig. 3-33 *Trichomonas vaginalis* in urine. *(From Stepp CA, Woods M:* Laboratory procedures for medical office personnel, *Philadelphia, 1998, Saunders; Zakus SM:* Mosby's clinical skills for medical assistants, *St Louis, 1998, Mosby.)*

Fig. 3-36 Hair fiber in urine. *(From Ringsrud KM, Linne JJ:* Urinalysis and body fluids: a color text and atlas, *St Louis, 1995, Mosby.)*

Fig. 3-35 Fecal contamination in urine. *(From Ringsrud KM, Linne JJ:* Urinalysis and body fluids: a color text and atlas, *St Louis, 1995, Mosby.)*

Fig. 3-37 Diaper fiber in urine. *(From Ringsrud KM, Linne JJ:* Urinalysis and body fluids: a color text and atlas, *St Louis, 1995, Mosby.)*

Table 3-2 Calculating a Microscopic Urinalysis

	PER LOW POWER FIELD				PER HIGH POWER FIELD						
Field	Casts	Mucus	WBCs	RBCs	Squamous Epithelial	Transitional Epithelial	Round Epithelial	Bacteria	Crystals	Other
1	0	Few	16	1	1	0	0	Moderate (rods)	Calcium oxalate (few) Uric acid (few)	—
2	1 hyaline	Few	32	0	3	0	0	Many	Calcium oxalate (few)	Yeast
3	1 coarse granular	Moderate	21	2	3	0	0	Many	Calcium oxalate (few)	Yeast
4	1 coarse granular	Few	12	1	5	0	1	Moderate	Uric acid (few)	—
5	0	Few	25	0	4	0	0	Many	—	—
Total	1 hyaline 2 coarse granular	Few	106	4	16	0	1	Many	Calcium oxalate (few) Uric acid (few)	Yeast
Average	0.2 hyaline 0.4 coarse granular	Few	21.2	0.8	3.2	0	0.2	Many	Calcium oxalate (few) Uric acid (few)	Yeast
Report	Hyaline 0-1 coarse granular	Few	20-30	0-1	Few	0	Occasionally	Many (rods)	Calcium oxalate (few) Uric acid (few)	Yeast

RBCs, Red blood cells; WBCs, white blood cells.

From Proctor D, Adams A: Kinn's the medical assistant: an applied learning approach, ed 12, St Louis, 2014, Saunders.

✳ **PROCEDURE 3-6** Procedure for the Preparation and the Microscopic Examination of Urine

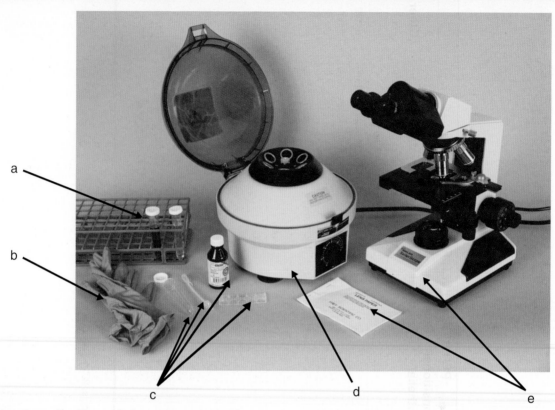

a
b
c
d
e

A, *(a)* Specimen (freshly voided urine) in tube holder, *(b)* gloves, *(c)* Kova system (cap and tube, pipette, stain, slide), *(d)* centrifuge, *(e)* microscope and lens paper.

B, Place a centrifuge tube with urine and a centrifuge tube with the same amount of water or urine directly opposite each other to balance the centrifuge. Spin for 5 minutes at 1500 rpm.

C, After centrifuging, place the pipette in the spun specimen to hold back the sediment and pour off the supernatant.

PROCEDURE 3-6 Procedure for the Preparation and the Microscopic Examination of Urine—cont'd

D, Add stain to the sediment and mix well.

E, Fill the slide wells with the well-mixed stained sediment.

Objective

To prepare a urine microscopic examination slide

Equipment and Supplies

Specimen (freshly voided urine), Kova system (cap, pipette, slide, stain), test tube holder, centrifuge, microscope (Figure A)

Preanalytical: Microscopic Setup

1. Sanitize your hands, and collect the equipment.
2. Put on gloves, and mix the urine. Allow it to come to room temperature if needed.
3. Pour the well-mixed urine specimen to the 12-mL mark in a urine centrifuge tube, and cap it.
4. Centrifuge the tube for 5 minutes at 1500 rpm, which will cause the solid particles in the urine to settle to the bottom of the tube (Figure B).
5. After centrifugation is completed, carefully remove the spun tube from the centrifuge so that the sediment is not disturbed.

6. After removing the cap, place the Kova pipette into the bottom of the tube. Seat the tube firmly, hooking the clip on top of the pipette over the outside of the tube.
7. Pour off (decant) the supernatant by inverting the tube (Figure C). With the Kova pipette method, approximately 1 mL of sediment will remain in the tube.
8. Remove the pipette from the tube, and add a drop of stain so that the structures may be seen more easily (Figure D). Reinsert the pipette into the tube, and mix the urine sediment and stain by gently squeezing on the pipette bulb.
9. Transfer a drop of the stained sediment mixture to the Kova slide by placing the tip of the pipette onto the open area of one of the sections and squeezing the bulb until the well is filled (Figure E). Do not overfill or underfill the well. Return the pipette to the urine tube after the well is filled. To allow the sediment to settle, let the filled well sit for 1 minute before performing the microscopic examination. NOTE: An alternative method is to place a drop of mixed sediment onto a glass slide and place a glass coverslip over the drop of urine (as seen on the Evolve website in the video entitled "Preparation for microscopic examination" in the *Video – Saunders Clinical Skills On-Line* section.)
10. Place the filled well (or slide) on the mechanical stage of the microscope and focus on low power with the coarse adjustment. With the fine adjustment knob, bring the specimen into sharp focus. Adjust the light source as needed for low power.

Analytical Interpretation of the Sediment on the Slide – Performed by Physician or Laboratory Technician

11. Scan the specimen under low power for casts, particularly at the edge of the slide.
12. Change the objective to high power by rotating the nosepiece and clicking it into place. Bring the specimen into sharp view by focusing with the fine adjustment. The coarse adjustment should not be used for focusing the high power objective because the objective could strike the slide. The intensity of the light source will need to be adjusted for the high power objective.
13. Use high power to examine the specimen, viewing 10 to 15 fields. Casts are counted on low power but identified on high power. All other substances seen should be counted and identified on high power.
14. Record the results for each field.

(Continued)

3-6

PROCEDURE 3-6 Procedure for the Preparation and the Microscopic Examination of Urine—cont'd

Postanalytical: Cleanup and Recording of Results

15. The medical assistant may be asked to turn off the microscope and discard the plastic Kova slide, pipette, and capped centrifuge tube in the biohazard waste container. Rinse the remaining urine down the sink, and place the container in a biohazard waste container.

16. Remove the gloves and discard them in a biohazard waste container. Sanitize your hands.

17. Record the calculated results of each finding on the patient's requisition form and chart.

Photos A and B by Zack Bent.

Review Questions

1. A patient's urine specimen is orange-yellow (or greenish). Which of the following substances would be found in the urine?
   a. glucose
   b. ketones
   c. bilirubin
   d. nitrate

2. Which substance would be found in normal urine that gives the urine its yellow color?
   a. hemoglobin
   b. urochrome
   c. porphyrin
   d. myoglobin

3. Which four conditions are conducive to cast formation?
   a. high pH, increased plasma proteins, increased rate of urine flow, and low specific gravity
   b. low pH, increased plasma proteins, decreased rate of urine flow, and low specific gravity
   c. low pH, decreased plasma proteins, decreased rate of urine flow, and high specific gravity
   d. low pH, increased plasma proteins, decreased rate of urine flow, and high specific gravity

4. In a 24-hour urine specimen collection method, which of the following is correct?
   a. All the urine for a 24-hour period is collected, including the first morning sample of the first day.
   b. When the patient is collecting a urine sample, the first third should go into the toilet.
   c. The first specimen of a 24-hour urine is collected.
   d. The last specimen of a 24-hour urine is collected.

5. Which of the following values would represent a dilute specific gravity?
   a. 1.015
   b. 1.005
   c. 1.020
   d. 1.025

6. The correct flow of urine is
   a. glomerulus, glomerular capsule, renal tubules, urinary bladder, renal pelvis, ureter, urethra, and urinary meatus.
   b. glomerulus, glomerular capsule, renal pelvis, renal tubules, ureter, urinary bladder, urethra, and urinary meatus.
   c. glomerulus, glomerular capsule, renal tubules, renal pelvis, urinary bladder, ureter, urethra, and urinary meatus.
   d. glomerulus, glomerular capsule, renal tubules, renal pelvis, ureter, urinary bladder, urethra, and urinary meatus.

7. Which of the following substances is observed and counted on low power?
   a. crystals
   b. casts
   c. yeasts
   d. bacteria

8. Which casts are occasionally found in healthy people?
   a. renal epithelial casts
   b. white blood cell casts
   c. hyaline casts
   d. waxy casts

9. Triple phosphate crystals resemble
   a. envelopes.
   b. dumbbells.
   c. rosettes.
   d. coffin lids.

10. Which is the most common parasite found in the urine?
   a. *Candida albicans*
   b. *Trichomonas vaginalis*
   c. *Enterobius vermicularis*
   d. *Escherichia coli*

Educating a female patient in the correct midstream clean-catch method of collection includes some of the steps below. Write "C" if the step is correct and "I" if the step is incorrect. If the step is incorrect, explain why.

11. The patient should wash her hands.

12. The patient should spread the labia and hold them apart during the procedure with her nondominant hand.

13. The patient should clean one side with a towelette, wiping from back to front.

14. The patient should repeat step 3 (step 13 above) on the other side with the same towelette.

15. The patient should urinate the first third of the urine into the toilet, catch the second third in the sterile cup, and urinate the last third in the toilet.

16. The medical assistant should disinfect the outside of the container.

Websites

National Kidney Foundation:
www.kidney.org/

National Institute of Diabetes & Digestive & Kidney Diseases (NIDDK):
www.niddk.nih.gov/

National Kidney Disease Kidney Education Program (NIH):
www.nkdep.nih.gov/index.htm

"Bladder Diseases" from Medline Plus (NIH and the U.S. National Library of Medicine):
www.nlm.nih.gov/medlineplus/bladderdiseases.html

4 Blood Collection

OBJECTIVES *After completing this chapter, you should be able to do the following:*

1. Define and match key terms and abbreviations in this chapter.

Fundamental Concepts—Theory, Safety, and Patient Preparation

2. Identify the cardiovascular anatomical structures, and state their functions and each of their relationships to blood collection.
3. Discuss the Needlestick Safety and Prevention Act, and list the ways an employer complies with the Act.
4. Perform the appropriate steps for patient preparation, emphasizing the importance of correctly identifying the patient.

Blood Collection Procedures—Capillary Puncture and Venipuncture

5. Do the following regarding capillary puncture procedures:
   - Perform the proper procedure for capillary puncture according to the stated task, conditions, and standards listed in the Learning Outcome Procedure Sheets in the student workbook, demonstrating an understanding of site selection, equipment, and complications of this procedure.
   - Perform or describe a simulated heel stick and neonatal blood screening collection onto a card according to the stated task, conditions, and standards listed in the Learning Outcome Evaluation in the student workbook.
   - Relate the most current OSHA safety guidelines for capillary puncture methods and maintain a safe work environment by following the most

current guidelines for disposing used equipment and cleaning and disinfecting the work area.

6. Do the following regarding venipuncture procedures:
   - Evaluate a patient's venipuncture site availability, and determine the correct venipuncture method that should be performed.
   - Describe the vacuum tube, syringe, and butterfly venipuncture equipment and explain the order of draw for multiple-tube orders.
   - Perform a Vacutainer venipuncture, syringe venipuncture, and butterfly venipuncture according to the stated task, conditions, and standards listed in the Learning Outcome Evaluation in the student workbook.
   - Relate the most current OSHA safety guidelines for the various venipuncture methods and maintain a safe work environment by following the most current guidelines for disposing used equipment and cleaning and disinfecting the work area.

Advanced Concepts—Specimen and Patient Care

7. Describe or perform the proper way to process blood specimens including how to centrifuge a serum specimen and a plasma specimen in a serum separator tube (SST) and a plasma separator tube (PST).
8. Identify patient issues and complications that may occur during phlebotomy procedures and discuss the appropriate steps to take when they occur; also discuss the importance of risk management as it pertains to blood collection procedures.

KEY TERMS

antecubital space area in front of the elbow

anticoagulant a natural or synthesized chemical that prevents blood from clotting

arteries blood vessels with a pulse that carry blood away from the heart

blood culture a test to detect bacteria or organisms growing in the blood

buffy coat narrow middle layer of white blood cells and platelets in a centrifuged whole blood specimen

capillaries microscopic blood vessels that contain a mixture of arterial and venous blood

capillary action process by which blood flows freely into a capillary tube in microcollection procedures

capillary puncture skin puncture or "stick" (typically finger sticks on adults and heel sticks on infants)

cyanotic a condition in which the skin and mucous membranes are blue; caused by an oxygen deficiency

edema abnormal collection of fluid in interstitial spaces that causes swelling

EDTA a synthesized anticoagulant that also preserves the blood cells (ethylenediaminetetraacetic acid)

evacuated tubes tubes with air removed to produce a vacuum (e.g., Vacutainer tubes used in collecting blood)

hematoma tumor or swelling of blood in the tissues (resulting in bruising during blood collection procedures)

hemoconcentration condition in which the blood concentration of large molecules such as proteins, cells, and coagulation factors increases

hemolysis the breaking open of red blood cells and the release of hemoglobin

heparin a natural anticoagulant that prevents the blood from clotting

humors fluid or semifluid substances found in the body

interstitial fluid all the fluid except blood that is found in the space between tissues; also referred to as tissue fluid

lancets capillary puncture devices

lumen inner tubular space of a needle, vessel, or tube

mastectomy removal of the breast

microcollection collecting a small amount of blood

neonate a newborn child

osteomyelitis inflammation of the bone; caused by bacterial infection

palpating gently touching and pressing on an area to feel texture, size, and consistency

petechiae tiny purple or red skin spots caused by small amounts of blood under the skin; found in patients with coagulation problems; condition can lead to excessive bleeding during phlebotomy procedures

phlebotomy blood collection; derived from the Greek words *phlebo,* meaning vein, and *tomy,* meaning to cut

plasma liquid part of whole blood

serum liquid part obtained when blood is clotted; lacks the clotting factors

stat needed immediately

syncope fainting

tourniquet a band placed above the venipuncture site to make the vein more prominent

veins blood vessels with valves that carry blood toward the heart

ABBREVIATIONS

CLSI	Clinical Laboratory Standards Institute	**PST**	plasma separator tube
PKU	phenylketonuria (an inherited metabolic disorder)	**SST**	serum separator tube

Fundamental Concepts— Theory, Safety, and Patient Preparation

One of the skills that medical assistants perform routinely is blood collection, or **phlebotomy**. The word *phlebotomy* means cutting into a vein, and *phlebotomist* is the term for the professional who performs phlebotomy. The history of blood collection dates to before the fifth century BC. At that time all medical treatment was based on four body **humors** (fluid or semifluid substances found in the body): blood, phlegm, yellow bile, and black bile. To reestablish health, techniques such as purging, starving, vomiting, and bloodletting were used. By the Middle Ages, barbers, along with surgeons, practiced the art of bloodletting. The red stripe on the barber's pole represented blood, the white stripe represented the tourniquet, and the pole symbolized the stick squeezed by the patient to dilate the vein. Bloodletting flourished into the eighteenth and early nineteenth centuries. In 1799 George Washington died after 9 pints of blood were taken in a 24-hour period in an attempt to cure his throat infection.

Today phlebotomy is primarily performed by trained professionals. Before studying the procedures involved with blood collection, the function and structures of blood vessels must be understood.

Function and Structures of Blood Vessels

Blood vessels are part of the cardiovascular system. They make up a *closed circuit system* (Figure 4-1) in which blood is pumped from the heart to the blood vessels and then returns to the heart. In general, all blood vessels except capillaries have three layers (Figure 4-2). These layers surround the area through which the blood flows and are called the *outer (tunica adventitia), middle (tunica media),* and *inner layers (tunica intima).*

Types of Blood Vessels

Blood vessels are classified as arteries, arterioles, capillaries, venules, and veins. **Arteries** have all three layers, and their function is to carry blood away from the heart. Each artery has a thick middle muscle layer that allows the vessel to expand and contract as blood pressure rises and falls. Arteries have a pulse and are located deeper than veins. They branch into

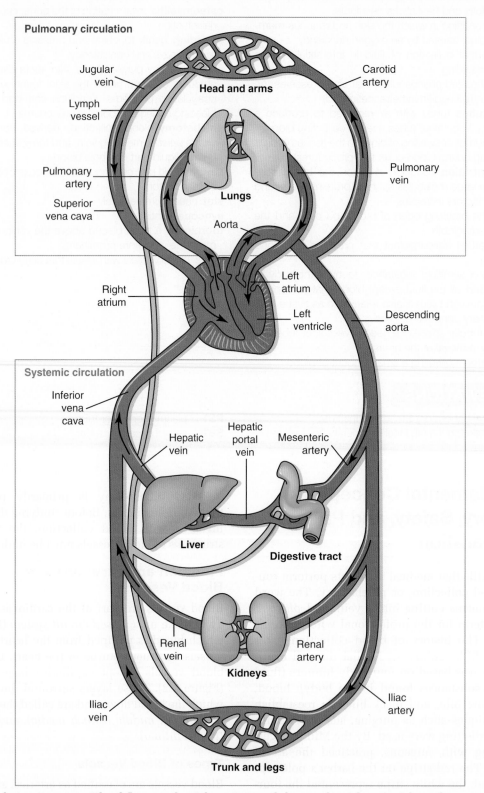

Pulmonary circulation

Jugular vein

Lymph vessel

Pulmonary artery

Superior vena cava

Carotid artery

Head and arms

Lungs

Pulmonary vein

Aorta

Right atrium

Left atrium

Left ventricle

Descending aorta

Systemic circulation

Inferior vena cava

Hepatic vein

Hepatic portal vein

Mesenteric artery

Liver

Digestive tract

Renal vein

Renal artery

Kidneys

Iliac vein

Iliac artery

Trunk and legs

Fig. 4-1 Closed circuit system. Blood flows to the right atrium and then to the right ventricle, pulmonary artery, lungs, and pulmonary veins; then it flows to the left atrium, left ventricle, aorta, arteries, arterioles, capillaries, venules, veins, superior vena cava and inferior vena cava, then back into the right side of the heart to repeat the sequence. *(From Warekois R, Robinson R:* Phlebotomy: worktext and procedures manual, *ed 3, St Louis, 2012, Saunders.)*

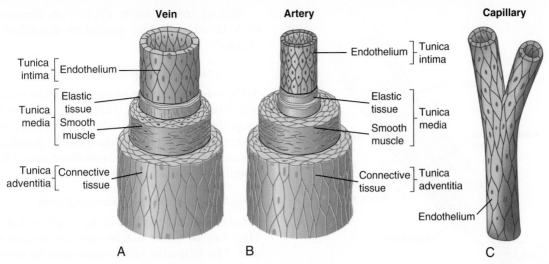

Fig. 4-2 Layers of the vein **(A)**, artery **(B)**, and capillary **(C)**. *(From Warekois R, Robinson R:* Phlebotomy: worktext and procedures manual, *ed 3, St Louis, 2012, Saunders.)*

arterioles, which are smaller blood vessels. Arterioles also have three layers, but the layers are thinner than those found in arteries. Arterioles then branch into capillaries. **Capillaries** are microscopic blood vessels composed of one layer of simple squamous epithelial cells. Substances are exchanged between blood and the surrounding tissue in the capillaries. Capillary blood is a mixture of arterial and venous blood. Capillaries join venules, which are composed of three thin layers, and the venules unite to form veins. **Veins** carry blood toward the heart and contain valves that prevent backflow of blood. Veins have three layers but thinner walls and less muscle than arteries.

A difference in the feel of veins and arteries can be detected when **palpating** (gently touching and pressing on an area to feel texture, size and consistency, and movement). Arteries will have palpable pulses that when counted for 1 minute provide the patient's pulse rate (which is the patient's heart rate in beats per minute). Veins feel spongy and do not have a pulse. Veins are the vessels most often used in blood collection because they are closer to the surface than arteries *and* are safer and easier to access.

Most blood tests are performed on venous or capillary blood. The differences in the blood composition of these vessels should be understood.

Comparison of Blood Substances

The composition of capillary blood is different from that of venous blood. Some of the differences are listed in Table 4-1. Capillary blood has higher amounts of hemoglobin and glucose than venous blood, whereas venous blood has higher amounts of potassium, calcium, and total protein.

Because capillary and venous blood specimens may yield different test results, performance of a capillary

technique must always be reported. In addition, if an analyte from Table 4-1 needs to be retested, the same blood collection technique must be used (e.g., venipuncture versus capillary). This is especially significant when comparing glucose concentration results during a glucose tolerance test, which requires the completion of multiple glucose tests during a 2- to 3-hour time frame.

Table 4-1	Comparison of Capillary and Venous Blood Analyte Values	
Capillary Blood Results	**Venous Blood Results**	
Hemoglobin: higher	Potassium: higher	
Glucose: higher	Total protein: higher	
	Calcium: higher	

Most Commonly Used Veins

The veins most commonly used when performing venipuncture are found in the **antecubital space** of the arm, the area in front of the elbow (Figure 4-3). There are three veins to locate. They are the median cubital vein, the cephalic vein, and the basilic vein. The median cubital is large and is the most commonly used vein. It is located in the middle of the arm and is well anchored above the lower arm muscle. The second vein of choice is the cephalic vein, on the thumb side of the arm. This vein is not well anchored and may move, but in an obese person it may be the only vein that can be found. (NOTE: When locating the cephalic vein, it helps to turn the lower arm so that the thumb of the hand is turned up, causing the

Fig. 4-3 The veins of the forearm. *(From Hunt SA: Saunders medical assisting, St Louis, 2002, Saunders.)*

cephalic vein to be on the upper surface of the arm, rather than on the lateral side.) The basilic vein is the least well anchored and is the last choice of the three. It is located on the little-finger side near the brachial artery. Its position increases the risk of puncturing the artery if the needle is inserted too deeply.

Federal Law Concerning Safety Equipment

According to the Centers for Disease Control and Prevention, health care workers receive approximately 600,000 percutaneous injuries annually from contaminated sharps. Because of concern over this issue and the development of technologies for protection, the Needlestick Safety and Prevention Act was passed by Congress, which directed the Occupational Safety and Health Administration (OSHA) to revise the Bloodborne Pathogens Standard to require employers to identify and use safer medical devices. Federal Bill HR 5178 was signed by President Bill Clinton on November 6, 2000, with an April 18, 2001, compliance date. An employer is in compliance with this law by performing the following actions:

- Creating and updating a bloodborne pathogen exposure control plan
- Evaluating and implementing safer medical devices for eliminating or minimizing occupational exposures
- Including health care workers who are using the devices in the evaluation and selection process
- Consistently monitoring the effectiveness of devices
- Maintaining a detailed sharps injury log, which gives a description of each exposure incident

Various current safety devices are discussed with each blood collection procedure described in this chapter.

Procedure Preparation

All blood-collecting procedures have the same preparation steps in common. These steps include having a properly completed requisition form, correctly identifying the patient, and appropriately positioning the patient. Understanding the role these steps play in the overall procedure is important.

Proper Completion of Requisitions

Requisitions are generated by a physician's order. They can be either handwritten or computer generated. The following information must be verified and included on a requisition and/or electronic record before obtaining the blood specimen:

- Patient's name
- Patient's identification number
- Patient's date of birth
- Name of the test ordered
- Name of the physician ordering the test
- Timing of the test (e.g., routine, stat, timed test)
- Other information, such as whether the patient is in a fasting state
- Insurance or billing information (e.g., if it is being sent to a laboratory for testing)

The requisition and/or electronic record must be entirely completed because it is used to correctly identify the patient and to determine how and when the specimen sample is to be collected.

Proper Identification of the Patient

The patient should always be greeted in a professional manner, and the medical assistant should introduce himself or herself to the patient. A brief explanation of the procedure being performed should be given. If the patient has any questions concerning the tests that have been ordered, the medical assistant should tactfully direct the patient to the physician.

One of the most critical steps in any phlebotomy procedure is to identify the patient correctly. The most serious laboratory error is the misidentification of a patient. To avoid this error, a three-way identification system should be used. This system consists of matching the patient's name and date of birth with the information on the test requisition, plus one more type of identification, such as a driver's license, address and/or zip code, phone number, or a chart number (outpatient) or hospital identification number on the patient's wrist (inpatient). When determining the patient's name, do not ask, "Are you Mrs. Smith?" Often patients may not hear the question, or they may be taking medication and mistakenly answer yes to the wrong name. It is better to ask, "Will you please spell your last name for me?"

For some tests the patient needs to be fasting. The proper way to determine this is to ask if the patient has had anything to eat or drink for 12 to 14 hours before the phlebotomy procedure. Do not ask patients if they have fasted. Some patients do not understand this concept and may answer yes even if they have had coffee, chewed gum, or done other things that could affect the testing. If the patient is not in a fasting state, it is important to note on the requisition and the patient's chart the time and the type of food constituting the patient's last intake. Also, the physician or lab should be consulted to determine if the test will need to be rescheduled for a time when the patient is in the proper fasting state needed for the ordered test.

A patient has the right to refuse a blood collection procedure, in which case the physician should be notified.

Proper Patient Positioning

The patient must be properly positioned for a phlebotomy procedure. A semireclining position on an examination table is preferred. However, having the patient sit in an elevated chair with an armrest (Figure 4-4, *A, B*) is also appropriate. This position can help protect the patient from falling forward if he or she faints, and it allows the vessels in the arm to expand to their maximum volume when the arm is extended downward. This position is also the best way to collect multiple tubes that need to be filled from the bottom up. Never have the patient sit on a stool or stand up when drawing blood. In these positions the patient could be injured if fainting occurs.

Blood Collection Procedures—Capillary Puncture and Venipuncture

Capillary Puncture

Although venipuncture is usually the most common blood collection method used, the capillary puncture is becoming very common in point-of-care testing procedures. The physician typically determines if this method should be used based on the test ordered on the requisition.

Capillary puncture, also called *skin puncture* or "stick," is a method of collecting blood by puncturing the skin through the epidermis into the dermal layer. The composition of blood analytes from a skin puncture is not the same as that of venous blood. Because capillaries are the bridge between arteries and veins, a skin puncture draws blood from arterioles, venules, and capillaries as well as **interstitial fluid** (all the fluid except blood found in the space between tissues, also called *tissue fluid*). Blood from skin punctures is also more like arterial blood than venous blood because arteries exert more pressure into the capillaries than the veins. Because of these differences in composition (venous blood compared to capillary blood), the requisition must state that a capillary puncture procedure was performed.

Fig. 4-4 A, Elevated phlebotomy chair allows phlebotomist to ergonomically stand upright. **B,** Patient extending arm downward allows the tubes to fill from the bottom up. *(Photos by Zack Bent.)*

The capillary puncture method is the method of choice in the following situations:

- When only a small amount of blood is needed as in point-of-care, CLIA-waived testing
- When the patient has burns, skin irritation, or small or fragile veins on the arms
- With cancer, geriatric, or obese patients, whose blood may be difficult to draw
- With children, because the risk of venipuncture removing excessive amounts of blood may cause anemia
- When minimal blood volume reduction is critical for **neonate** (a newborn child) safety (e.g., a 10-mL sample of blood is 5% to 10% of the total blood volume in a neonate's body)

The capillary puncture method should *not* be used in the following circumstances:

- If the test requires a large amount of blood, as in a sedimentation rate or a **blood culture** (a test to detect bacteria or organisms growing in the blood)
- If the patient has poor peripheral circulation in the hands and feet
- If interstitial fluid from **edema** (swelling) could dilute the test, causing inaccurate results

Equipment Used in Capillary Puncture

Capillary Puncture Devices

Many types of capillary puncture devices, **lancets**, are available. The safest and most current are *retractable nonreusable lancets* (Figure 4-5) that are made with locks that prevent reuse. These retractable devices are color coded by their manufacturers according to the depth of the puncture. Punctures performed on neonates and infants are implemented with the lancet color coded for infants. The National Committee for Clinical Laboratory Standards (now **CLSI**, Clinical Laboratory Standards Institute) made a change in the standard that applies to the depth of a heel stick

for an infant. The depth should not exceed 2 mm to prevent infection caused by puncturing a bone. For adults the average skin puncture depth should be 2 to 3 mm.

Automatic capillary puncture devices are used in home monitoring tests, but these usually do not result in a puncture sufficiently deep to collect the necessary amount of blood for point-of-care testing. Laser devices are also now available. They are used for glucose, hematocrit, and cholesterol screening. The laser concentrates on a small portion of the skin, makes an indentation 1 to 2 mm deep, and draws approximately 100 mcg/L of blood. All capillary puncture devices must be discarded in a biohazard sharps container.

Point-of-Care Testing Collection Devices

Point-of-care testing (POCT) refers to testing that has expanded beyond the laboratory to include the hospital bedside, the home, the nursing home, and any other direct-contact patient setting. Examples of POCT capillary blood collection supplies in Figure 4-6 consist of the following:

- Capillary tubes for four different test methods (see Figure 4-6, *A*)
- Critoseal (Sherwood Medical) plastic sealant for capillary tubes (see Figure 4-6, *B*)
- Microtainers with color-coded lids (see Figure 4-6, *C*)
- Microtainers with capillary tubes to aid in filling (see Figure 4-6, *D*)
- Cuvette for collecting the blood specimen and placing it in the analyzer (see Figure 4-6, *E*)
- Collection cup on the end of a lancet for a specific protime test method (see Figure 4-6, *F*)

Capillary Tubes

Capillary tubes are one type of device used to collect blood from a skin puncture site (see Figure 4-6, *A*). These tubes can be glass or plastic, but the plastic tubes or plastic-covered glass tubes are recommended for safety reasons. Blood moves freely into the capillary tubes during **microcollection** (collecting a small amount of blood). The blood is pulled into the tube by a process called **capillary action**. Red-marked capillary tubes contain **heparin**, a natural **anticoagulant**, which keeps the blood from clotting. Mixing these tubes by rolling them back and forth after collection is important. Blue-marked capillary tubes do not contain anticoagulants, allowing the blood to clot naturally.

The following guidelines should be followed when using capillary tubes:

1. Air bubbles in a capillary tube may cause erroneous results. The best way to prevent bubbles is to start with a large drop of blood and then hold the capillary tube horizontally to the puncture site. Figure 4-7 shows the tube incorrectly held downward, which results in bubbles.

Fig. 4-5 Adult and pediatric safety lancets before and after use.

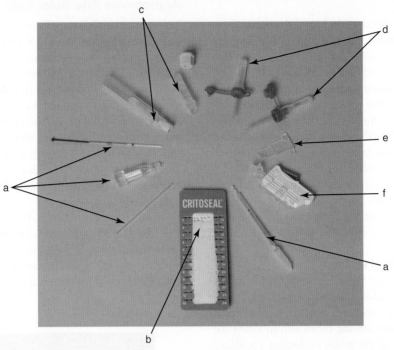

Fig. 4-6 Point-of-care testing equipment. *a,* Capillary collecting tubes; *b,* sealant for capillary tubes; *c,* Microtainers with color-coded lids; *d,* Microtainers with capillary tubes; *e,* cuvette; *f,* collection cup and lancet for protime testing.

Fig. 4-7 The capillary tube is *improperly* held downward, resulting in air bubbles. *(Photo by Zack Bent.)*

Fig. 4-8 Self-sealing capillary tube will seal itself when the specimen flows down the tube and connects with the clay seen on the right end of the tube. NOTE: The tube must then be held vertically for 15 seconds so that sealing can take place. *(Photo by Zack Bent.)*

2. Capillary tubes may be sealed so that the specimen is less likely to be lost. Sealants may be clay, as seen in Figure 4-6, *B,* and in the on-line video, or the specimen may be contained in a self-sealing tube, as seen in Figure 4-8. NOTE: The blood specimen must then be held vertical for 15 seconds against the self-sealant so that sealing can take place.
3. Capillary tubes are difficult to label. The recommended procedure is to place the sealed capillary tube into an empty vacuum tube and then label the vacuum tube. *Tip:* If the sealed capillary specimen is to be tested on-site, a sticky note with the patient's identification, technician's initials, and date may be used to hold the specimen against the adhesive portion while transporting the specimen from the collection area to the testing area. Another method is to thread the sealed capillary tube through two slits in a paper with the patient information written on it.

Microcollection Tubes

Microcollection tubes hold more blood than capillary tubes. Some tubes have a lip that allows the drop of blood to flow into the tube (see Figure 4-6, *C*). The lids on these tubes are coded with various colors corresponding to the anticoagulant present (or absent) in the container. Collect the specimen into the Microtainer tube by allowing the blood to run down the collection lip while holding the tube at a 30- to 45-degree angle. Do not scrape the tube across the blood specimen. Another type of collection tube consists of a plastic capillary tube inserted into a microtube receptacle (see Figure 4-6, *D*). Blood flows into the container because of the same capillary action that takes place within the capillary tube.

Order of Draw for Capillary Puncture

Because of the different types of anticoagulants in microcollection tubes, CLSI has recommended a specific order of draw for capillary punctures to prevent the transfer of substances among tubes and to allow for the clotting that takes place while collecting capillary specimens. According to NCCLS Standard H4-A3, "Procedures for the Collection of Diagnostic Blood Specimens by Skin Puncture," the order of draw for capillary skin puncture is as follows (also see Table 4-2):

1. Lavender Microtainer tubes used for hematology tests are filled first to avoid any microclots from forming, which distort the blood cells.
2. Other tubes with anticoagulation additives (i.e., green, blue, and gray)—These microcontainers also prevent blood from clotting and produce "whole blood" samples.
3. Nonadditive tubes (red-topped Microtainer tubes that contain no anticoagulants) are filled last because the capillary blood will clot in these tubes. Blood normally clots in 2 to 6 minutes. Nonadditive tubes are filled last because clotting always occurs in these tubes.

Appropriate Site Selection

The best site for capillary punctures is fleshy and vascular (pink not blue). A vascular site consists of a large capillary area without scars or calluses. Fleshiness helps protect against puncturing the bone. A bone puncture could lead to **osteomyelitis**, inflammation of the bone caused by bacterial infection. Sites that are swollen or callused should be avoided for skin puncture. **Cyanotic** sites, where the skin and mucous membrane are blue because of oxygen deficiency, should be warmed before use. A cyanotic site will not produce a good blood sample if it is not warmed or massaged.

In adults and children, the appropriate skin puncture site is the middle or ring finger (Figure 4-9). The little finger should be avoided because it is thinner and less fleshy than the other fingers. The index finger and thumb are also not recommended. The index

Fig. 4-9 Appropriate capillary puncture sites on the fingers. *(From Proctor D, Adams A: Kinn's the medical assistant: an applied learning approach, ed 12, St Louis, 2014, Saunders.)*

Table 4-2	Order When Collecting More than One Microtainer by Capillary Puncture	
Order	**Microtainer Color**	**Rationale**
First	Lavender	EDTA specimen is drawn first to ensure adequate volume and accurate hematology test results (e.g., CBC). There cannot be any microclots in the specimen to interfere with the blood cell counts and blood smears.
Second	Green, blue (two), gray	These "whole blood" tubes also prevent clotting using various anticoagulants. The blue top needs two numbered tubes to prevent any anticoagulant from the lavender or green tubes from entering the second blue tube, which will be used for coagulation studies. Label them #1 & #2.
Last	Gold (two), red	The clotted blood in these tubes is used to test the serum. Two gold tubes containing a gel barrier are needed to ensure that sufficient blood is collected to run the blood chemistry tests.

CBC, Complete blood count; *EDTA*, ethylenediaminetetraacetic acid.

Fig. 4-10 Appropriate capillary puncture sites for infant. *(From Proctor D, Adams A:* Kinn's the medical assistant: an applied learning approach, *ed 12, St Louis, 2014, Saunders.)*

finger could be more sensitive or callused, making it difficult to obtain blood, and the thumb has a pulse. With the middle or ring finger, the puncture should be made on the lateral part of the fingertip (slightly to the side of the center) and perpendicular to the whorls of the fingerprint. A puncture performed parallel to the fingerprint whorls will cause the blood to travel down the troughs of the fingerprint, preventing the blood from forming a drop.

The appropriate skin puncture site for newborns and infants who are not yet walking is the medial or lateral plantar surface of the heel of the foot (Figure 4-10). The puncture depth should be less than or equal to 2 mm to prevent puncturing the child's bone or connective tissue.

Site Preparation

Blood flow can be increased seven times by warming the site. This can be accomplished by massaging the area five or six times or by applying a warmed towel, an exam glove filled with warm water and tied at the wrist, a preemie diaper, or a commercially available device to the site for 3 to 5 minutes. The temperature of the warmed device should not be higher than 42° C. Microwave heating is not advisable because heating may be uneven.

The site should be cleaned with a 70% aqueous solution of isopropyl alcohol. Allow the cleaned site to dry thoroughly because alcohol may cause hemolysis, contaminate glucose determinations, or prevent drops of blood from forming. Always follow the manufacturer's directions regarding how to cleanse the site before puncturing the site. Cleaning the site with povidone-iodine (Betadine) is not recommended because it may cause a false elevation of potassium, phosphorus, or uric acid measurements. After the site

has been prepared, the skin puncture procedure can be performed.

Additional Information

When performing a capillary puncture, always remove the first drop of blood because it contains tissue fluid that could dilute the sample. (NOTE: Some tests will not require removal of the first drop; therefore, check the manufacturer's directions.)

If the blood has stopped flowing and insufficient blood was obtained, the entire procedure should be repeated at a new site with a new sterile puncture device. Never stick the same puncture site more than once.

Bandages are not recommended for small children because they can irritate the skin and cause choking if swallowed. If an adhesive bandage must be used to control bleeding, inform the parent that it should be removed as soon as the bleeding has stopped. Adhesive strips should not be used on infants because their skin is very delicate and could macerate when this type of bandage is used or be damaged when the bandage is removed. (See the Evolve capillary puncture video demonstration on-line and refer to Procedure 4-1 at the end of this section.)

Newborn Screening (Formerly PKU)

Neonatal (pertaining to a newborn) screening for two genetically transferred diseases, **PKU** (*phenylketonuria*) and *hypothyroidism,* is federally mandated in the United States for all newborns. These are conditions in which the newborn lacks the enzyme or hormone needed for certain metabolic reactions. If these conditions are not discovered and treated early, abnormalities as severe as mental retardation could develop. Some states require screening for other conditions as well, such as galactosemia, sickle cell anemia, cystic fibrosis, and human immunodeficiency virus (HIV). More about these requirements can be found at www. mchb.hrsa.gov, the website of the Maternal and Child Health Bureau of the Health Resources and Services Administration, and at www.aap.org, the website of the American Academy of Pediatrics.

The newborn screening blood collection must be performed between 24 and 72 hours after birth. If screening is done before the child is 24 hours old, it must be repeated before the child is 14 days old, because many newborns have not yet had enough feedings to determine if a metabolic condition is present. The collection of blood for these tests is generally performed in the hospital, but sometimes the test samples are required in the outpatient setting. Be sure to read and follow the instructions for collecting these specimens properly and note the following guidelines.
1. After warming the newborn's heel, a capillary puncture (no deeper than 2 mm) is done on the

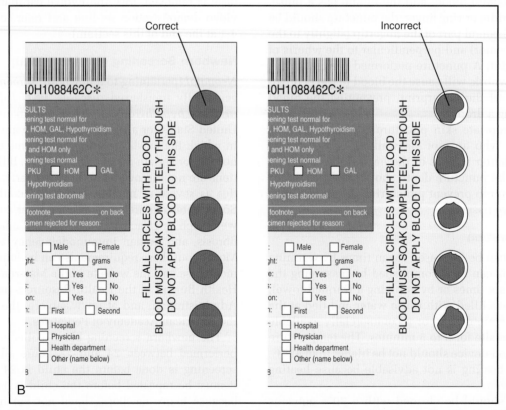

Fig. 4-11 A, Blank neonatal screening filter paper. **B,** Correct and incorrect completed screening forms. *(Modified from Warekois R, Robinson R: Phlebotomy: worktext and procedures manual, ed 3, St. Louis, 2012, Saunders.)*

medial or lateral plantar surface of the heel of the foot.

2. Remove the first drop of blood, and then collect the blood in the appropriate microcontainer or on the screening card.

3. Apply a drop of blood to each circle on the screening filter paper form, making sure to apply the blood to only one side of the paper (Figures 4-11 and 4-12).

4. All circles must be filled and completely saturated while the blood is extracted onto the circle. You may add a second drop to the same circle immediately if it soaks into the paper without sitting on top. Do not return to a circle that has started to dry.

5. Do not massage the foot of an infant with excessive force because this can cause bruising.

6. Allow the screening forms to dry in a horizontal position for a minimum of 3 hours.

7. Do not stack wet forms.

8. Mail the forms to the testing center (the state health department) in the provided envelopes within 24 hours of collection.

Becoming Proficient at Capillary Puncture

Now that you have learned about the equipment, appropriate sites, site preparation, and the procedure for capillary punctures and neonatal screenings, you will want to reinforce your knowledge by doing the following:

1. Answer the capillary puncture questions in Chapter 4 of the workbook using your structured notes and text.

2. View the Evolve videos on-line to see demonstrations of the finger stick and the heel stick.

3. Perform the Evolve on-line Chapter 4 exercises designed to reinforce your knowledge of terminology and capillary puncture.

4. Study Procedure 4-1: Capillary Puncture Procedure at the end of this section before your lab.

5. Also study Procedure 4-2: Heel Stick for Neonatal Screening Test Procedure before your lab.

Venipuncture

Another method of collecting blood samples is venipuncture, which involves extracting blood from a vein. Venipuncture can be accomplished in three ways: by the **evacuated tube** (or vacuum tube) method, the syringe method, and the butterfly method.

Equipment Used in Venipuncture

Vacuum Collection Tubes

The collection containers for venipuncture are called *vacuum tubes* (Figure 4-13). These tubes are **evacuated** (the air has been removed to create a vacuum) so that a preset amount of blood will be collected. They are available in different sizes, ranging from 2 to 15 mL (5, 7, and 15 mL for adults and 2, 3, and 4 mL for children). The tubes are available in glass or plastic, but OSHA recommends that plastic tubes be used for safety reasons. The manufacturer's label on each tube indicates the type of anticoagulant or additive that is present, the expiration date of the tube, and the amount of blood it will hold. Hemogard (Becton Dickinson, Franklin Lakes, NJ) plastic-covered tubes are designed with a special rubber stopper surrounded by a color-coded plastic closure that hangs over the outside of the tube and reduces the risk of blood splattering when the stopper is removed.

The expiration date on the tubes should always be checked and the tubes examined for cracks and other damage before use. If air enters the tube, the tube would be rendered useless because no blood would flow into it as a result of the lack of vacuum pressure.

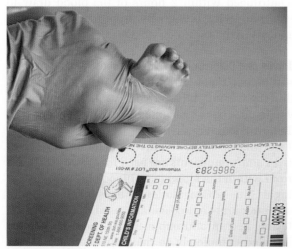

Fig. 4-12 Technique for placing a drop of blood from an infant's foot on the neonatal screening filter form. *(Photo by Zack Bent.)*

Fig. 4-13 Vacutainer Hemogard tubes in the proper order of draw. *(Photo by Zack Bent.)*

Each tube has a colored stopper and a label that indicate whether anticoagulants or additives are present and, if so, what type. When blood is extracted from the body and nothing is added to the specimen, the cells automatically clot, yielding a liquid called **serum** and clotted cells. When anticoagulants are added to the collection tubes to prevent the blood from clotting, a "whole blood" sample is produced in which the cells are suspended in liquid that is referred to as **plasma**.

Figure 4-14, *A*, shows a blood specimen collected in the left gold-topped tube that allows the blood to clot. The recommended time to allow blood to clot is 30 to 45 minutes, no longer than 1 hour, in an upright position at room temperature. NOTE: Tubes may also contain additives that accelerate clotting, such as silicone and glass beads. If the appropriate amount of time is not allowed for clotting, insufficient liquid serum will be obtained. Also, fibrin clots could form in the serum if the clotting factors do not have time to settle into the clot. When the blood has clotted, the tube is then spun

A

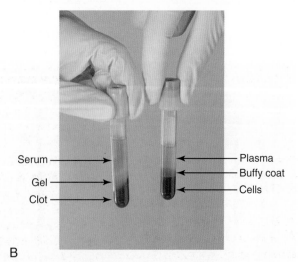

B

Fig. 4-14 **A,** Gold tube with clotted blood and lavender tube with whole blood before centrifuging. Note the composition of each. **B,** Clotted and whole blood after centrifuging. Note the layers in each tube.

in a centrifuge for 15 to 20 minutes. The clot becomes compressed on the bottom of the tube with the serum on top (see Figure 4-14, *B*, left tube). The white gel in the tube acts as a barrier between the *serum* and the clot.

Blood collected in an anticoagulant tube, as seen in the right lavender tube in Figure 4-14, *A*, will not clot and can be used for testing when *whole blood* is needed. When whole blood is centrifuged, the red cells pack into the bottom of the tube. The **buffy coat** is the narrow middle layer of white blood cells and platelets in the centrifuged whole blood specimen, and the liquid layer on top is referred to as *plasma* (see Figure 4-14, *B*, right tube).

Anticoagulation occurs by using a variety of additives, such as oxalates, citrates, EDTA, and heparin. Oxalates, citrates, and EDTA bind with calcium, which is needed for clotting to occur. Heparin prevents clotting by inactivating thrombin and thromboplastin, the proteins needed in the blood-clotting mechanism.

Both serum and plasma are straw colored and contain essentially the same substances. The main difference between the two is that serum no longer has its clotting factors because they were used to form the fibrin clot.

Another common additive is the white gel that forms a barrier between the cells and the liquid (serum or plasma, depending on the tube) to stop further interaction between these layers. The gel has a lower density than that of the red blood cells or the clot and a higher density than that of the liquid part. After the blood is centrifuged, the clot or red blood cells will be on the bottom of the centrifuged tube, the gel in the middle, and the liquid portion on top. When this gel is in a "clot" tube, it is referred to as **SST**, which is "serum separator tube." When the gel is in a whole blood tube with anticoagulant it is referred to as **PST**, or plasma separator tube. In both cases the tubes must be centrifuged within 2 hours of the blood draw to prevent the living blood cells from metabolizing the chemicals in the serum or plasma.

Additives and Color-Coded Vacuum Tubes

The different types of anticoagulants and additives within the vacuum tubes are differentiated by the following color-coded plastic and rubber stoppers seen in Table 4-3 and described next:

1. Pale yellow—"Sterile" tubes containing preservatives and/or nutrients are used for growing bacteria from within the blood (e.g., blood cultures).
2. Light blue—"Coagulation" tubes contain liquid sodium citrate anticoagulant, used for coagulation testing (e.g., prothrombin time). These tubes must be filled completely to maintain the ratio of one part liquid sodium citrate to nine parts of blood.
3. Red—"Clot" tubes contain no anticoagulants, which means the blood will automatically clot.

Table 4-3 List of Common Hemogard™ and Rubber Tube Stoppers

BD Hemogard™ Plastic Colors	Rubber Stopper Colors	Additive	Number of Inversions to Mix During Blood Draw	Laboratory Use
Yellow, Sterile	Yellow, Sterile	Sodium polyanetholsulfonate (SPS)	8	Blood cultures
Light blue	Light blue	Sodium citrate	3-4	Coagulation studies
Red	Red	None or clot activator to produce clot and serum	0	Chemistries Serology Blood bank
Gold	*Marbled red and gray	Thixotropic gel to separate serum from clot and clot activators	5	Most chemistry testing Not suitable for blood bank testing
Light green	* Marbled green and gray	Thixotropic gel to separate plasma and cells and lithium Heparin	8	Potassium determinations
Dark Green	Dark Green	Sodium heparin, or lithium heparin, or ammonium heparin	8	Stat Plasma chemistries electrolytes
Lavender	Lavender	EDTA	8	Whole blood hematology cell count, CBC
Gray	Gray	Sodium fluoride and potassium oxalate	8	Glucose testing (usually) Glucose tolerances

*Note the mixing requirements.
CBC, complete blood count; *EDTA,* ethylenediaminetetraacetic acid.
(BD Hemogard™ plastic covers and rubber stopper colors from BD Diagnostics, Preanalytical Systems, 1 Becton Drive, Franklin Lakes, NJ, 07417, USA. **www.bd.com/vacutainer.** BD, BD Logo and all other trademarks are property of Becton, Dickinson, and Company. © 2014.)

(NOTE: *Red plastic* tubes contain a clot activator to accelerate the clotting process.)

4. Gold and tiger-topped (marbled red and gray)—"*SST*" *(serum separating tubes)* contain a silicone coating to accelerate clotting and a gel barrier to separate the serum from the cells (SST tube). They contain no anticoagulant. The serum is typically used for blood chemistry tests.

5. Green—"Heparin" tubes contain a heparin anti-coagulant: sodium heparin, lithium heparin, or ammonium heparin; they are used for chemistry specimens, especially when a test is **stat** (needed immediately), because waiting for the blood to clot is not necessary as it is with serum tubes. It is important to note the type of anticoagulant substance that is in a heparin tube (e.g., a sodium heparin tube would not be used if sodium testing, and a lithium heparin tube would not be used for a lithium test because the sodium and lithium would falsely increase the patient's test results). Lithium heparin tubes are often used with the separating gel and are referred to as *PST (plasma separating tubes).* The *PST tubes* are distinguished from the non-gel heparin tubes by a lighter shade of green.

6. Lavender—**EDTA** tubes contain an anticoagulant and preservative for blood cells; they are used for hematology studies and molecular diagnostic testing. EDTA prevents platelet aggregation and allows preparation of blood smears with minimal distortion of white blood cells.

7. Gray—"Glucose" tubes contain potassium oxalate, which removes calcium to prevent clotting, and sodium fluoride, which is used for glucose studies because the fluoride inhibits glycolysis (sugar breakdown).

Figure 4-15 shows additional tubes that might be ordered for the following special tests:

- Yellow topped with acid citrate dextrose (ACD) is used in blood banks, paternity testing, and genetic testing.
- Black is used for erythrocyte sedimentation rate (ESR).
- White Hemogard over blue is a non–liquid citrate–coated tube used for coagulation studies.
- Royal blue is used for toxicology and detection of trace minerals in the blood (e.g., lead).
- White Hemogard over lavender is a PST tube for testing molecular diagnostics and viral load detection such as human immunodeficiency virus (HIV) and hepatitis C virus (HCV) levels.

Vacuum Tube Method Using the Vacutainer Collection System

The most commonly performed venipuncture method involves the use of vacuum tubes, which automatically fill with blood during the procedure. This method requires Vacutainer tubes, Vacutainer holders, and Safety Vacutainer needles, as seen in Figure 4-16.

Equipment Used in the Vacutainer Method

Vacutainer Needle. The *Vacutainer needle* is pointed at both ends (Figure 4-17). The shorter end punctures the vacuum tube, and the longer end has a bevel that is inserted into the vein. For a smoother and less painful puncture, the bevel end should always be turned upward. Safety needles are now required by law. Some types of safety needles are activated by a one-hand thumb mechanism (Figure 4-18, *A* and *B*); another type is activated by pressing against a hard surface (Figure 4-18, *C*).

The Vacutainer needle ranges in length from 1 to 1.5 inches. The space inside the needle is referred to as the **lumen** or *bore*. The diameter of the needle is called the *gauge*. The higher the gauge number, the

Fig. 4-15 Additional color-coded tubes for special tests.

Fig. 4-16 Vacutainer safety needles with pink safety devices *(left, middle).* Vacutainer holder with orange safety device *(right).*

smaller the diameter. The most frequently used gauges are 20 to 22. A high-gauge needle (e.g., 25) could cause hemolysis of the cells because the lumen is too small.

Vacutainer Holder. The *Vacutainer holder* is a plastic sleeve that allows the tube to connect to the needle (Figure 4-19). The Vacutainer double needle screws into one end of the holder. After the needle has been inserted into a patient's vein, the tube is pushed all the way into the holder. The needle must be in the vein before pushing the vacuum tube all the way into the holder. An indentation is present approximately ½ inch down from where the needle attaches to the holder. Pushing the vacuum tube within this ½-inch space *before* the needle is in the vein will result in the tube being filled with air.

Two types of Vacutainer holders are available: one for adults and one for children. A plastic extension, or flange, is located at the large-opening end of the Vacutainer. The design of the flange prevents the holder from rolling and provides a lip on which to position the fingers as the tube is inserted and removed.

OSHA recommends that Vacutainer needles not be removed from the holder after use but instead be disposed with the holder attached because the rubber-stoppered needle can expose health care workers to needle sticks.

Tourniquet. A **tourniquet** is a band placed above the venipuncture site to make the vein more prominent and easier to puncture. The average tourniquet is approximately 1 inch wide and 15 to 18 inches long and should be placed 3 to 4 inches above the venipuncture site. A tourniquet that is too tight is uncomfortable for the patient and can give inaccurate results. It should be tight enough to restrict venous flow but not so tight that it stops arterial flow. It should be looped so that it can be easily released with one hand. Do not place a tourniquet over sores or burned areas on the skin.

Multiple sample needle - short needle covered with rubber sleeve to prevent escape of blood when tubes are changed.

Multiple sample needle when penetrating rubber stopper - rubber sleeve compressed between hub and stopper.

Fig. 4-17 Vacutainer multisample needles with rubber sleeves that allow blood to flow only when the sleeved needle is pushed into the vacuum tube. *(From Hunt SA: Saunders fundamentals of medical assisting, Philadelphia, 2002, Saunders.)*

Fig. 4-18 A, One-hand thumb safety activation. **B,** One-hand spring device. **C,** One-hand surface activation.

Fig. 4-19 Vacuum tube system. *(From Hunt SA: Saunders fundamentals of medical assisting, Philadelphia, 2002, Saunders.)*

The recommended time to leave a tourniquet in place is 1 minute. If it is left on too long, results may be inaccurate because of **hemoconcentration**, a condition in which the blood concentration of large molecules (such as proteins, cells, and coagulation factors) increases. The recommended tourniquet procedure is to remove the tourniquet after a vein has been chosen, clean the site, prepare the equipment, and then reapply the tourniquet before making the incision. Tourniquets should be cleaned after use or discarded if they are disposable. See Procedure 4-3 for the proper application of the tourniquet.

Site Preparation

Have the patient place his or her arm in a downward position to prevent reflux (backward flow of blood). For patients who do not want to feel the needle stick (e.g., children), a eutectic mixture of local anesthetics (EMLA) can be used to anesthetize the puncture area. EMLA is a topical cream that is a mixture of lidocaine and prilocaine. It is applied as a cream or patch and requires approximately 60 minutes for optimal anesthesia to occur. It may last as long as 2 or 3 hours. Some of the limitations to its use are the cost of the product, the need to wait 60 minutes, and the need to repeat the anesthetizing procedure if the venipuncture is not successful. Another topical anesthesia, IOMED "Numby Stuff" (IOMED, Inc., Salt Lake City, Utah), contains lidocaine hydrochloride 2% with epinephrine. It penetrates to a depth of 10 mm and takes 10 minutes to take effect.

See Procedure 4-3: Vacutainer Method at the end of this section for the pictorial sequence and step-by-step instructions on how to perform a successful venipuncture using the Vacutainer method.

Syringe Method

The syringe method is used on fragile veins that might collapse under the pressure of the Vacutainer method. The procedure is the same as the Vacutainer procedure, except that when the syringe needle is in the arm, the phlebotomist pulls *back* on the syringe plunger, creating back-pressure and drawing blood into the syringe. The syringe method allows control over the pressure exerted on the vein. This control helps keep the vein from collapsing, which makes the syringe method particularly useful for small, fragile veins.

Equipment Used in the Syringe Method

Syringe. The *syringe* consists of a barrel and a plunger (Figure 4-20). The barrel is graduated into milliliters in sizes ranging from 2 to 20 mL and larger. The plunger should always be loosened by moving it back and forth several times before use, and then pushed in before connecting the needle. (Figure 4-21, *A* and *B*).

Fig. 4-20 Parts of a syringe and a hypodermic needle. *(From Hunt SA:* Saunders fundamentals of medical assisting, *Philadelphia, 2002, Saunders.)*

Fig. 4-21 **A,** The plunger should always be loosened by pulling it back *(a)* and pushing it in *(b)* several times before use. **B,** Make sure it is pushed in completely before connecting the needle and drawing blood from the patient. *(Photos by Zack Bent.)*

When the plunger is pulled back after the attached needle is in the vein, a back-pressure is produced and blood fills the syringe.

Syringe Needle. The *syringe needle* is also called a *hypodermic needle*. Like the Vacutainer needle, it has a shaft and a hub, but the hub attaches directly to the syringe with no opposing sheathed needle. Blood can be seen entering the tip of the syringe as soon as the needle enters the vein. Syringe needles must have a safety section that allows the needle to be covered or blunted when the procedure is completed. The most commonly used needle gauge is 20 to 22, with a length of 1 to 1.5 inches. See Procedure 4-4: Syringe Method at the end of this section for a pictorial and written description of how to properly draw blood using a syringe.

Butterfly Method

The *butterfly method* is used on very small veins, such as those in the hand, and for pediatric draws. Hand veins collapse and bruise more easily because they have thin walls. More nerves are also present in this area, which makes a hand puncture more uncomfortable for the patient. The equipment for this method consists of a uniquely designed needle with a safety sheath and plastic wings (used to grip the needle as it is inserted into the vein), tubing, and devices to attach to either a syringe or a Vacutainer collection system. Figure 4-22 shows the push-button butterfly needle, tubing, and connecting devices.

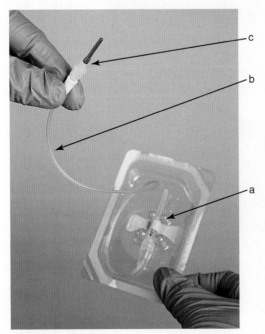

Fig. 4-22 The push-button butterfly needle *(a)*, tubing *(b)*, and connecting devices *(c)*. Also note the black button just below the "wings." When pushed, the needle instantly retracts into the body of the butterfly. *(Photo by Zack Bent.)*

In the butterfly method, a crucial safety issue arises when the needle is pulled out of the vein. Two recommended safety methods are described in Procedure 4-5. Laboratory professionals should stay informed of the most current safety devices and how they are activated. It is also wise to practice on a training model before using a new safety device on a patient. (The student workbook contains a form to evaluate various safety devices.)

If the Vacutainer method is used, a small adapter device (Luer adapter) is attached to the end of the butterfly tubing that will allow the tubing to attach to a Vacutainer holder. If the syringe method is used, the Luer adapter is removed and the end of the butterfly tubing fits directly onto the tip of the syringe. The syringe method allows more control of the pressure, which is necessary when working with fragile veins.

See Procedure 4-5 to learn the steps for performing the butterfly method using both a Vacutainer method and a syringe method. Also, both butterfly safety devices will be presented: the safety lock and the push button.

Figure 4-23 displays all the supplies used in the three venipuncture procedures: Vacutainer, syringe, and butterfly methods. The vacuum tubes have also been placed in their correct order of draw from left to right.

Order of Draw for All Venipuncture Methods and Other Quality Assurance Considerations

When performing each of the aforementioned venipuncture methods, keep in mind that there is a recommended order of draw regarding which colored tube needs to be drawn up first, second, and so on. Based on the requisition order, the proper colored tubes will need to be set in their proper order of draw. NCCLS (now CLSI) has recommended a specific order of draw for venipuncture as it has for capillary puncture. NOTE: The venipuncture order of the vacuum tubes is very different from the capillary order of Microtainers. This is because the sheathed needle that enters each Vacutainer tube is exposed to the additives in one tube that might affect the test result in a subsequent tube. Tests adversely affected by *additive contamination* from one tube to another are listed in Table 4-4.

The following pictures of the color-coded tubes in Figure 4-24 reflect the national recommendations on the order of drawing multiple tubes ("Order of Draw," NCCLS H3-A6). The following list of corresponding descriptions provides important quality assurance information:

1. *Yellow* "blood culture tube" is drawn first. The **SPS tubes** are used for blood culture specimen collection in microbiology, which are always drawn first to maintain sterility. NOTE: Chapter 8: Microbiology also discusses the drawing of both anaerobic and aerobic cultures. It is important to note that the anaerobic tube must always be drawn first, except when using the butterfly method. The aerobic tube is drawn first

Fig. 4-23 Venipuncture supplies. *a,* Gloves; *b,* tourniquet; *c,* sterile gauze and alcohol; *d,* Vacutainer holder; *e,* Vacutainer needle with pink safety device; *f,* syringe needle with spring safety device; *g,* butterfly needle assembled to connect directly to tip of syringe; *h,* syringe; *i,* safety transfer device for transferring blood from syringe to vacuum tube; *j,* butterfly needle assembled to connect directly to Vacutainer holder; *k,* nonlatex (COFLEX) pressure bandage and gauze to control bleeding; *l,* the six most commonly used Hemogard Vacutainer tubes in the recommended order of draw.

Table 4-4 Tests Adversely Affected by Anticoagulant Additive Contamination from a Previously Drawn Tube

	Additive	Tests Adversely Affected
Lavender stopper	EDTA	Chemistry: calcium, iron, sodium, potassium
		Coagulation: APTT, PT
Green stopper	Heparin	Coagulation: PT, APTT, ACT
Gray stopper	Potassium oxalate	Chemistry: potassium
		Coagulation: APTT, ACT

ACT, Activated clotting time; *APTT,* activated partial thromboplastin time; *EDTA,* ethylenediaminetetraacetic acid; *PT,* prothrombin time.

Fig. 4-24 The order of draw, according to Standard H3-A6. *1,* Yellow, sterile; *2,* light blue; *3,* red; *4,* gold Hemogard closure or red-gray rubber stopper; *5,* green; *6,* lavender; *7,* gray. *(From Warekois R, Robinson R:* Phlebotomy: worktext and procedures manual, *ed 3, St Louis, 2012, Saunders.)*

with butterfly needles because the air from the butterfly tubing should not enter the anaerobic bottle.

2. *Light blue* **"coagulation tube" (sodium citrate)** is drawn next because anticoagulants and additives from the other tubes will interfere with coagulation testing. This tube must be completely filled to achieve accurate clotting results. In the past, when a coagulation study (light blue tube) was ordered, a plain red glass tube with no additives was drawn first to absorb the tissue thromboplastin released from the traumatized tissue that could interfere with coagulation testing. The red tube was referred to as the "waste tube" because its only purpose was to collect the tissue thromboplastin caused by the venipuncture. However, the new recommendations no longer require this. The new standard does, however, recommend that a plain red waste tube be drawn before a light blue tube when the butterfly method is being used. The tubing in the butterfly system has dead space in the line that reduces the volume of blood drawn, thereby resulting in an underfilled tube. An alternative, if a plain red tube is not available, would be to use two blue tubes, with the first tube considered a waste tube whose only function is to clear the butterfly tubing of air. Neither the red nor the blue waste tubes need to be filled completely because they will not be sent to the laboratory. Their only purpose is to pull the blood through the tubing before connecting the blue tube that will then be filled accurately (with no air from the tubing) and sent to the laboratory.

3. *Red* **"clot tube,"** with or without clot activators, yields a serum/clot specimen. A glass red top tube has nothing in it, whereas a plastic red top tube often contains a clot activator because blood does not clot well in plastic tubes.

4. *Gold* **"SST tube"** contains gel and clot activators and is also considered a "clot tube" that is able to separate the serum from the clotted cells. Some laboratories may also order a **"tiger"** rubber-topped tube that appears marbled with red and gray. This SST tube also contains gel and is similar to the Hemogard gold tube. In all three cases (red, gold, and tiger topped tubes), it is important to follow the

laboratory's designated serum tube choice based on the tests they will be running.

5. **Green "heparin tube"** (dark green plain and light green gel PST) must be drawn *before* the EDTA tubes because the EDTA interferes with some heparin tube chemistry tests, such as electrolyte testing. EDTA is usually bound to potassium or sodium. If an EDTA tube is drawn before a heparin tube for electrolyte testing, some of the EDTA potassium and sodium would be mixed in with the green tube's specimen and cause inaccurate electrolyte results (see Table 4-4).

6. **Lavender "hematology tube"** (EDTA) is drawn next and is most commonly used for hematology testing.

7. **Gray "glucose tube"** (potassium oxalate/sodium fluoride) is drawn last, after the EDTA tube, because the anticoagulant, potassium oxalate, also affects potassium results and red blood cell morphology. It is commonly used for glucose testing.

Table 4-5 details the correct order of drawing using the most common plastic Vacutainer (Becton Dickinson) tubes, their additives, and uses, plus the two marbled rubber stopper tubes. A helpful way to remember the proper order is to visualize the picture in Table 4-5. Start at the top of the picture, and work your way down.

Becoming Proficient at Venipuncture

Now that you have learned about the equipment, appropriate sites, site preparation, four methods of obtaining venous blood (Vacutainer, syringe, and two butterfly methods), and proper order of draw, you will want to reinforce your knowledge by doing the following:

1. Answer the venipuncture questions at the end of this chapter and in Chapter 4 of the workbook using your structured notes and text.

2. Perform the Chapter 4 exercises on-line to reinforce your terminology and venipuncture theory skills, and order of draw.

3. View the Evolve animated interactive venipuncture lesson and videos on-line to see Venipuncture with a Vacuum Tube and Venipuncture with Winged Infusion Set and Syringe.

4. Study the pictures and text in the following procedures:

   a. Procedure 4-3: Vacutainer Method before your lab.

   b. Procedure 4-4: Syringe Method before your lab.

   c. Procedure 4-5: Two Butterfly Needle Methods before your lab.

Table 4-5	Order of Draw and Data for Seven Common Tubes

a. Blue sky is usually the first plastic tube to draw for coagulation studies. (Do not forget the waste tube if using a butterfly needle and tubing.)

b. The *red* and *gold* rays of the sun are on the horizon. Both of these "clot" tubes (along with the tiger topped tubes) must be drawn *after* the blue but *before* the remaining anticoagulant tubes.

c. The *green* grassy hill is below the red and gold rays of the sunset. *Light green* is the PST heparin tube, and dark green is typically the lithium heparin tube.

d. *Lavender* flowers are at the base of the hill below the green grass near the bottom of the picture.

e. *Gray* rocks are at the bottom of the picture because the gray "glucose" tube is the last tube to draw.

Table 4-5 Order of Draw and Data for Seven Common Tubes—cont'd

	Plastic Hemogard™ tube	Rubber topped tube	Additive or Lab Descriptors	Laboratory Uses
Blue sky	Light blue	Light blue	"Citrate tube"	Coagulation studies such as prothrombin time
Red and gold rays of sun coming from above the grassy hill	Red	Red	"Clot tube" Clot activator in plastic tubes (NOTE: Red glass tubes do not have clot activator.)	All yield serum commonly used for testing blood chemistry analytes
	Gold	Marbled red and gray	"SST tube" Clot activator and gel to separate the serum from the clot	
Green grass of the hill	Light green	Marbled green and gray	"PST tube" contains heparin plus gel to separate the plasma from the cells	Special tests such as electrolytes and chemistry stat tests that need to be run immediately
	Dark green	Dark green	"Heparin tubes" (with lithium, ammonium, or sodium)	
Lavender flowers at the bottom of the hill	Lavender	Lavender	"EDTA tube"	Hematology tests such as CBC
Gray rocks under the flowers	Gray	Gray	"Oxalate tube"	Glucose testing

CBC, complete blood count; EDTA, ethylenediaminetetraacetic acid; PST, plasma separator tube; SST, serum separator tube.
(BD Hemogard™ plastic covers and rubber stopper colors from BD Diagnostics, Preanalytical Systems, 1 Becton Drive, Franklin Lakes, NJ, 07417, USA. www.bd.com/vacutainer. BD, BD Logo and all other trademarks are property of Becton, Dickinson, and Company. © 2014.)

✳ PROCEDURE 4-1 Capillary Puncture Procedure

A, Capillary puncture setup. *a,* Sterile gloves; *b,* sterile gauze; *c,* 70% isopropyl alcohol pads in sterile packages; *d,* sterile, disposable, retractable, nonreusable lancet; *e,* latex-free bandage.

B, Warm the puncture site.

C, Disinfect with alcohol.

D, Perform the puncture with an incision-type safety lancet.

E, Alternatively, perform the puncture with a Tenderlett (ITC, Edison, NJ) safety lancet.

F, A puncture-type Safe-T-Pro lancet (Roche Diagnostics, Indianapolis, Ind) can also be used.

G, Wipe away the first drop of blood, and then gently massage the finger to produce a large drop of blood.

PROCEDURE 4-1 Capillary Puncture Procedure—cont'd

H, Collect the specimen in a Microtainer.

I, Alternatively, collect the specimen in a plastic pipette from a CLIA-waived test kit.

J, Alternatively, use a capillary tube for a hematocrit test.

K, Alternatively, place the blood on a slide for a blood smear.

L, After 3 to 5 minutes of applying pressure to the puncture site, check for bleeding and apply a latex-free bandage.

Equipment and Supplies (Figure A)

- Gloves (preferably nonlatex for latex-sensitive patients)
- Sterile gauze
- 70% isopropyl alcohol pads in sterile packages
- Sterile, disposable, retractable, nonreusable lancets (varying lengths for the appropriate depth)
- Latex-free bandage

Additional supplies for collecting and processing the specimen (not pictured) are appropriate, including microcollection containers based on tests ordered, plastic capillary tubes (with and without anticoagulants) and sealers, glass slides to make hematology slides, biohazard puncture-resistant sharps container, warming devices (optional), and a marking pen.

Preparation—Preanalytical

1. Wash the hands if they are visibly soiled. If not, use an alcohol-based rub for routine decontamination. Apply the hand rub to the palm of one hand, and rub the hands together, covering all surfaces until dry.
2. Correctly identify the patient by using the three-way match. The patient should be sitting or lying.
3. Choose the appropriate site for a finger stick according to the guidelines.
4. Put on gloves, first determining if the patient is allergic to latex. Nonlatex gloves should be worn if the patient is latex-sensitive.
5. Warm the site, if needed, by massaging the area or applying a warming device to the site for 3 to 5 minutes (Figure B).
6. Clean the site with 70% isopropyl alcohol (Figure C). Allow the alcohol to dry, and do not fan or blow on the cleansed site.

(Continued)

PROCEDURE 4-1 Capillary Puncture Procedure—cont'd

Blood Collection Procedure—Analytical

7. Determine the appropriate lancet device (Figures D, E, F) according to the age of the patient and the amount of blood needed.

8. Open the lancet package, and keep the lancet sterile until used. Tell the patient, "You will feel a stick." Firmly hold the finger below the cleansed site, and puncture the site in the appropriate place. When making the puncture, be sure to press hard to get a good blood flow so that the patient does not have to be stuck again. Observe the hand positioning with each of the lancet devices in Figures D, E, and F. Immediately after the puncture, discard the lancet into a biohazard sharps container placed nearby.

9. Wipe away the first drop of blood, which contains tissue fluid that could dilute the sample.

10. Gently massage the finger from the base of the finger to just below the puncture site to get a uniform drop of blood. Apply intermittent pressure below the site. You should be able to obtain an adequate drop to fill at least a capillary tube (Figure G). NOTE: Do not squeeze excessively at the tip of the finger. Squeezing with too much force near the site could cause the blood sample to be contaminated with tissue fluid.

11. Collect the sample in the appropriate container for the test ordered: a Microtainer (Figure H), a plastic pipette from a CLIA-waived test kit (Figure I), a capillary tube for a hematocrit test (Figure J), or a slide for a blood smear (Figure K). When collecting blood in a microcollection tube, do not scrape or scoop the container against the site because it could cause tissue fluid to contaminate the sample. Collect only free-flowing drops of blood. The microcollection tube should be collected in the order of draw for capillary puncture. If a capillary tube is being filled, hold it horizontally to prevent air bubbles from getting into the tube. Tubes with additives should be gently tapped or mixed during the collection procedure to prevent microclots from forming. Cap or seal the container when full.

12. Place gauze on the puncture site, and ask the patient to apply pressure to it.

Follow-Up—Postanalytical

13. Immediately invert the microtube 8 to 10 times to mix the specimen with any anticoagulants that may be present. Always follow the manufacturer's instructions.

14. Recheck the puncture site. If the patient has stopped bleeding, apply an adhesive bandage to the puncture site as necessary (Figure L). Make sure the patient is not allergic to the bandage material. If bleeding does not subside after 5 minutes, contact the physician.

15. Label the tubes with the patient's name and identification number, the date and time the specimen was drawn, and your name (initials are sufficient in some facilities). When using capillary tubes, the recommended procedure is to place the filled tubes into unfilled vacuum tubes and label the vacuum tubes.

16. When the procedure is completed, discard blood-contaminated items in appropriate biohazard containers including gloves.

17. Remove gloves and sanitize hands.

18. Document the procedure on the specimen log sheet and in the patient's record making sure to include the following six items:

    When: date and time of collection

    Where: location on the body where the blood was collected (e.g., right antecubital space, hand, finger) and where the specimen is being sent (e.g., reference lab, hospital, in office)

    What: types of tubes collected (e.g., gold and lavender)

    Why: what tests were ordered (e.g., blood chemistry profile, complete blood cell count)

    How: did the patient respond to the procedure (tolerated well? experienced pain? fasting state? difficult draw?)

    Who: person who collected the specimen (your name, credentials)

    Patient's name

    Date, time: Performed finger stick and collected a lavender-topped microtainer of blood for hemoglobin testing in our lab. There were no complications --First initial, Last name, Credentials

✳ PROCEDURE 4-2 Heel Stick for Neonatal Screening Test Procedure

A, Neonatal safety lancets are the lower green and pink lancets designed to puncture the heel at a depth equal to or less than 2 mm.

DO NOT WRITE IN BLUE SHADED AREAS–DO NOT WRITE ON BARCODE

CC040H1088462C

ALL INFORMATION MUST BE PRINTED

Birthdate: ☐☐ ☐☐ ☐☐ MM/DD/YY Time ☐☐ ☐☐ (Use 24 hr time only)

Baby's name: ☐☐☐☐☐☐☐☐☐☐☐☐☐☐☐☐☐☐☐☐
(last, first)

Hospital provider number: ☐☐☐☐☐☐☐ (mandatory)

Hospital name: ☐☐☐☐☐☐☐☐☐☐☐☐☐☐☐☐☐☐☐☐

Mother's name: ☐☐☐☐☐☐☐☐☐☐☐☐☐☐☐☐☐☐☐☐
(last, first, Initial)

Mother's ID: ☐☐☐☐☐☐☐☐☐ Baby's ID: ☐☐☐☐☐☐☐☐☐

Mother's address: ☐☐☐☐☐☐☐☐☐☐☐☐☐☐☐☐☐☐

Mother's phone: (☐☐☐) ☐☐☐ – ☐☐☐☐

Specimen date ☐☐ ☐☐ ☐☐ MM/DD/YY Time ☐☐ ☐☐ (Use 24 hr time only)

Physician's name: ☐☐☐☐☐☐☐☐☐☐☐☐☐☐☐☐☐☐

Physician's address: ☐☐☐☐☐☐☐☐☐☐☐☐☐☐☐☐☐☐

City: ☐☐☐☐☐☐☐☐☐☐☐☐☐☐ Ohio zip ☐☐☐☐☐ – ☐☐☐☐

Physician's phone: (☐☐☐) ☐☐☐ – ☐☐☐☐   **ODH COPY**

Physician's provider number: ☐☐☐☐☐☐☐ (mandatory)

ODH COPY: ☐ SPECIAL:

TEST RESULTS
☐ Screening test normal for
PKU, HOM, GAL, Hypothyroidism
☐ Screening test normal for
PKU and HOM only
☐ Screening test normal
☐ PKU ☐ HOM ☐ GAL
☐ Hypothyroidism
☐ Screening test abnormal
_____
See footnote _____ on back
☐ Specimen rejected for reason:
_____

Baby sex: ☐ Male ☐ Female
Birth weight: ☐☐☐☐ grams
Premature: ☐ Yes ☐ No
Antibiotics: ☐ Yes ☐ No
Transfusion: ☐ Yes ☐ No
Specimen: ☐ First ☐ Second
Submittor: ☐ Hospital
☐ Physician
☐ Health department
☐ Other (name below)

HEA 2518 _____

FILL ALL CIRCLES WITH BLOOD
BLOOD MUST SOAK COMPLETELY THROUGH
DO NOT APPLY BLOOD TO THIS SIDE

○
○
○
○
○

B, Neonatal screening filter paper with five circles to saturate with the neonate's blood.

(Continued)

PROCEDURE 4-2 Heel Stick for Neonatal Screening Test Procedure—cont'd

C, A commercial warming device designed for infant heels. After 3 to 5 minutes, the blood flow will increase 7 times. NOTE: A disposable glove half-filled with warm water and tied off at the wrist also works well to warm the heel.

D, Note the hand position for holding the foot while the other hand performs the heel puncture on the lateral plantar portion of the heel.

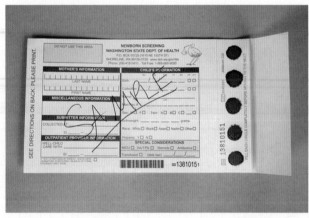

E, Apply gentle pressure with the thumb and forefinger and ease intermittently as drops of blood form.

F, Example of a thoroughly dried card with all five circles saturated.

Equipment and Supplies (see Figure A)

- Gloves (preferably nonlatex for latex-sensitive patients)
- Sterile gauze
- Warming device
- 70% isopropyl alcohol pads in sterile packages
- Sterile, disposable, retractable, nonreusable neonatal lancets with no more than 2 mm depth (Figure A)
- Neonatal screening filter paper (Figure B)

Preparation—Preanalytical

1. Wash the hands if they are visibly soiled. If not, use an alcohol-based rub for routine decontamination. Apply the hand rub to the palm of one hand, and rub the hands together, covering all surfaces until dry.
2. Correctly identify the newborn by using the three-way match, and fill out all the information required on the card.
3. Choose the appropriate site for the heel stick according to the guidelines.
4. Put on gloves.
5. Warm the site by applying a warming device to the site for 3 to 5 minutes (Figure C).

PROCEDURE 4-2 Heel Stick for Neonatal Screening Test Procedure—cont'd

Blood Collection Procedure—Analytical

6. Clean the site with 70% isopropyl alcohol. Allow the alcohol to dry, and do not fan or blow on the cleansed site.
7. With a gloved hand, place the lancet against the medial or lateral plantar surface of the heel of the foot.
8. Place the blade slot area securely against the heel, and firmly and completely depress the lancet trigger (Figure D).
9. After triggering the lancet, remove the lancet and discard it into a biohazard sharps container.
10. Gently wipe away the first drop of blood with sterile gauze or a cotton ball.
11. Apply gentle pressure with the thumb and ease intermittently as drops of blood form. Be sure to apply pressure in such a way that the incision site remains open. Note the position of the hand in Figure E.
12. The filter paper should be touched gently against the large blood drop, and a sufficient quantity of blood should penetrate to completely fill a pre-printed circle on the filter paper before going to the next circle. Do not go back and reapply additional drops in the same circle after you have left.
13. The paper should not be pressed or smeared against the puncture site of the heel. Simply hover the heel very close to the filter paper and allow the blood to fill the circle.
14. Blood should be applied only to one side of the filter paper, but both sides of the filter paper should be examined to ensure that the blood uniformly saturated the paper.
15. After all five circles of blood have been collected from the heel of the newborn, the foot should be elevated above the body. NOTE: A minimum of three successful circles is needed by the laboratory to test for multiple metabolic disorders.
16. A sterile gauze pad or cotton swab should be pressed against the puncture site until the bleeding stops.
17. It is not advisable to apply adhesive bandages over skin puncture sites on newborns.

Follow-Up—Postanalytical

18. Wash the hands.
19. Document the procedure on the specimen log sheet and in the patient's record making sure to include the following six items:

    When: date and time of collection

    Where: location on the body where the blood was collected (e.g., right antecubital space, hand, finger) and where the specimen is being sent (e.g., reference lab, hospital, in office)

    What: types of tubes collected (e.g., gold and lavender)

    Why: what tests were ordered (e.g., blood chemistry profile, complete blood cell count)

    How: did the patient respond to the procedure (tolerated well? experienced pain? fasting state? difficult draw?)

    Who: person who collected the specimen (your name, credentials)

    Patient's name

    Date, time: Performed heel stick on a warmed right heel and collected five full samples of blood for neonatal screening. Specimen card was sent to the health department. There were no complications ----------First initial, Last name, Credentials
20. Allow filter paper to dry thoroughly on a horizontal, level, nonabsorbent open surface for 3 hours at ambient temperature and away from direct sunlight.
21. Do not touch or smear blood on the filter paper, and do not contaminate the specimen card with cleaning chemicals or other substances.
22. Mail the thoroughly dried card (Figure F) in the envelope provided by the health department.

Photos C through F by Zack Bent.

✳ PROCEDURE 4-3 Vacutainer Method

A, Apply the tourniquet. Pull the two ends of the tourniquet taut, and then cross them in the front of the arm.

B, While holding the crossed area, tuck the top strap under the bottom strap from above so that the ends hang upward.

C, Palpate across the antecubital area, and visualize the size, depth, and direction of the vein.

D, After removing the tourniquet, disinfect the area and assemble equipment on the appropriate side of the arm.

E, Reapply the tourniquet, apply alcohol to the finger if you need to recheck the position of the vein by palpation just above the insertion area, and remove the needle cover.

F, Anchor the vein with the nondominant hand, and insert the needle with the dominant hand.

PROCEDURE 4-3 **Vacutainer Method—cont'd**

G, Push the Vacutainer tube into the needle holder with the thumb of the nondominant hand. Apply counterpressure on the flange of the Vacutainer holder with the fingers of the nondominant hand.

H, Pull out the tube with the fingers of the nondominant hand while applying counterpressure against the flange with the forefinger.

I, Mix the specimen by gently tilting the tube back and forth allowing the blood to flow from one end of the tube to the other.

J, Insert the second tube with the nondominant hand.

K, Remove the tourniquet as the last vacuum is filling.

L, Remove the final tube from the holder.

(Continued)

PROCEDURE 4-3 Vacutainer Method—cont'd

4-3

M, Have the patient relax his or her fist.

N, Hold sterile gauze over the site with the nondominant hand. Remove the needle, then apply pressure using the gauze, and activate the needle safety device with the dominant hand.

O, Immediately dispose of the needle/holder assembly in a biohazard sharps container.

P, Label the tubes while the patient applies pressure to the puncture site.

Q, After 3 to 5 minutes, check for bleeding and apply a pressure bandage.

PROCEDURE 4-3 Vacutainer Method—cont'd

Equipment and Supplies

- Disposable gloves
- Tourniquet
- 70% isopropyl alcohol
- Vacutainer double-pointed needle
- Vacutainer holder
- Correct vacuum tubes for the requested tests
- Sterile gauze pads
- Adhesive bandages
- Test tube rack
- Biohazard sharps containers and bags

Preparation—Preanalytical

1. Wash the hands if they are visibly soiled. If not, use an alcohol-based hand rub. Apply the rub to the palm of one hand, and rub the hands together, covering all surfaces until dry.
2. Correctly identify the patient by using the appropriate three-way match for your facility (spell name, date of birth, last four digits of their social security number, phone number, hospital identification number, or driver's license number).
3. Position the patient properly, such as in a semireclining position or sitting in a chair with an arm support. Have the patient place his or her arm in a downward position to prevent reflux.
4. Determine if the patient is allergic to latex. Put on the appropriate type of gloves.
5. Apply the tourniquet, and determine the appropriate site (Figures A and B). Have the patient make a fist, and palpate the arm for a vein. Ask the patient to clench and unclench the fist a few times and then hold the fist to push the blood from the lower arm to the veins, but the patient should avoid vigorous pumping, which could cause hemoconcentration.
6. Begin on one side of the antecubital space, and palpate across to the other side with the index finger (Figure C). The vein will feel spongy. When the vein is found, determine its size and depth and follow it up and down to determine its direction.
7. Remove the tourniquet and have the patient release his or her fist.
8. Clean the arm with 70% isopropyl alcohol (Figure D). Rub the chosen site with the alcohol, working in concentric circles from the inside out, making sure not to backtrack. Allow the alcohol to dry without fanning or blowing on the cleansed site.
9. While the site is drying, assemble the equipment. Take the sheath off the holder end of the Vacutainer needle, and screw it into the holder (while leaving the puncturing needle covered). Determine which vacuum tubes are needed for the testing, and place them in a rack in the order of draw. Check the expiration date of the tubes and look

for cracks. Be sure to tap the tubes that contain additives to release any additives that may be on the lids. Place the gauze, tubes, and all equipment close to the drawing station so they can be easily reached during the procedure.

Blood Collection Procedure—Analytical

10. The collection process begins after the alcohol has dried. Reapply the tourniquet, being careful not to contaminate the cleansed site. Have the patient make a fist again. If you need to palpate the site again, clean your gloved finger(s) with 70% alcohol (Figure E) and palpate the vein just above the area where you will be entering. Remove the needle sheath, exposing the needle.
11. Anchor the vein with the nondominant thumb, placing it approximately 1 to 2 inches below and to the side of the puncture site so that it is not in the way of the entry of the needle into the vein (Figure F). Make the skin over the vein taut by pulling toward the patient's hand. This will help keep the vein from moving and allow the needle to enter more easily.
12. Approximately ¼ to ½ inch below the site and with the bevel up, insert the needle at a 15-degree angle with one swift, continuous motion to prevent tissue damage. Phlebotomist and needle should be positioned in the same direction as the vein. The correct angle will vary depending on the depth of the palpated vein. The common angle is 15 degrees. If the angle is less than 15 degrees, the needle may go above the vein; conversely, if the angle is greater than 15 degrees, the needle may go through the vein. Never stick unless a vein has been determined. The holder should be held steady with the dominant hand during the procedure so that the needle does not move through the vein or pull out.
13. Push the tube into the needle holder (Figure G). Put the index and middle fingers of the nondominant hand on both sides of the flange of the holder, and push the tube into the Vacutainer needle with the thumb of the same hand.
14. Follow the order of draw for vacuum tubes when filling the tubes. If possible, fill the tubes from the bottom up, so that the sheathed needle inside of the collecting tube does not make contact with additives in one tube and cross-contaminate the next tube. To remove a tube from the holder, put the forefinger of the nondominant hand against the flange of the holder and pull the tube out with the fingers of the nondominant hand (Figure H). Gently invert the tube a few times to start mixing the blood with the additives (Figure I).

(Continued)

PROCEDURE 4-3 Vacutainer Method—cont'd

15. Insert the next tube into the holder, and use the same method of pushing the tube into the holder (Figure J). (NOTE: Once the second tube is filling, you may tilt the previous tube to reach the required five to eight times.)

16. While the *last* tube is filling, remove the tourniquet (Figure K). When the last tube is filled, remove it (Figure L) and mix it by tilting. The last tube must be removed before removing the needle from the arm to prevent blood from dripping out of the needle.

17. Make sure the patient's hand is relaxed (Figure M) and that the tourniquet is removed *before* you take the needle out of the arm. If this is not done, blood may leak into the tissues from the venous puncture site, causing a hematoma (literally, a tumor or swelling of blood in the tissues).

18. Hold a sterile gauze or cotton ball over the needle as the needle is swiftly pulled out to prevent tissue damage. Do not press down on the gauze until the needle has been removed (Figure N). Pressure on the needle is painful for the patient.

19. After exiting the vein, activate the needle safety device and discard the entire Vacutainer device (holder with attached needle) in a biohazard sharps container (Figure O). Never recap a needle.

Follow-Up—Post Analytical

20. With the gauze over the site, ask the patient to apply pressure for 3 to 5 minutes with the arm straight or elevated above the heart. This pressure will help prevent a hematoma from forming. Bending the arm at the elbow can cause blood flow from the puncture site to increase.

21. While the patient is applying pressure, gently continue to mix the tubes 5 to 8 times. Label them with the patient's name, identification number, the date and time that the specimen was drawn, and your initials, if appropriate (Figure P). NOTE: Never prelabel tubes before the actual specimen is obtained—a prelabeled tube may end up with someone else's specimen!

22. During the entire process, assess the patient for signs of fainting. Check the site for bleeding after 3 to 5 minutes. If bleeding has subsided, first determine if the patient is allergic to any type of bandage, then apply a pressure bandage if appropriate (Figure Q). Tell the patient not to lift any heavy objects for approximately 1 hour. If the site is still bleeding, continue to apply pressure. If bleeding has not stopped after 5 minutes, contact the physician. During the entire process, make sure that the patient is feeling well.

23. Discard all materials in the appropriate containers.

24. Remove gloves in the appropriate manner discussed in Chapter 1, and discard in a biohazard bag.

25. Wash the hands.

26. Document the procedure on the specimen log sheet and in the patient's record making sure to include the following six items:

When: date and time of collection

Where: location on the body where the blood was collected (e.g., right antecubital space, hand, finger) and where the specimen is being sent (e.g., reference lab, hospital, in office)

What: types of tubes collected (e.g., gold and lavender)

Why: what tests were ordered (e.g., blood chemistry profile, complete blood cell count)

How: did the patient respond to the procedure (tolerated well? experienced pain? fasting state? difficult draw?)

Who: person who collected the specimen (your name, credentials)

Patient's name

Date, time: Performed venipuncture on the left arm and collected a lavender tube for CBC and a gold tube for a Chemistry Profile. Tubes were processed and picked up by the ABC lab. There were no complications --

--First initial, Last name, Credentials

✳ PROCEDURE 4-4 Syringe Method

A, Assemble the sterile syringe and safety needle. NOTE: Pull and push the plunger back and forth in the barrel, and then make sure the plunger is pushed all the way into the barrel to remove all air.

B, Apply the tourniquet as in the Vacutainer method, disinfect the site, and have supplies ready.

C, Anchor the vein with the nondominant hand, and insert the needle.

D, Withdraw blood by pulling back on the plunger. Note the thumb is placed against the flange to provide counter-pressure while the other fingers pull the plunger.

E, Instruct the patient to unclench the fist, and remove the tourniquet before collecting the last blood specimen.

F, Hold the sterile gauze over the puncture site while removing the needle. After the needle is removed, immediately apply pressure.

(Continued)

4-4

PROCEDURE 4-4 Syringe Method—cont'd

G, Immediately activate the needle safety device.

H, Remove the protected needle from the syringe, and discard the needle in a biohazard sharps container.

I, Attach the yellow safety transfer device to the tip of the syringe.

J, Invert the syringe above the device, and connect the vacuum tubes in their proper order of draw by pushing them into the transfer device from below. Mix each tube after it is filled.

K, When the transfer is finished, discard the entire syringe/transfer device assembly in the biohazard sharps container.

PROCEDURE 4-4 Syringe Method—cont'd

Equipment and Supplies

- Disposable gloves
- Tourniquet
- 70% isopropyl alcohol
- Syringe and needle in correct sizes
- Correct vacuum tubes for the requested tests
- Safety transfer device
- Sterile gauze pads
- Adhesive bandages
- Test tube rack
- Biohazard sharps containers and bags

Preparation—Preanalytical

1. Follow steps 1 through 8 of Procedure 4-3.
2. While the site is drying, assemble the equipment. Remove the sterile syringe and needle from their packages, keeping them sterile (Figure A). Move the plunger back and forth several times to break the seal on the syringe. Make sure the plunger is fully pushed into the barrel to remove all air. Screw the hub of the needle tightly onto the syringe. Determine which vacuum tubes are needed for the testing, and place them in a rack in the order of draw for vacuum tubes. Check the expiration date of the tubes, look for cracks, and tap the tubes that contain additives to release any additives that may be on the lids. Place all equipment close to the draw station so it is easily reached during the procedure.

Blood Collection Procedure—Analytical

3. Follow steps 10 through 12 of Procedure 4-3, including applying the tourniquet, disinfecting the site (Figure B), and anchoring the vein while inserting the needle (Figure C).
4. When the needle is in the vein, blood may be seen in the hub of the syringe. Gently pull back on the plunger to pull blood into the syringe (Figure D). If the plunger is moved too fast, the blood may be hemolyzed or the vein may collapse. Be careful not to move the needle while it is in the vein, which could be painful for the patient. Also, do not withdraw the needle prematurely from the patient's arm while pulling back on the plunger.

5. When the syringe has filled with the required amount of blood, have the patient unclench his or her fist and release the tourniquet (Figure E). Place sterile gauze over the puncture site as you remove the needle (Figure F). Be careful to remove the needle in the same path it was inserted. Do not press down on the gauze until the needle has been removed; such pressure would be painful for the patient.
6. Activate the syringe needle safety device after the needle has been removed from the arm (Figure G). Detach the needle from the syringe, and discard the protected needle in the sharps biohazard container (Figure H).

Follow-Up—Postanalytical

7. With the gauze on the site, ask the patient to apply pressure for 3 to 5 minutes with the arm straight or elevated above the heart.
8. The blood must be transferred into the vacuum tubes as quickly as possible so that it does not clot in the syringe. While the patient applies pressure to the puncture site, transfer the blood from syringe to vacuum tubes with a *safety transfer device*. This device looks like a Vacutainer holder with only the inner sheathed needle in the holder. One end of the safety transfer device attaches to the end of the syringe (Figure I). The inside of the holder containing the rubber-sheathed needle then pierces the Vacutainer tube when the syringe and holder are inverted (Figure J). The blood in the syringe is drawn automatically into the tubes because of the vacuum in these tubes. To keep from hemolyzing the red blood cells, never push on the syringe plunger while transferring blood with this device.
9. Mix the tubes 8 to 10 times, and label them with the patient's name and identification number, the date and time that the specimen was drawn, and your name (or initials, if appropriate).
10. Discard the entire connected syringe/transfer device into the sharps container (Figure K). Discard all other potential biohazard materials in a biohazard bag.
11. Follow steps 20 through 24 of Procedure 4-3.

4-4

✳ PROCEDURE 4-5 Two Butterfly Needle Methods: Butterfly Safety Lock and Push-Button Needles

I. Butterfly Safety Lock Needle Using Vacutainer Tube System

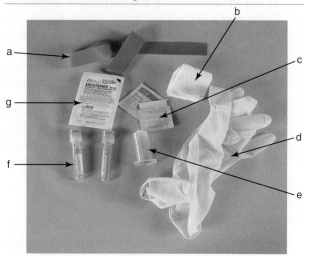

A, Butterfly setup. a, Tourniquet; b, sterile gauze pads; c, 70% isopropyl alcohol; d, disposable gloves; e, Vacutainer holder; f, Vacutainer tubes; g, winged infusion Safety Lock butterfly set with Vacutainer adapter to connect to Vacutainer holder.

Equipment and Supplies (Figure A)

- Tourniquet
- Sterile gauze pads
- 70% isopropyl alcohol
- Disposable gloves
- Vacutainer holder
- Vacutainer tubes
- Winged butterfly with safety lock needle and Vacutainer adapter to connect to Vacutainer holder
- Biohazard sharps containers and bags

Preparation—Preanalytical

1. Follow steps 1 through 4 of Procedure 4-3. The procedure for entering a vein in the arm is the same as those for the syringe and vacuum tube methods. If blood is being drawn from the hand, apply the tourniquet above the wrist and have the patient make a half-fist.
2. Beginning on one side of the puncture area, palpate across to the other side with the index finger. The vein will feel spongy. When the vein is found, determine its size and depth and follow it up and down to determine its direction.
3. Remove the tourniquet.
4. Clean the hand with 70% isopropyl alcohol. Allow the alcohol to dry without fanning or blowing on the cleansed site.

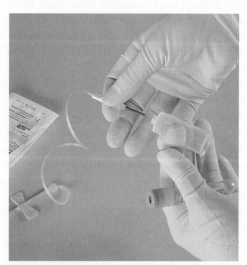

B, **Firmly** attach the rubber-sheathed multineedle Vacutainer adapter to the butterfly tubing, and then screw the needle into the Vacutainer holder. Reaffirm that the adapter is firmly attached to avoid air leaks during the blood draw.

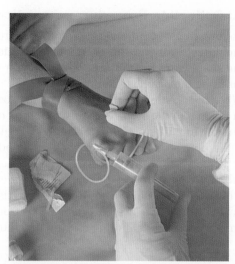

C, After disinfecting the hands, apply the tourniquet and anchor the vein. Insert the butterfly needle into the vein. Push the vacuum tubes into the holder, which will draw the blood through the tubing into the tubes. NOTE: When possible, angle the Vacutainer tube with the stopper up allowing the blood to flow to the bottom of the tube.

4-5

PROCEDURE 4-5 Two Butterfly Needle Methods: Butterfly Safety Lock and Push-Button Needles—cont'd

D, Activate the safety device using the "OK" method making sure both hands are behind the exposed needle.

5. While the site is drying, assemble the equipment. Remove the winged infusion set from the package, and stretch the tubing to straighten it. If you are using the Vacutainer method, attach a Luer adapter to the end of the tubing of the winged infusion, and then screw the other end into a Vacutainer holder. Double check to affirm there is a tight seal where the Luer adapter fits onto the sheathed needle to prevent air from entering the Vacutainer tubes (Figure B).

6. Determine which vacuum tubes are needed for the testing, and place them in a rack in the order of draw. NOTE: If a blue top is ordered, it is necessary to draw a waste tube first to remove the dead space in the tubing. A red tube with no additives or an additional blue top may be used to clear the air in the tubing with blood. The waste tubes do not need to be filled because they will be discarded after the procedure. Check the expiration date of the tubes, look for cracks, and tap the tubes that contain additives. Place all equipment close to the draw station so it can be easily reached during the procedure.

Blood Collection Procedure—Analytical

7. When the alcohol has dried, reapply the tourniquet. If you need to determine the puncture site again, clean the gloved finger(s) you will use with 70% alcohol. Remove the needle sheath from the needle.

8. Anchor the vein by placing the nondominant thumb 1 to 2 inches below and to the side of the puncture site. Make the skin over the vein taut by pulling toward the patient's knuckles.

9. Grip the folded plastic wings to guide the needle into the vein (Figure C). At approximately ¼ to ½ inch below the site and with the bevel up,

quickly insert the bevel of the needle into the vein at a 15-degree angle or less when drawing from a hand. Continue to "thread" the needle with one continuous, swift motion to keep the needle from twisting out of the vein.

10. If you are using the Vacutainer holder/system, push the vacuum tubes into the holder (Figure C). After each tube has filled with blood, remove it and gently mix it.

11. After the required amount of blood has been obtained, have the patient unclench his or her fist and release the tourniquet. Place a piece of sterile gauze over the puncture site, and remove the needle by holding the tail of the needle device with the thumb and forefinger of the dominant hand forming the "OK" sign. Swiftly pull the needle out and to the side. NOTE: Do not press down on the gauze until the needle has been removed.

12. Immediately activate the safety device by using the nondominant hand to grab the tubing with its thumb and forefinger forming the "OK" sign, and then pull on the tubing. The needle will retract into the butterfly body. Use the remaining fingers to apply pressure to the site as seen in (Figure D). (NOTE: Always keep both hands behind the needle tip to prevent an accidental stick.) After the safety device has been activated with the butterfly/Vacutainer method, the entire Vacutainer holder and butterfly apparatus should be discarded in a biohazard sharps container.

13. With the gauze on the site, ask the patient to apply pressure for 3 to 5 minutes with the arm straight or elevated above the heart.

Follow-Up—Postanalytical

14. Follow steps 20 through 26 of Procedure 4-3.

(Continued)

PROCEDURE 4-5 Two Butterfly Needle Methods: Butterfly Safety Lock and Push-Button Needles—cont'd

II. Butterfly Push-Button Needle Using a Syringe

This procedure is basically the same as the previously described safety lock butterfly procedure, with a few changes. The push-button butterfly needle is considered safer than the safety lock needle when used properly. The best way to learn any new safety device is to practice first on a training model. Figures E through M demonstrate the ways in which this method differs from the previous procedure.

Photos E through M by Zack Bent.

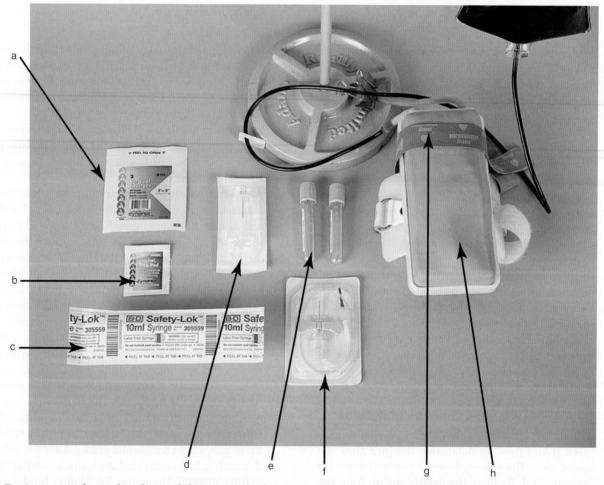

E, Equipment and supplies for push-button method using a syringe: *a*, Sterile gauze pads; *b*, 70% isopropyl alcohol; *c*, sterile syringe; *d*, transfer device; *e*, Vacutainer tubes; *f*, butterfly with push-button safety needle; *g*, tourniquet; *h*, training model with artificial blood for practicing.

PROCEDURE 4-5 **Two Butterfly Needle Methods: Butterfly Safety Lock and Push-Button Needles—cont'd**

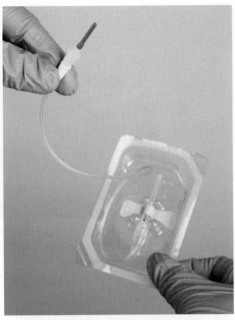

F, Proper removal of the butterfly from its container consists of pulling out the entire assemble using the adapter end of the tubing to prevent accidental activation of the black push button located just under the blue "wings."

G, When using a syringe, remove the Luer-Lok Vacutainer holder adapter (seen in the left hand) and place the syringe adapter tightly onto the tip of the syringe. Also, remember to move the plunger back and forth several times to break the seal on the syringe, and then push the plunger all the way in to remove all air from the syringe.

H, While anchoring the vein with the nondominant hand, quickly insert the bevel of the butterfly needle at a 15-degree angle (or less if drawing from a hand) and observe the flash of blood entering the tail of the butterfly. Continue to thread the needle along the lumen of the vein to anchor the needle.

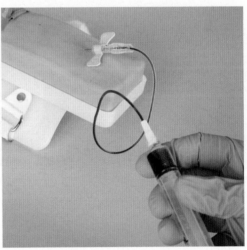

I, With the needle in place, both hands may be used to slowly pull the blood into the syringe. It may be necessary to pull back the plunger a little at a time to keep the vein from collapsing.

(Continued)

PROCEDURE 4-5 Two Butterfly Needle Methods: Butterfly Safety Lock and Push-Button Needles—cont'd

J, After you have collected enough blood in the syringe, grasp the body of the butterfly using the thumb and forefinger of the dominant hand to stabilize the needle. Place gauze over the needle to safely prevent splattering of the blood during the retraction of the needle. NOTE: Tell the patient to expect a snapping sound that will indicate the procedure is over. The nondominant hand uses the side of the thumb to push down the black button located just below the wings. The needle then instantly retracts inward and juts out the back end of the butterfly body.

K, After the snap has been heard and the needle is safely tucked into the body of the butterfly, the nondominant hand immediately applies pressure to the site.

L, Remove the hub of the butterfly from the syringe, and throw the tubing into the sharps container.

M, Using the transfer device, transfer the blood into the appropriate tubes in their correct order of draw. Hold the syringe above and the vacuum tubes below in an upright position. NOTE: It is still wise to draw a waste tube before filling the blue top tube because the syringe will contain the air that was first removed through the butterfly tubing. Also, keep pushing on the tubes as they are filling so they do not slip off the sheathed needle in the transfer device, causing an incomplete fill.

4-5

Advanced Concepts— Specimen and Patient Care

Preparing Blood Specimens for Laboratory Pickup

The last step in blood collection is the processing of the blood before the laboratory retrieves the specimen for testing. Each laboratory and/or CLIA-waived test procedure has a specific protocol regarding how to process the blood for the test they will be performing. Therefore, it is important to check the lab manual provided by the laboratories that will be picking up the specimens and to perform the following steps:

- Log each collection on the laboratory log sheet, indicating date, time, patient identification, tubes drawn, tests ordered, lab where tests will be performed, and the phlebotomist's initials. (See Chapter 2 appendix for logging lab specimens in workbook.)
- Allow 30 minutes for gold, red, and tiger rubber-topped tubes to clot in an upright position in a test tube rack. They should then be centrifuged within 2 hours of collection to separate the liquid from the clotted cells (Figure 4-25):
- Place the closed tubes in the centrifuge, creating a balanced load. Opposing centrifuge holders must be equally weighted with loaded samples that are the same size and equal in fill.
- Fill a tube with water to match the weight of any unpaired sample, and place it across from the sample.
- The tubes should remain closed with their tops on at all times during the centrifugation process.

- Centrifuge the clotted specimens for 15 to 20 minutes depending on centrifuge speed (usually 3000 rpm) and laboratory recommendations (Figure 4-26).
- PSTs should also be centrifuged for 15 to 20 minutes within 2 hours of collection, according to laboratory protocol.
- Store all specimens at room temperature or refrigerate, according to laboratory guidelines.
- Place specimens in a biohazard specimen bag with their corresponding requisition placed in the front pocket of the bag.

Centrifuge Safety

- Do not spin uncovered specimen tubes, and always have the centrifuge lid cover closed when the centrifuge is running to prevent the vaporization of hazardous droplets.
- If an abnormal noise, vibration, or sound is noted while the centrifuge is in operation, immediately stop the unit by turning off the switch, and check for a possible load imbalance.
- Centrifuges must never be slowed or stopped by grasping any part of the device with your hand or applying another object against the rotating equipment.
- Broken tubes or liquid spills must be cleaned according to OSHA standards. Clean the centrifuge daily with a disinfectant and paper towel.

NOTE: Watch the on-line Evolve video: Preparing a Serum Specimen Using a Serum Separator Tube.

Fig. 4-25 Place the capped tubes in the centrifuge, creating a balanced load. Opposing centrifuge holders must be equally weighted with loaded samples that are the same size and equal in fill. *(Photo by Zack Bent.)*

Fig. 4-26 Observe the settings for spinning a clotted blood specimen: 3.0 × 1000 = 3000 rpm for 20 minutes. *(Photo by Zack Bent.)*

Patient Issues When Locating a Suitable Vein

Patient issues and complications may occur before, during, and after a phlebotomy procedure. It is important to understand the following complications and learn ways to prevent them, when possible.

Obesity

The veins on obese patients may be difficult to visualize and palpate, making them a challenge to find and penetrate. The following are some possible solutions to this challenge:

- Ask the patient if he or she has had their blood drawn previously and if there is a "favorite" vein of choice.
- Have the patient warm the antecubital space for several minutes and then use a blood pressure cuff as a tourniquet on the patient's downward extended arm.
- First palpate for the median vein by feeling between the creases in the antecubital space while the patient makes a fist.
- If the median vein is not palpable, then have the patient turn his or her extended lower arm with the thumb up, which may then expose the cephalic vein when a fist is made.
- If the cephalic vein is not palpable, apply the tourniquet above the wrist and check the hand for visible or palpable veins on the back of the hand (Figure 4-27) or on the thumb side of the hand.
- Currently, there is an instrument that trans illuminates the surface of the skin with infrared light to assist in locating difficult to find veins (Figures 4-28 and 4-29).
- Caution must be taken not to probe the area excessively if a vein is missed.

Complications During Blood Collection

Hematomas

Hematoma is a swelling or tumor of blood under the skin causing a bruise. It results from an open break in a blood vessel. It can occur around a puncture site when blood leaks from the vein into the surrounding tissue. A hematoma may result when any of the following occurs:

- The needle penetrates the vein.
- The needle is only partially in the vein (Figure 4-30, *A*).
- Insufficient pressure was applied to the puncture site after the procedure was completed.
- The patient has lifted heavy objects with the arm too soon after the draw, causing the puncture site to reopen.

If a hematoma occurs during the procedure, remove the tourniquet and needle immediately followed by applying direct pressure for 3 to 5 minutes. If the bleeding continues, call for assistance.

Fig. 4-28 The vein finder. Venoscope II Model VT 03 infrared light source displays vein. *(Photo by Zack Bent.)*

Fig. 4-27 Drawing blood from a hand when veins are difficult to find in the antecubital space. Note how the vacuum tube is held to allow the blood to flow down to the bottom of the tube. Also note the specialized tourniquet at the wrist which improves patient comfort. *(Photo by Zack Bent.)*

Fig. 4-29 Attaching Venoscope to arm for assisting in blood draw. *(Photo by Zack Bent.)*

Failure to Obtain Blood When Needle Is in the Arm

If blood is not seen after connecting the vacuum tube, one of the following problems may have occurred as seen in Figure 4-30, *B-E*:

- The bevel is against the upper wall of the vein and the vein has collapsed (Figure 4-30, *B*). Adjust by slightly tipping the needle downward.
- The needle pierced all the way through the vein (Figure 4-30, *C*). Insertion of the needle at an angle greater than 15 degrees is a likely cause. Adjust by slightly pulling back and correcting the angle.

- The needle is inserted above the vein, possibly because the needle is inserted at less than a 15-degree angle (Figure 4-30, *D*). Adjust by slightly correcting the angle and pushing forward.
- The needle has missed the vein entirely (Figure 4-30, *E*). Do not probe excessively if the vein is missed because this bruises the arm and could hemolyze the red blood cells.
- A defective vacuum tube has been used. Always inspect tubes before using them, and never reuse a tube from a failed blood draw. It must be discarded.

Fig. 4-30 Complications when searching for a vein. **A,** Hematoma caused by blood escaping into the tissue from partially inserted needle. **B,** The needle bevel is on the wall of a collapsed vein. **C,** The needle bevel has gone entirely through the vein. **D,** The needle is above the vein due to incorrect angle. **E,** The needle has completely missed the vein. **F,** A successful insertion at the correct angle and the proper depth. *(Art provided by Gala Bent.)*

If none of these issues are resolved, remove the tourniquet and needle, observing the same safety techniques as a successful draw and repeat the procedure on the other arm. A patient should never be stuck more than two times by the same phlebotomist.

Mastectomy

Do not perform a venipuncture on the arm adjacent to a **mastectomy** (removal of the breast) site. A patient who has undergone a mastectomy may have no lymph flow to that arm because the axillary lymph nodes on the mastectomy side may have been removed. This condition carries a potential risk for infection, along with alterations in the levels of body fluids and blood analytes in that arm. In addition, the tourniquet may injure the patient's arm.

Intravenous Therapy

Drawing blood from a patient's arm in which there is an intravenous (IV) fluid running is not recommended because the fluid could dilute or influence the results of the tests. A glucose drip, for example, could falsely increase glucose values. If an arm with an IV tube must be used, always draw on the arm *below* the IV insertion area (e.g., from the hand).

Edema

Areas affected by *edema* (abnormal accumulation of fluid in interstitial spaces) should not be used for venipuncture because the extra tissue fluid may contaminate and dilute the test results. An example of an edematous arm would be one that is in a cast.

Areas to Avoid

Veins that are obstructed in some way—such as when the skin is sclerosed (hardened), psoriatic with plaque, or scarred—should not be used. Sites with open wounds or that are burned and susceptible to infection should also be avoided.

Hemolysis

Hemolysis is the breaking open of red blood cells and the release of hemoglobin. Hemoglobin turns serum or plasma pink or red. Hemolysis can be caused by one of the following actions:
- Using a needle that is too small
- Collapsing the vein by putting too much pressure on it, either by using the Vacutainer method on a small vein or by pulling back the plunger too quickly with the syringe method
- Vigorously shaking the filled tubes
- Allowing hemolyzed blood to release chemicals into the plasma and serum that adversely affect the test results for the following analytes:
  - Potassium
  - Magnesium
  - Iron
  - Lactate dehydrogenase

- Phosphorus
- Ammonia
- Total protein

Excessive Bleeding

A patient typically stops bleeding in 2 to 6 minutes after applying pressure to the site. However, patients who take medications such as blood thinners and arthritis medications may bleed for a longer time. Even aspirin can act as a blood thinner. Patients may also have coagulation abnormalities such as platelet defects. In this case **petechiae** (small red or purple spots) may appear on the patient's skin. Petechiae are caused by small amounts of bleeding under the skin. Let the physician know if bleeding does not stop.

Neurological Problems

Syncope, or fainting, is not uncommon for some patients to experience during or after phlebotomy procedures. Signs of fainting include pallor, sweating, and hyperventilation. If a patient expresses concern about fainting, place him or her in a reclining position before starting the procedure.

If a patient feels faint during the procedure, release the tourniquet and remove the needle and apply pressure. Be sure to activate the safety device. Have the patient lower his or her head and breathe deeply. Place a cold or wet towel on the forehead and back of the neck. Do not attempt to put anything in the patient's mouth. If possible, place the patient in a reclining position and stay with the patient for at least 15 minutes after the patient has recovered. Instruct the patient not to drive for at least 30 minutes. Giving the patient a glass of juice may be helpful. An incident report from your health care facility should be completed describing the fainting incident and any follow-up action taken.

Seizure is another neurological problem that could occur during a phlebotomy procedure. If a patient has a seizure, remove the tourniquet and needle immediately and apply pressure to the puncture site. Call for help, and do not attempt to put anything in the patient's mouth unless authorized to do so.

Hitting a nerve during venipuncture is rare but serious. The patient will probably experience a tingling sensation radiating down the affected nerve. Immediately remove the tourniquet and needle, and apply pressure to the site. Notify an authorized person, and file an incident report.

Risk Management

OSHA regulates the Bloodborne Pathogens Standard by requiring all health care facilities to have an exposure control plan in place to help reduce employee exposure. The most common exposure to bloodborne pathogens in health care results from accidental puncture wounds with contaminated needles, glass, or

other sharp items. In an effort to reduce these percutaneous incidents in the workplace, the Bloodborne Pathogens Standard requires documentation of the selection and evaluation of any new safety technology used by employees. The goal is to determine the effectiveness of new safety devices in the following areas:
- Decreased risk of injuries
- Acceptance of the device by users
- Ability of the device to not affect patient care adversely

Two sample safety device evaluation forms from OSHA are included in the workbook appendix Chapter 4 forms: "Sample Device Preselection Worksheet" and "Sample Device Evaluation Form." All employees who are at risk of exposure must be alert and involved in finding ways to eliminate exposure to bloodborne pathogens. Be sure to take the time to complete the forms and answer the questions during the blood-collecting laboratory practice sessions.

Review Questions

1. What is the *most critical* error a phlebotomist can make before collecting a specimen?
   a. Not collecting enough blood
   b. Not releasing the tourniquet before removing the needle
   c. Misidentifying the patient
   d. Collecting the blood in the wrong tube

2. A certified medical assistant is in the process of collecting a blood sample by the Vacutainer method. During the procedure a hematoma begins to form. Which of the following scenarios could explain why this occurred?
   a. The bevel is against the wall of the vein.
   b. The bevel is in the middle of the vein.
   c. The bevel was inserted above the vein.
   d. The bevel is only partially inserted in the vein.

3. Which of the following tubes is used for coagulation studies?
   a. Lavender
   b. Light blue
   c. Green
   d. Gray

4. A capillary puncture is performed on a newborn. All the following steps are correct *except*
   a. the puncture site is warmed before the puncture is made.
   b. the medial or lateral section of the plantar surface of the foot is the site of the puncture.
   c. a lancet no deeper than 3 mm is used for the puncture.
   d. the first drop of blood is wiped away.

5. A certified medical assistant is performing a Vacutainer blood collection. Which of the following techniques is *incorrect*?
   a. The tourniquet is placed 3 inches above the puncture site.
   b. The puncture site is cleaned with 70% isopropyl alcohol in a concentric circular motion, starting with the puncture site and spreading outward.

   c. The tourniquet is removed after the last tube and the needle are removed.
   d. The tubes are mixed 8 to 10 times after being filled with blood.

6. If the angle of needle insertion is lower than 15 degrees during a venipuncture procedure, which of the following may occur?
   a. The needle may enter above the vein.
   b. The needle may pierce completely through the vein.
   c. The vein may collapse.
   d. The needle bevel may stick to the bottom of the vein wall.

7. You are in the process of drawing blood when you notice that the patient is looking pale and sweating. Which of the following steps should you *not* do?
   a. Continue with the procedure until all the required blood is drawn.
   b. Call for help.
   c. Try to get the patient into a reclining position.
   d. Apply cold compresses to the patient's head and back of the neck.

8. What is the recommended maximum time to apply a tourniquet?
   a. 4 minutes
   b. 3 minutes
   c. 2 minutes
   d. 1 minute

9. Which of the following tests should *not* be done by the capillary puncture method?
   a. Glucose
   b. Complete blood count
   c. Blood cultures
   d. Cholesterol

10. The following tubes are being used in a Vacutainer venipuncture procedure: green, lavender, red (plastic), and light blue. Place them in the correct order of draw.

Websites

Newborn screening:
www.nlm.nih.gov/medlineplus/newbornscreening.html
http://kidshealth.org/parent/medical/genetic/newborn_screening_tests.html
www.marchofdimes.com/pnhec/298_834.asp
www.cincinnatichildrens.org/health/info/newborn/procedure/infant-screening.htm

American Academy of Pediatrics:
www.aap.org

Becton Dickinson site for safety needle and lancet supplies:
www.bd.com

Clinical and Laboratory Standards Institute (formerly NCCLS):
www.clsi.org/

Occupational Safety and Health Administration:
www.osha.gov

Phlebotomy:
www.phlebotomypages.com/phlebotomist_skills.htm
www.marketlabinc.com/products/details/806
www.phlebotomy.com/index.html
www.cdc.gov/niosh/topics/bbp/safer/default.htm
www.bd.com/safety/products/b_collect/index.asp#b3

Maternal and Child Health Bureau of the Health Resources and Services Administration:
www.mchb.hrsa.gov

Website for vein finder:
www.venoscope.com

5

Hematology

OBJECTIVES *After completing this chapter you should be able to do the following:*

1. Define and match terms and abbreviations in this chapter.

Fundamental Concepts

2. Identify the proper specimen collection for hematology testing.
3. Identify the blood components found in bone marrow and peripheral blood. Describe their functions, characteristics, and their basic formation in the bone marrow.
4. Perform a blood smear and stain and identify typical blood cells from the smear.
5. Observe selected abnormal cells from visual aids.
6. Describe the basic principles of hemostasis (including the involvement of blood vessels, platelets, clotting factors, and anticoagulants).

CLIA-Waived Tests

7. Identify equipment and supplies used in waived hematology and coagulation tests.
8. Follow the most current OSHA safety guidelines when performing hematology and coagulation

tests, and apply the correct quality control for the CLIA-waived hematology tests.

9. Perform the following FDA-approved waived tests according to the stated task, conditions, and standards listed in the Learning Outcome Procedure Sheets in the student workbook: hemoglobin, hematocrit, erythrocyte sedimentation rate, and prothrombin time.
10. Describe the role of prothrombin in blood coagulation and explain the major use of the prothrombin time test.

Advanced Concepts

11. Describe the seven tests involved in the complete blood count.
12. Identify the red blood cell indices, and explain their significance in determining anemia.
13. Explain the significance of the white blood cell count and differential.

KEY TERMS

anemia condition in which the red blood cell or hemoglobin level is below normal

anisocytosis abnormal variances in red blood cell size

band immature neutrophil whose nucleus has not segmented (also called stab)

baso- prefix meaning alkaline

basophil white blood cell with large granules that stain dark blue

cytoplasm fluid within cells between the nucleus and the outer cell membrane

differential count procedure for determining the distribution of the five types of leukocytes based on their staining characteristics, shapes, and sizes

embolus traveling clot

eosino- prefix meaning acid

eosinophil white blood cell with large granules that stain red

erythroblasts immature red blood cells (also called rubriblasts)

erythrocyte sedimentation rate (ESR) rate at which red blood cells settle out of an anticoagulated blood specimen after 60 minutes

fibrinogen (factor I) one of two plasma proteins involved in clotting

formed elements cells and cell fragments that can be viewed under the microscope

granulocytes white blood cells that contain granules in their cytoplasm: neutrophils, basophils, and eosinophils

hematocrit test that measures percentage of packed red blood cells compared with total blood volume

hematologist person who evaluates the cellular elements of blood microscopically and analytically by using a variety of test methods

hematology study of the visible cellular components in the bloodstream and bone marrow

hematopoiesis blood production

hemocytoblast stem cell that differentiates (changes) and becomes any of the seven visible blood elements found in circulating blood

hemoglobin oxygen-carrying reddish pigment in red blood cells

hemolysis (hemolyzing) destruction of the red blood cells

hemostasis body's ability to initiate a clotting response to stop bleeding and at the same time prevent the blood from forming an unwanted stationary clot

hyperchromia increase in color (based on hemoglobin concentration)

hypochromia lacking (or low) in color

hypochromic pertaining to less than normal color

hypoxemia lack of oxygen in the blood

immunoglobulins antibodies that destroy or render harmless foreign invaders containing antigens

leukemia various cancers of the white blood cells

leukocytosis abnormal increase in number of white blood cells

leukopenia abnormal decrease in number of white blood cells

lymphocyte small, nongranular white blood cell that develops from lymphoblasts in bone marrow

macrophages large, engulfing cells that come from monocytes when they enter the tissues

megakaryocyte large nuclear cell in the bone marrow that fragments its cytoplasm to become platelets

monocytes large, nongranular white blood cells that develop from monoblasts in bone marrow

myeloblasts stem cells that develop into the three kinds of granulocytes

neutro- prefix meaning neither acidic nor alkaline

neutrophil white blood cells with fine granules that stain lavender/pink

nongranulocytes (agranulocytes) white blood cells that may have a few or no granules in their cytoplasm; lymphocytes and monocytes

normocytes young red blood cells that shed their nuclei before entering the bloodstream

nucleus central controlling structure in the cell

-phil suffix meaning attraction

poikilocytosis abnormal shapes in red blood cells

polychromia increase in color variation (based on hemoglobin concentration)

polycythemia abnormal condition of increased number of red blood cells

polymorphonuclear having a multishaped, segmented nucleus; sometimes abbreviated as PMN or seg

prothrombin (factor II) one of two plasma proteins involved in clotting

protime test test for monitoring coagulation times for patients taking anticoagulants

RBC indices mathematic ratios of the three red blood cell tests (hemoglobin, hematocrit, and red blood cell count)

reticulocytes newly released red blood cells in the blood that still contain some nuclear DNA

rouleaux formation arrangement of red blood cells resembling stacked chips

thrombocytes platelets; cellular fragments that gather at the site of a damaged blood vessel and release clotting chemicals to form a clot

thrombosis abnormal condition of clotting

thrombus unwanted stationary clot

vitamin K critical element in the production of prothrombin

ABBREVIATIONS

ALL	acute lymphocytic leukemia	**Hgb**	hemoglobin
AML	acute myelocytic leukemia	**INR**	international normalized ratio (for protime test results)
CBC	complete blood count		
CLL	chronic lymphocytic leukemia	**MCH**	mean cell hemoglobin
CML	chronic myelocytic leukemia	**MCHC**	mean (average) cell hemoglobin concentration
ESR	erythrocyte sedimentation rate	**MCV**	mean cell volume
g/dL	grams per deciliter, which represents the weight of a substance (g) per volume (dL)	**PMN**	polymorphonuclear
		PT	prothrombin time (protime)
HCT	hematocrit		

Fundamental Concepts

Overview of Hematology and Blood

Hematology is the study of the visible cellular components in the bloodstream and bone marrow. The complete blood count (**CBC**) is one of the most commonly ordered "routine" tests for evaluating a person's internal health status. **Hematologists** work in the hematology departments of hospitals, reference labs, and private practices, where they evaluate the blood's cellular elements microscopically and analytically by using a variety of test methods. Hematologists may also evaluate **hemostasis**, the body's ability to initiate a clotting response to stop bleeding and at the same time prevent the blood from forming an unwanted stationary clot.

In the ambulatory setting, basic CLIA-waived hematology tests and coagulation (clotting) tests are performed on capillary blood. If a reference laboratory does the testing, the requisition and laboratory protocol must be checked to ensure the proper tubes are drawn and correctly processed. The blood for hematology tests is usually collected in lavender-topped vacuum tubes containing the anticoagulant

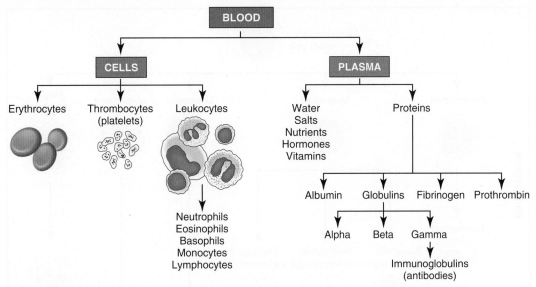

Fig. 5-1 Blood components. *Left,* Formed cellular elements; *right,* liquid plasma and its chemical divisions. *(From Chabner D: The language of medicine, ed 10, St. Louis, 2014, Saunders.)*

ethylenediaminetetraacetic acid (EDTA), which also preserves cellular elements in their natural state.

The blood for coagulation studies is usually collected in blue-topped vacuum tubes that must be allowed to fill accurately because the blood and the liquid anticoagulant in the tube must be in the proper ratio. This is why a "waste" tube is needed when using the butterfly needle and tubing.

Blood is a complex liquid connective tissue that is constantly circulating through the blood vessels. The **formed elements** within blood can be viewed under the microscope as cells and cell fragments (Figure 5-1, *left*). These formed elements (erythrocytes, or red blood cells [RBCs]; thrombocytes, or platelets; and leukocytes, or white blood cells [WBCs]) are suspended in the watery liquid called *plasma,* which contains hundreds of dissolved biochemical substances (see Figure 5-1, *right*). (Note: Chapters 6 and 7 will focus on the biochemical substances located in the plasma.)

Blood cells are produced in the red bone marrow found in flat bones and at the ends of long bones (Figure 5-2). All the cells originate from a stem cell, or **hemocytoblast**, that differentiates (changes) and becomes any of the following seven formed elements that are seen in circulating blood:

- Red blood cells (RBCs, also called *erythrocytes*)
- Five types of white blood cells (WBCs, also called *leukocytes*):
  - Basophils
  - Neutrophils
  - Eosinophils
  - Monocytes

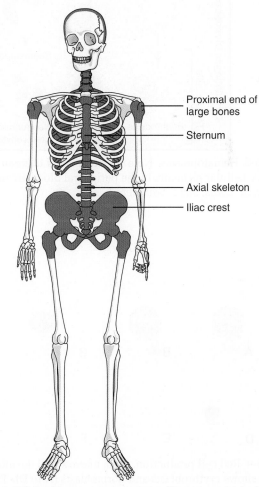

Fig. 5-2 Red bone marrow sites of hematopoiesis. *(From Rodak BF: Hematology: clinical principles and applications, ed 4, St. Louis, 2012, Saunders.)*

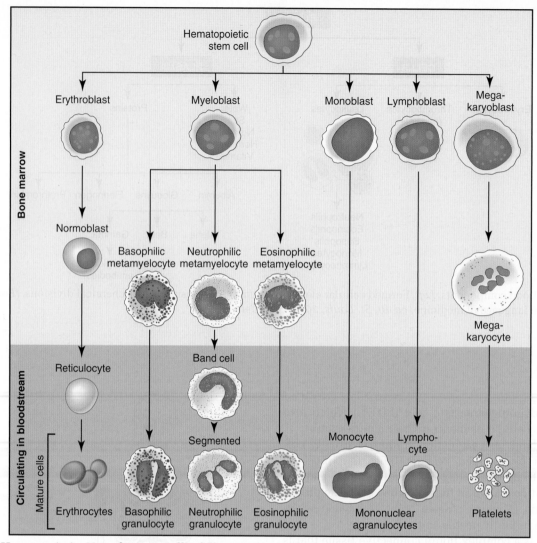

Fig. 5-3 Hematopoiesis. Note the stem cell's differentiation in the bone marrow *(top yellow area)* and immature and mature cellular elements in the peripheral bloodstream *(bottom tan area). (From Chabner D:* The language of medicine, *ed 10, St. Louis, 2014, Saunders.)*

Fig. 5-4 Red cell production. Bone marrow cell development shows erythroblasts and normoblasts **(A to D).** The bloodstream contains the immature reticulocytes **(E)** and mature erythrocytes **(F).** *(From Rodak BF, Carr JH:* Clinical hematology atlas, *ed 4, St. Louis, 2013, Saunders.)*

Fig. 5-5 Stained reticulocytes showing nuclear remains. *(From Rodak BF:* Hematology: clinical principles and applications, *ed 4, St. Louis, 2012, Saunders.)*

- Lymphocytes
- Platelets (also called *thrombocytes*)

Figure 5-3 is a simplified flow chart illustrating blood production, or **hematopoiesis**. Each of the seven formed elements is viewed and discussed as it is developed in the bone marrow and then released into the bloodstream or tissue, where it fulfills its function.

Red Blood Cells (Erythrocytes)

The bone marrow is constantly producing new RBCs. The beginning stages of RBC production in the bone marrow are shown in Figure 5-4. **Erythroblasts** (immature RBCs), also called *rubriblasts,* become **normocytes** that shed their nuclei before entering the bloodstream. In the bloodstream the young RBCs, which still contain some nuclear deoxyribonucleic acid (DNA), are called **reticulocytes** (Figure 5-5). The average amount of reticulocytes found in peripheral blood is approximately 1%. A percentage higher than 3% indicates that the individual is actively producing new red cells because of a loss of RBCs, such as when hemorrhaging occurs. As the reticulocytes continue to mature, they shed their remaining intracellular nuclear material while retaining millions of **hemoglobin (Hgb)** molecules (reddish pigment capable of carrying oxygen).

Mature red cells are biconcave disks filled with a reddish pigment called *hemoglobin* (Figure 5-6). Hgb consists of an iron (heme) and a protein (globin) molecule. Hgb has a strong affinity for oxygen that it picks up and carries from the lungs to the cells of the body. This oxygen-carrying capacity of RBCs is critical to sustaining life energy throughout the body. Because of their critical role, RBCs account for almost half of the blood volume. After 80 to 120 days, RBCs disintegrate, releasing the iron (heme) portion, which goes back to the bone marrow to make new RBCs (Figure 5-7). The remaining elements convert to bilirubin, which is further processed through various stages in the liver, intestines, and kidneys (Figure 5-8).

White Blood Cells

WBCs fall into two general categories: granulocytes, consisting of neutrophils, basophils, and eosinophils; and nongranulocytes, consisting of lymphocytes and monocytes.

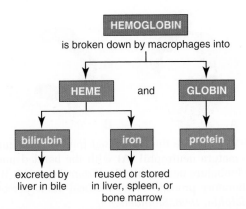

Fig. 5-6 Dimensions and shape of a mature red cell. (Note: Micron is another name for micrometer (one millionth of a meter.) *(From Stepp CA, Woods M:* Laboratory procedures for medical office personnel, *Philadelphia, 1998, Saunders.)*

Fig. 5-7 Breakdown of hemoglobin into heme and globin and their further breakdown into bilirubin, iron, and protein. *(From Chabner D:* The language of medicine, *ed 10, St. Louis, 2014, Saunders.)*

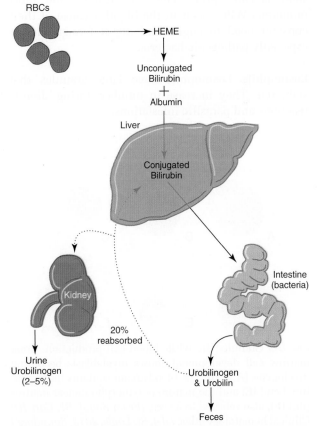

Fig. 5-8 Bilirubin metabolism in the liver, intestines, and kidney. *(From Rodak BF:* Hematology: clinical principles and applications, *ed 4, St. Louis, 2012, Saunders.)*

Granulocytes

Myeloblasts are the stem cells in the bone marrow that become myelocytes (see Figure 5-3). The myelocytes develop into the three kinds of granulocytes: neutrophils, eosinophils, and basophils. Figure 5-9 illustrates a myeloblast becoming a myelocyte and metamyelocyte within the bone marrow. The granulocyte enters the bloodstream with its **nucleus** (the central controlling structure in the cell) in an elongated "**band**" shape. The maturing nuclei of the eosinophils and basophils become segmented into two lobes. The mature neutrophil's multisegmented nucleus is referred to as **polymorphonuclear (PMN)** or as a *seg* (Figure 5-10).

The three mature **granulocytes** in the bloodstream are distinguished from one another by the staining characteristics of the granules located in their **cytoplasm** (fluid within cells between the nucleus and the outer cell membrane). When a drop of whole blood is smeared onto a slide and then stained, the three different granulocytic WBCs show an affinity, or attraction, to either the *red* acid dye (**eosino**), the *blue* alkaline dye (**baso**), or *both* colors (**neutro**). The WBCs are named on the basis of their *attraction* to the dyes (indicated by the suffix **phil**) and have distinct purposes in aiding the body during infection and inflammation.

Neutrophils. **Neutrophils** have small granules that stain lavender/pink. They are usually the most numerous WBCs seen in the blood because of their constant need to engulf and digest foreign matter, especially pathogenic bacteria.

Eosinophils. **Eosinophils** have large granules that stain red. They increase in number during allergic reactions and parasitic infestations.

Basophils. **Basophils** have large granules that stain dark blue. They are the rarest WBCs in the blood and are involved in preventing blood from excessive clotting by producing the anticoagulant heparin. They also mediate the inflammatory response.

Nongranulocytes (Agranulocytes)

Bone marrow also produces the following two **nongranulocytes**, or **agranulocytes**, which may have a few or no granules in their gray and sky-blue cytoplasm:

1. **Monocytes** in the blood originate as monoblasts (immature monocytes) in the bone marrow. They are the largest WBCs and can leave the bloodstream to enter the tissues as **macrophages** (large, engulfing cells). Their numbers increase during the recovery stage of infection and during the healing of traumatized tissue when debris needs to be cleared.

2. **Lymphocytes** are the smallest, nongranular WBCs that develop from lymphoblasts (immature lymphocytes) in the bone marrow. They further differentiate into B and T cells, as seen in Figure 5-11.
   - *T lymphocytes* are stimulated by the thymus gland to develop a variety of immune responses toward invaders.
   - *B lymphocytes* become plasma cells capable of producing specific antibodies (**immunoglobulins**) that destroy or render harmless foreign invaders, especially viruses. (The immune response involving T and B lymphocytes is covered in Chapter 7.)

Lymphocytes are the smallest WBCs in the bloodstream. They move freely among the blood vessels, lymph vessels, and tissues as they constantly survey for and respond to foreign invaders.

Fig. 5-9 Granulocytic white blood cell production. Bone marrow cell development shows myeloblasts becoming myelocytes **(A to D).** The bloodstream contains the immature band **(E)** and the mature polymorphonuclear neutrophil **(F),** also referred to as *seg. (From Rodak BF, Carr JH: Clinical hematology atlas, ed 4, St. Louis, 2013, Saunders.)*

Fig. 5-10 Compare the segmented (multilobed) nucleus in the mature neutrophil **(A)** with the banded nucleus in the immature neutrophil **(B).** *(From Stepp CA, Woods M: Laboratory procedures for medical office personnel, Philadelphia, 1998, Saunders.)*

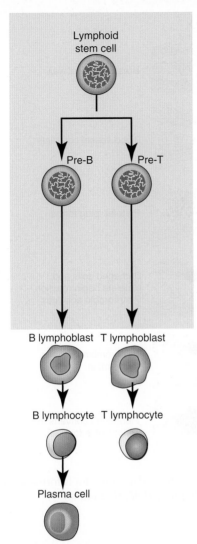

Fig. 5-11 Lymphocytic flow chart showing the lymphoblast differentiating into B and T lymphoblasts and cells. The B cells become plasma cells when they leave the bloodstream and enter body tissues. *(From Rodak BF, Carr JH:* Clinical hematology atlas, *ed 4, St. Louis, 2013, Saunders.)*

Fig. 5-12 Megakaryocyte in the bone marrow **(A)** and cytoplasmic platelets in the peripheral bloodstream **(B)**. *(From Rodak BF, Carr JH:* Clinical hematology atlas, *ed 4, St. Louis, 2013, Saunders.)*

Platelets (Thrombocytes)

The seventh formed element also comes from the stem cell (hemocytoblast) after it differentiates into a megakaryoblast and then into a **megakaryocyte** (large nuclear cell) in the bone marrow (Figure 5-12). This very large cell releases fragments of its cytoplasm into the bloodstream, which are seen as small **thrombocytes**, or platelets.

Platelets also release clotting chemicals that activate the formation of sticky fibrin strands that entangle the blood cells and form a clot (Figure 5-13). They gather around the site of a damaged blood vessel in an effort to "plug" the leak (Figure 5-14).

Fig. 5-13 Fibrin strands enmesh the cells and form a clot that plugs the bleeding vessel. *(From Chabner D:* The language of medicine, *ed 10, St. Louis, 2014, Saunders. Originally from Page J et al:* Blood: the river of life, *Washington, DC, 1981, New Books.)*

Capillary

Arteriole

Break in vessel wall

Blood vessel contracts

Platelet plug forms

Damaged cells and
platelets begin reaction.
Prothrombin activates

Prothrombin converts
to thrombin

Fibrinogen converts to
fibrin; clot is formed

Fig. 5-14 Hemostasis. The damaged blood vessel constricts, platelets congregate, and a fibrin clot is formed. *(From Stepp CA, Woods M:* Laboratory procedures for medical office personnel, *Philadelphia, 1998, Saunders.)*

Preparing a Blood Smear to Be Viewed by the Physician or Laboratory Technician

A blood smear can be made by using fresh blood from a gently mixed lavender-topped EDTA Vacutainer tube (Becton Dickinson, Franklin Lakes, NJ) or from a fresh capillary puncture. A drop of blood is placed on the end of a clean slide with a Diff safety device (Becton Dickinson) inserted into the lavender EDTA tube. This device is a convenient and safe way to obtain a drop of blood from the Vacutainer tube without removing the sealed top of the tube. Push the white device into the top of the EDTA lavender tube; then invert the tube and press the device against the slide (Figure 5-15). The pressure on the slide causes a drop of blood to flow onto the slide. A drop of blood can also be obtained from a finger capillary puncture. Next, the drop of blood is spread across the slide by bringing a clean "pusher" slide back into the drop at a 30- to 35-degree angle. As soon as the blood spreads approximately three fourths along the edge, quickly move the pusher slide forward (Figure 5-16). Allow the slide to air-dry.

Fig. 5-15 **A,** One way to apply a drop of blood to a slide for smearing is to push a Safety Diff device into a lavender-topped Vacutainer tube. **B,** Press the device against the slide to deliver a drop of blood. **C,** Another method is to apply the drop of blood directly from a finger stick.

Fig. 5-16 Proper blood smear technique. **A,** Pull upper slide back into the drop of blood. **B,** Allow blood to spread along the edge of the slide. **C,** Then, with downward pressure, quickly push the slide to the other end until stopped by the fingers. *(From Rodak BF: Hematology: clinical principles and applications, ed 4, St. Louis, 2012, Saunders.)*

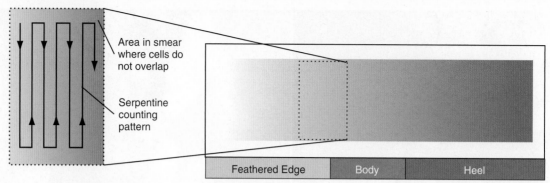

Fig. 5-17 Ideal smear, showing the thinning out of the "feathered edge" on the left with the "body" of the slide for viewing the cells. The "heel" is the thick area of blood cells that were pulled from the drop of blood. Note the serpentine pattern of moving the slide up and over and down and over the body of the smear to observe many different fields without duplicating an area. *(From Stepp CA, Woods M:* Laboratory procedures for medical office personnel, *Philadelphia, 1998, Saunders.)*

Fig. 5-18 Improper smears resulting from dirty slides and improper pushing techniques. *(From Rodak BF:* Hematology: clinical principles and applications, *ed 4, St. Louis, 2012, Saunders.)*

A properly performed smear will look like the one illustrated in Figure 5-17. Improper, unacceptable smears resemble those depicted in Figure 5-18.

Evaluate the smear to see if the following are present:

1. A feathered edge
2. A well-distributed "body" with margins on each side
3. Smooth, thick-to-thin spreading of the smear with no ridges or tails

The smeared blood slide is then stained with either Wright's stain or a Diff-Quick (Becton Dickinson) stain. Both of these staining methods use three ingredients: a methanol fixative, a red acid dye, and a blue alkaline dye. The Wright's stain also uses a buffer solution to change the pH. Refer to the material safety data sheets in the workbook and the labels on the bottles when working with stains, and take appropriate precautions. The simple Diff-Quick staining procedure used in ambulatory settings is provided in the workbook and is demonstrated in Procedure 5-1 at the end of this section.

Stained blood smears must be observed by the physician, a trained hematologist, or a laboratory technician.

White Blood Cell Identification and Differential

The hematologist scans stained blood smears to identify the distribution of the five types of leukocytes on the basis of their staining characteristics, shapes, and sizes. This procedure is called a **differential count**. See the WBC atlas, which lists and shows the distinguishing characteristics that are observed for each of the leukocytes.

Note the following facts found in the atlas for each of the following:

- Segmented neutrophil—most prevalent WBC; fine lavender or pink granules in the cytoplasm and a segmented nucleus *(A)*
- Immature banded neutrophil; nucleus has a banded shape *(B)*
- Small (mature) lymphocyte—second most prevalent WBC: dense circular nucleus and scant blue cytoplasm *(C)*
- Monocyte—largest of the leukocytes; has large, lacy nucleus *(D)*
- Eosinophil—has large red granules *(E)*
- Basophil—rarest; has large, dark-blue or black granules *(F)*

The WBC atlas is presented in on pp. 144-145.

Each time a leukocyte is found, the hematologist identifies it and presses the corresponding key on a differential counter (Figure 5-19). After identifying 100 leukocytes, the counter sounds a bell. Each of the 5 leukocytes is then displayed as a percentage of the total 100 cells identified.

Fig. 5-19 Differential counter showing keys for counting: *eos, bands, segs, lympho,* and *mono.* (NOTE: *baso* is missing because it is so rare. The tech mentally remembers when a *baso* is seen.) *(From Rodak BF: Hematology: clinical principles and applications, ed 4, St. Louis, 2012, Saunders. Courtesy Beckman Coulter.)*

White Blood Cell Atlas

	Cell Type	Cell Size (μm)	Nucleus	Chromatin in Nucleus	Cytoplasm
A	Polymorphonuclear neutrophil (poly, PMN), segmented neutrophil (seg)	10-15	Two to five lobes connected by thin filaments	Coarsely clumped	Pale blue to pink
B	Band neutrophil (band)	10-15	C or S shaped, constricted but no thread-like filaments	Coarsely clumped	Pale blue to pink
C	Lymphocyte (lymph)	7-18*	Round to oval; may be slightly indented; occasional nucleoli	Condensed to deeply condensed	Scant to moderate; sky blue; vacuoles may be present
D	Monocyte (mono)	12-20	Variable; may be round, horse-shoe, or kidney shaped; often has folds producing "brainlike" convolutions	Lacy	Blue-gray; may have pseudopods; vacuoles may be absent or numerous
E	Eosinophil (eos)	12-17	Two to three lobes connected by filaments	Coarsely clumped	Pink; may have irregular borders
F	Basophil (baso)	10-14	Usually two lobes connected by thin filaments	Coarsely clumped	Lavender to colorless

A, **Segmented neutrophils,** the most prevalent white blood cell, have fine lavender/pink granules throughout the cytoplasm.

B, **Banded neutrophils** show immature nonsegmented nuclei.

C, **Lymphocytes** are typically the second most frequently seen white blood cell. Note the dense nucleus with scanty cytoplasm.

D, **The large monocytes** contain a convoluted nucleus and abundant cytoplasm.

E, **The eosinophils** have large red granules.

F, **The basophils** have large, dark-blue granules.

Illustrations modified from Carr JH, Rodak BF: *Clinical hematology atlas, ed 4, St. Louis, 2013,* Saunders.

*The difference in size from small to large lymphocytes is primarily caused by a larger amount of cytoplasm.

Granules	Reference Range	Microscopic View
Abundant lavender/pink granules	50-70%	A
Abundant lavender/pink granules	0-5%	B
±Few	20-40%	C
Many fine granules frequently giving the appearance of ground glass	3-11%	D
Granules are large red to orange, round	0-7%	E
Large dark blue/black; variable in number with uneven distribution	0-1%	F

Red Blood Cell Identification and Description

Next, the hematologist observes and reports the appearance of the RBCs. Normal RBC appearance and distribution are shown in Figure 5-20.

In a diseased state, the RBCs may become altered in appearance. The three columns in the flow chart (Figure 5-21) located in the RBC atlas show how RBCs can vary in size (**anisocytosis**), shape (**poikilocytosis**), and color (**polychromia**, **hypochromia**, and **hyperchromia**). The hematologist reports the degree of these variances by using +1, +2, and so on. The following abnormal RBC sizes, colors, and shapes are also shown in the RBC atlas:

- Macrocytes (large cells) (Figure 5-22)
- Microcytes and hypochromic RBCs (small cells and faded color cells) (Figure 5-23)
- Polychromatic RBCs (multicolored cells) (Figure 5-24)
- Dacryocytes (tear-shaped cells) (Figure 5-25)
- Ovalocytes (elliptical-shaped cells) (Figure 5-26)
- Spherocytes (ball-shaped round cells) (Figure 5-27)
- Sickle cells (collapsed, C-shaped cells) (Figure 5-28)

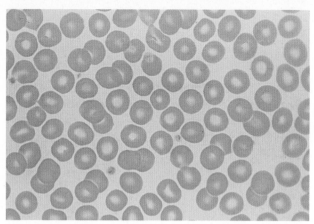

Fig. 5-20 Normal red blood cell appearance and distribution in the body of the smeared slide. This slide contains predominantly red blood cells with a few platelets. *(From Rodak BF:* Hematology: clinical principles and applications, *ed 3, St Louis, 2007, Saunders.)*

Red Blood Cell Atlas

Fig. 5-21 Flow chart with the terms relating to variations in red blood cell size *(left)*, shape *(middle)*, and color *(right)*. *(From Stepp CA, Woods M:* Laboratory procedures for medical office personnel, *Philadelphia, 1998, Saunders.)*

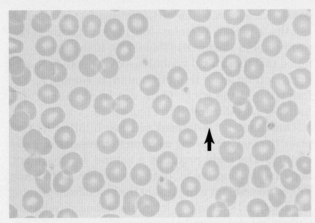

Fig. 5-22 Macrocytic red blood cell. *(From Rodak BF: Hematology: clinical principles and applications, ed 4, St. Louis, 2012, Saunders.)*

Fig. 5-23 Microcytes; hypochromic red blood cells. *(From Rodak BF: Hematology: clinical principles and applications, ed 4, St. Louis, 2012, Saunders.)*

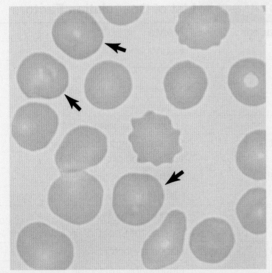

Fig. 5-24 Polychromatic red blood cells. *(From Carr JH, Rodak BF: Clinical hematology atlas, ed 4, St. Louis, 2013, Saunders.)*

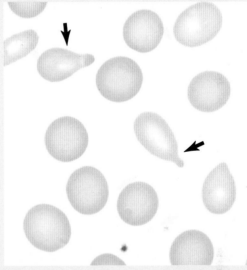

Fig. 5-25 Tear drop (dacryocytes). *(From Carr JH, Rodak BF: Clinical hematology atlas, ed 4, St. Louis, 2013, Saunders.)*

Fig. 5-26 Ovalocytes. *(From Carr JH, Rodak BF: Clinical hematology atlas, ed 4, St. Louis, 2013, Saunders.)*

Fig. 5-27 Spherocytes. *(From Rodak BF: Hematology: clinical principles and applications, ed 4, St. Louis, 2012, Saunders.)*

Fig. 5-28 Sickle cells. *(From Rodak BF: Hematology: clinical principles and applications, ed 4, St. Louis, 2012, Saunders.)*

Platelet Description

Platelets (thrombocytes) are also assessed while scanning the slide (Figure 5-29). Their quantity is approximated by the hematologist while observing various fields under oil immersion.

Theory of Hemostasis

The cardiovascular system is equipped with a remarkable mechanism that swiftly stops blood from escaping out of a damaged blood vessel. First the blood vessel constricts, slowing the rate of blood flow. Then platelets concentrate around the damaged site and initiate a clot made of a sticky fibrin mesh (see Figures 5-13 and 5-14). The fibrin strands are the result of a complex chain reaction of 13 clotting factors, including the 2 plasma proteins—**fibrinogen (factor I)** and **prothrombin (factor II)** (Table 5-1). It should also be noted that the critical vitamin used by the liver to produce clotting factor II (prothrombin) is vitamin K. The formation of the sticky fibrin can be simplified into four steps, as illustrated in Figure 5-30.

Once the clot is formed and has fulfilled its purpose, the body stops the reaction to prevent excessive clotting. The body produces a natural anticoagulant, heparin, to keep the clotting mechanism in balance. The anticoagulant will prevent the blood from forming an unwanted stationary clot, or **thrombus**, or releasing a traveling clot, or **embolus**.

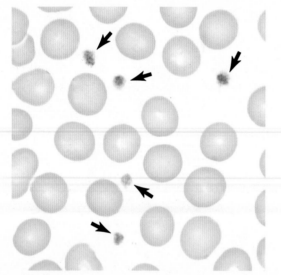

Fig. 5-29 Platelets among the red blood cells. *(From Carr JH, Rodak BF:* Clinical hematology atlas, *ed 4, St. Louis, 2013, Saunders.)*

Table 5-1	List of Coagulation Factors
Factor	**Name**
I	Fibrinogen
II	Prothrombin
III	Tissue factor; thromboplastin
IV	Calcium
V	Labile factor; proaccelerin
VII	Serum prothrombin conversion accelerator; proconvertin
VIII	Antihemophilic factor
IX	Plasma thromboplastin component
X	Stuart-Prower factor
XI	Plasma thromboplastin antecedent
XII	Hageman factor
XIII	Fibrin stabilizing factor
Platelet factor	Cephalin

From Stepp CA, Woods M: *Laboratory procedures for medical office personnel,* Philadelphia, 1998, Saunders.

Fig. 5-30 Four steps of the formation of fibrin. *(From Chabner D:* The language of medicine, *ed 10, St. Louis, 2014, Saunders.)*

Coagulation and Testing

Most coagulation tests are performed at the hospital or reference laboratory to help determine why a patient is bleeding, bruising, or forming clots abnormally. Table 5-2 lists reference values for selected coagulation tests.

A patient who is prone to **thrombosis** (an abnormal condition of clotting) may need to take anticoagulant drugs such as warfarin (Coumadin is the brand name). Patients receiving anticoagulant therapy must be monitored on a predetermined schedule, sometimes weekly and then moving to monthly over time. They are tested to see the amount of time a sample of their blood takes to coagulate. If their blood coagulates too rapidly, they may have an underdosage of their anticoagulant, which may lead to a life-threatening blood clot. If, on the other hand, the blood coagulates too slowly, it may indicate an overdosage of their anticoagulant, which may cause a fatal hemorrhage.

The CLIA-waived testing method for monitoring these patients' coagulation times is called the prothrombin time, or **protime test**. The result of the test is expressed as the number of seconds it takes for the prothrombin to form a fibrin clot in the laboratory. This result is then converted to an international normalized ratio (**INR**). The INR allows an accurate comparison of results from different methods of prothrombin testing. A normal INR reading will usually have a value of "1." The goal for a patient receiving anticoagulant therapy, on the other hand, is to keep the INR at a standardized 2 to 2.5 and occasionally higher. A therapeutic protime at this level prolongs the clotting time enough to prevent unwanted clotting but not so long that the patient is in danger of abnormal bleeding.

Summary of Fundamental Concepts

This section presented the function, formation, and distinguishing characteristics of the cells and coagulation factors in blood. Procedure 5-1 describes the steps involved in staining a smeared blood specimen. Once stained, the physician may identify the cells under the microscope using the white blood cell and red blood cell atlases as guides.

The next section, CLIA-Waived Hematology Tests, describes the most common hematology tests performed in physician office laboratories (POLs).

Table 5-2	Reference Values for Selected Coagulated Tests
Test	**Reference Values**
Bleeding time (Ivy)	1-8.5 min (average, 3-6 min)
Platelet count	150,000-400,000/mm^3 (average, 250,000/mm^3)
Platelet aggregation	Aggregation visible within <5 min
Capillary fragility	Normal: <10 petechiae/2 in circle
	Grade 1: 0-10 petechiae/2 in circle
	Grade 2: 11-20 petechiae/2 in circle
	Grade 3: 21-50 petechiae/2 in circle
	Grade 4+: >50 petechiae/2 in circle
Activated clotting time	70-120 sec
Partial thromboplastin time	30-45 sec
Prothrombin time	11.0-13.0 sec
Thrombin time	7.0-12.0 sec
Fibrinogen assay	200-400 mg/dL or 2.0-4.0 g/L
Clot retraction	50% in 2 hr; 90% in 4 hr

Modified from Stepp CA, Woods M: *Laboratory procedures for medical office personnel,* Philadelphia, 1998, Saunders.

✳ PROCEDURE 5-1 Diff-Quick Staining Procedure

A, Slide is dipped in fixative three times and *allowed to dry completely.*

B, Slide is dipped into the red eosin dye three to five times.

C, The excess dye is allowed to run off onto an absorbent paper.

D, The slide is dipped into the blue baso dye three to five times.

E, After the blue dye is blotted away, the slide is gently and thoroughly rinsed with water on both sides and dried, and then brought to the microscope for viewing under the oil immersion lens.

Equipment and Supplies

Diff-Quick stain: fixative, red eosin dye, blue baso dye; staining rack; water source (bottled or running water); bibulous paper

Procedure

1. Dip the slide in fixative three times, and allow it to dry completely (Figure A).
2. Dip the slide into the red eosin dye three to five times (Figure B).
3. Let the excess dye run off and blot the rest away with absorbent paper (Figure C).
4. Dip the slide into the blue baso dye three to five times (Figure D).
5. After the blue dye is blotted away, rinse the slide thoroughly with water on both sides hand allow it to air-dry (Figure E). It can also be pressed between two bibulous papers to help remove the water.

5-1

PROCEDURE 5-1 Diff-Quick Staining Procedure—cont'd

6. Observe the slide under the oil immersion lens of the microscope. Refer to the microscope skill sheet in Chapter 2 for the proper steps to bring the slide into focus under the oil immersion lens. The cells and platelets will be enlarged 1000 times (100× oil objective times the 10× ocular lens). The slide will show predominantly RBCs with some small platelet clumps throughout. The challenge is to find the WBCs. The two most commonly found WBCs are segmented neutrophils and small lymphocytes. See the White Blood Cell Atlas for assistance in identifying the WBCs.

CLIA-Waived Hematology Tests

The most common procedure associated with hematology is the CBC. A CBC generally consists of the following seven laboratory tests: RBC, WBC, platelet counts, Hgb, hematocrit (HCT), differential, and **RBC indices**. The Hgb and HCT are CLIA-waived tests. The other five tests are moderately or highly complex and are discussed at the end of this chapter.

Four hematology tests have been approved as CLIA-waived hematology tests and can be performed in Certificate of Waiver (CoW) offices: Hgb tests, HCT tests, erythrocyte sedimentation rates (**ESR**), and prothrombin time tests (protime). (Competency skill sheets for each procedure are provided in the workbook.)

Hemoglobin

The Hgb within the RBCs is measured by **hemolyzing** (destroying the RBCs) and allows the conversion of Hgb into cyanmethemoglobin. The new color reaction is then expressed as grams per deciliter (**g/dL**), which represents the weight of the Hgb (g) per the volume of blood (dL). The result is compared with the reference range. Expected Hgb values are as follows:

Adult men	14 to 18 g/dL
Adult women	12 to 16 g/dL
Children	10 to 15 g/dL (increases with age)
Newborns	17 to 21 g/dL

Notice that the Hgb level ranges in women are lower than those in men because women lose blood during menstruation each month during their reproductive years. Newborns are born with high Hgb levels that fall during early childhood and then build up to the adult levels. When any of the patient results drop below their reference range, it is referred to as *anemia*.

Hemoglobin Testing Methods

Common procedural steps in all Hgb tests include the following:
1. Collecting blood into an appropriate testing device.
2. Hemolyzing the RBCs to release their Hgb.
3. Analyzing the amount of released Hgb by sending a light source through the specimen. The instruments have highly sensitive optical readers that receive the light after it either passes through or reflects off the specimen; the resulting measurement of the light then allows the instrument to calculate the amount of Hgb within the specimen.
4. Reading and reporting the digital readout, expressed in grams per deciliter.
5. The instruments require daily optics checks and first-time operator verification of competency by using liquid controls. The workbook appendix has a generic quantitative competency check sheet that may be completed to meet the procedural requirements of these test methods. All the control results and patient results must be logged and evaluated by comparing them with their provided reference ranges.

Three common CLIA-waived Hgb test methods approved by the Food and Drug Administration (FDA) that are used in ambulatory care settings are: The HemoCue method (HemoCue Inc., Lake Forest, Calif), the Hgb meter method, and the i-STAT method (Abbott Laboratories, Abbott Park, Ill).

HemoCue Method

The HemoCue method procedure check sheet is provided in the workbook and is demonstrated in Procedure 5-2, at the end of this section.

Hgb Meter and i-STAT Methods

The Hgb meter and the i-STAT are hand-held point-of-care instruments that can be brought to the patient for a rapid assessment of Hgb level and other blood test results (Figure 5-31).

Hematocrit

Hematocrit (HCT) measures the percentage of packed RBCs that develop after centrifuging a specimen and comparing the volume of the packed cells with the total volume of the measured specimen. The packed RBCs are expressed as a percentage of whole blood. HCT expected values are the following:

Adult men	42% to 52%
Adult women	36% to 45%
Children	36% to 41% (increases with age)
Infants	30% to 40%
Newborns	44% to 64%

Fig. 5-31 **A,** Hemoglobin meter. **B,** i-STAT Point-of-Care blood analyzer. *(B from Rodak BF:* Hematology: clinical principles and applications, *ed 4, St. Louis, 2012, Saunders. Courtesy i-STAT Corp., East Windsor, NJ.)*

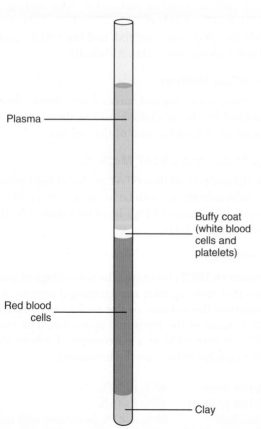

Fig. 5-32 HCT tube layers: plasma, buffy coat, red blood cell layer, clay sealant.

Notice that the RBCs occupy almost 50% of the total volume of blood in Figure 5-32. Also notice that the numerical values of Hgb are approximately one third the numerical values of the HCT. If a patient's results fall below the expected HCT range, this is considered anemia. A patient with an abnormally high HCT level is referred to as polycythemic.

General Spun Microhematocrit Procedures

Steps common to all microhematocrit procedures include the following:
- Collecting blood into two appropriate capillary tubes containing an anticoagulant to prevent clotting of the specimens (NOTE: OSHA safety precautions recommend using plastic capillary tubes, not glass, to prevent possible breakage and blood exposure incidents.)
- Sealing the capillary tubes with clay or a stopper at one end
- Centrifuging the specimens in a HCT centrifuge with the sealed end against the outer rubber gasket or down in the sleeved plastic holder for 5 minutes
- Observing the centrifuged layers: plasma, buffy coat, red cell layer, and sealant (see Figure 5-32)
- Determining the percent of RBC volume compared with the total blood volume by using a built-in scale or a variable volume scale

The results of the two capillary tubes should be within 2% of agreement, and the final result is recorded as the average of the two tubes. If the results of the two tubes are not within 2%, the test should be repeated. Also take note if the appearance of the

Fig. 5-33 Rouleaux formation causing a high ESR result. *(From Carr JH, Rodak BF:* Clinical hematology atlas, *ed 4, St. Louis, 2013, Saunders.)*

plasma is red, indicating hemolysis; white, indicating lipemia (fat in the blood); or dark yellow–brown, indicating jaundice.

Procedure 5-3, presented at the end of this section, describes the general HCT procedure, and its corresponding check sheet is provided in the workbook.

HemataSTAT Procedure

Procedure 5-4 describes an alternate method for measuring blood HCTs in which plastic-covered tubes are rapidly spun in a centrifuge for only 1 minute. The centrifuge has a built-in reading tray that provides a digital readout. A proficiency check sheet is provided in the workbook.

Erythrocyte Sedimentation Rate

The **erythrocyte sedimentation rate (ESR)** is the rate at which RBCs settle out of an anticoagulated blood specimen after 60 minutes. The result is reported in millimeters per hour. ESR expected values are as follows:

Adult men <50 years	0 to 15 mm/hr
Adult men ≥50 years	0 to 20 mm/hr
Adult women <50 years	0 to 20 mm/hr
Adult women ≥50 years	0 to 30 mm/hr

The ESR is a nonspecific screening test to help confirm and monitor changes in inflammatory diseases, autoimmune diseases, carcinomas, and certain forms of leukemia. Patients with these diseases will show sedimentation rates greater than the expected values in the preceding list depending on the amount of inflammation occurring when blood is drawn.

The principle of the ESR is based on the effect of plasma proteins (especially globulins and fibrinogen) produced during inflammatory conditions. These proteins cause the RBCs to become sticky and stack together in a **rouleaux formation** (resembling stacked chips) (Figure 5-33). The stacked RBCs fall (sediment) at an increased rate that is directly proportional to the increased amount of proteins that were produced during inflammation.

The shape and size of RBCs also affect ESR. For example, spherocytes fall and create an increased rate, whereas sickle cells fall at a slower rate, and macrocytes fall faster than microcytes.

Other technical factors, such as the following, can also interfere with obtaining accurate sedimentation rate results:

False Increased Rates

- Tilting the test tubes results in an erroneous increase in the sedimentation rate.
- Vibrations falsely increase the sedimentation rate.
- Extremely hot room temperatures falsely increase the sedimentation rate.
- Timing is critical; the results must be read at exactly 60 minutes because taking a reading after the specified time gives a result that is too high.

False Decreased Rates

- Extreme cold room temperatures falsely decrease the sedimentation rate.
- Taking a reading before the specified time gives a result that is too low.

Other Interferences

- Air bubbles in the tube interfere with sedimentation by breaking up the specimen and causing an erroneous lower value.
- The blood must be fresh, tested within 2 hours of collection or within 6 hours if the specimen has been refrigerated.

Sediplast ESR System

The Sediplast (Polymedco Inc., Cortlandt Manor, NY) ESR method uses a safe, disposable, calibrated plastic pipette that is inserted into a vial containing a mixture of transferred EDTA blood and a premeasured citrate solution. This closed-system test provides a sedimentation rate after allowing the pipette to stand in a vertical rack for 1 hour. The Sediplast procedure check sheet is provided in the workbook and is demonstrated in Procedure 5-5 at the end of this section.

Streck 30-Minute Manual ESR System

A new 30-minute test for ESR is now available. Blood may be collected directly into the black citrate tube or may be transferred from an EDTA tube to the citrate tube. The "Streck" tube is then suspended in the "Streck" rack for 30 minutes. The results are then manually read using the chart provided in the rack. See Procedure 5-6 in the workbook and demonstrated at the end of this section for this safe and timely way to test a patient's ESR.

Prothrombin Time

Prothrombin time (**PT**) is a commonly performed CLIA-waived test that measures the amount of time the blood takes to form a fibrin clot. The PT test uses thromboplastin as the active reagent to initiate the coagulation process by converting prothrombin to thrombin (refer back to Figure 5-30 under Fundamental Concepts).

The PT test is used as a *screening* test for patients who lack clotting factors, have a liver disease, or are deficient in **vitamin K** (a critical element in the production of prothrombin). The PT of these patients will be prolonged, indicating they will be prone to bleeding. The PT test is also widely used to *monitor* patients who require anticoagulant therapy. These patients are taking anticoagulant drugs (warfarin, Coumadin) because they have had a tendency to produce internal clots, which could lead to strokes and heart attacks. The anticoagulant drugs suppress the liver from synthesizing prothrombin. The PT test measures both normal and therapeutic PTs in fresh whole blood.

Results are displayed in PT seconds and INR value. The PT reference range will vary depending on the manufacturer's method of testing and the amount of thromboplastin used in the test.

The normal PT reference range is usually approximately 10 to 13 seconds. The INR value is the patient's PT in seconds divided by the normal control's PT in seconds. The control's PT rate is supplied by the manufacturer for each test lot of thromboplastin and/or it is built into the test system. A normal INR should be close to 1.0.

The INR is the coagulation value that more accurately compares to other PT test methods when a patient is monitoring his or her PT in a variety of settings. The therapeutic goal is to keep the patient's PT higher than normal at approximately 12 to 18 seconds (depending on the method used), or 2 to 2.5 INR (occasionally higher depending on therapeutic need).

Procedure 5-7, at the end of this section, presents the PT/INR method, and a proficiency check sheet is provided in the workbook. The PT/INR method uses a highly sensitive instrument that runs its optics check before each test and runs the normal and high controls alongside the patient's blood specimen. It will not give a patient's result unless all controls are accurate and precise (i.e., reliable).

Becoming Proficient at CLIA-Waived Hematology Tests

Now that you have learned about the significance of Hgb, HCT, ESR, and PT tests, take time to complete the following:

1. Answer the questions at the end of this chapter and the CLIA-waived portion in Chapter 5 of the workbook using your structured notes and text.
2. View the videos on-line to see Hgb and HCT testing performed.
3. Perform the Chapter 5 exercises on-line, which were designed to reinforce your knowledge of terminology and CLIA-waived test procedures.
4. Study Procedures 5-2 through 5-7 before your lab.

✳ PROCEDURE 5-2 Hemoglobin: *HemoCue Method*

After approximately 15–45 seconds the result is displayed.

A, HemoCue equipment and procedure. *a,* Hgb microcuvette; *b,* HemoCue instrument; *c,* digital readout; *d,* cuvette holder. *(From Zakus SM:* Clinical skills for medical assistants, *ed 4, St Louis, 2001, Mosby.)*

5-2

PROCEDURE 5-2 Hemoglobin: *HemoCue Method*—cont'd

B, HemoCue calibration with red control cuvette. (NOTE: Newer models now have the HemoCue internal controls.)

C, Fill the cuvette in one continuous process. It should never be topped up after the first filling.

D, Wipe off the excess blood on the outside of the cuvette tip. Make sure that no blood is drawn out of the cuvette in this procedure.

E, Place the filled cuvette into the cuvette holder immediately, and push it into measuring position.

Figure A shows the HemoCue system, which uses a blood-collecting device called the *hemoglobin microcuvette (a)*. After it has filled with blood from a finger puncture, it is placed on the black cuvette holder *(d)* and pushed into the red HemoCue instrument *(b)*, which then displays a digital result *(c)*. Figure B shows the manufacturer's control cuvette, which must be run daily, with the results logged to verify that the instrument's optical system is working correctly. Figures C to E show the following steps for obtaining a specimen: (C), Fill the cuvette in one continuous process. (D), Wipe away excess blood on the outside of the cuvette making sure no blood is drawn out of the cuvette. (E), Place the filled cuvette into the instrument

See the workbook for the analytical competency check-off sheet for Hemoglobin: HemoCue Method at the end of Chapter 5. Also see the workbook appendix pages for Chapter 5 with the following: Quality Control Flow Chart for HemoCue, Hemoglobin Quality Control Log, and Hemoglobin Patient Log.

5-2

✳ PROCEDURE 5-3 Hematocrit: *General Procedure*

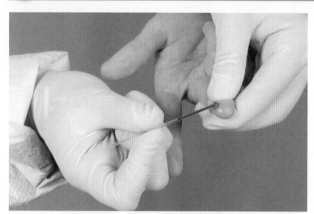

A, Hold the capillary tube in a horizontal position or slightly tipped downward to allow capillary action to pull blood into the tube.

B, When using a built-in hematocrit scale as seen in the illustration, the capillary tube must be filled to the designated line on the capillary tube. *(From Bonewit-West K: Clinical procedures for medical assistants, ed 9, St Louis, 2015.)*

C, The blood sample is being read on a variable reader to determine the percentage of total blood occupied by the red blood cells.

Equipment and Supplies

- Hematocrit centrifuge with locking cover for safety when spinning the specimens
- Plastic capillary tubes and sealing clay (or self-sealing plastic protected capillary tubes)
- Two liquid controls to check accuracy of high and low hematocrit readings
- Blood specimens used in test—either venous blood collected in **lavender EDTA tube** or **capillary blood** from finger using a lancet, alcohol, and sterile gauze

Preparation—Preanalytical

1. Sanitize the hands and put on a fluid-impermeable gown and gloves.
2. Check the expiration date and storage requirements of all supplies and controls.

D, This Micro-Capillary Reader is also able to adjust and read various volumes of blood collected and spun during the hematocrit test. *(From Rodak BF: Hematology: clinical principles and applications, ed 3, St Louis, 2007, Saunders.)*

3. All first-time operators should run and log results of the controls to check that their technique produces accurate results. Controls should also be run whenever new supplies are used and on days when patients will be tested.

PROCEDURE 5-3 Hematocrit: *General Procedure—cont'd*

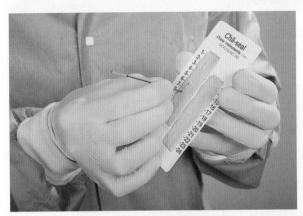

E, Seal the blood end of the tube with clay before centrifuging. *(From Bonewit-West K: Clinical procedures for medical assistants, ed 9, St Louis, 2015.)*

F, This is a safety tube that is coated with plastic and able to self-seal. The capillary collected blood is being tilted toward the sealing clay. When the blood reaches the clay, it automatically seals itself within 15 seconds of contact while holding it in a vertical position.

G, The filled tubes are placed opposite each other to balance the centrifuge while it spins the red cells to the bottom of the tube. *(From Bonewit-West K: Clinical procedures for medical assistants, ed 9, St Louis, 2015, Saunders.)*

Procedure—Analytical

4. Collect two heparin-anticoagulated capillary tubes with blood from a finger or an EDTA tube of blood.
   - Hold the capillary tube in a horizontal position or slightly tilted down to allow capillary action to pull the blood into the tube, as shown in Figure A.
   - Avoid allowing bubbles into your specimen, and fill exactly to the line if using a built-in centrifuge scale, as seen in Figure B.
   - If a variable scale reader that can adapt to any volume of blood is being used (Figure C or Figure D), the tubes may be filled approximately ½ to ¾ full.
5. Seal the clean end of both tubes with clay, as seen in Figure E, or tip the blood toward the presealed end of the tubes as seen in Figure F, and then hold the capillary tube vertical for 15 seconds to ensure a good seal.
6. Place the tubes opposite each other with their clay ends toward the outside of the hematocrit centrifuge to create a balanced centrifuge (Figure G).
7. Lock the cover firmly against the capillary tubes to prevent breaking, and centrifuge for 5 minutes.
8. Use the built-in scale or the variable scales to adjust your total volume (starting where the clay meets the cells and where the plasma meets the air at the top). Then determine the percentage of the total volume occupied by the red cells based on where they align with the plasma on the scale that is being used.
9. Check both readings to see if they are within 2% of each other, and then record the average of the two tubes. (NOTE: See the two readings in Figure C: Do their results fall within 2% of each other?)

Follow-Up—Postanalytical

10. Results of control and patient should be logged, and the patient results should be charted in the patient record.
11. Properly dispose of the lancets and capillary tubes in the biohazard sharps container and any other blood-contaminated supplies in the biohazard waste container. Disinfect the work area.
12. Remove personal protective equipment, and sanitize the hands.

Photos C and F by Zack Bent.

5-3

✳ PROCEDURE 5-4　Hematocrit: *HemataSTAT Method*

The HemataSTAT (Separation Technology, Inc., Altamonte Springs, Fla) is a rapid portable microhematocrit system that uses replaceable plastic holders and plastic capillary tubes for increased operator safety. It has a built-in reading system that supplies a digital readout.

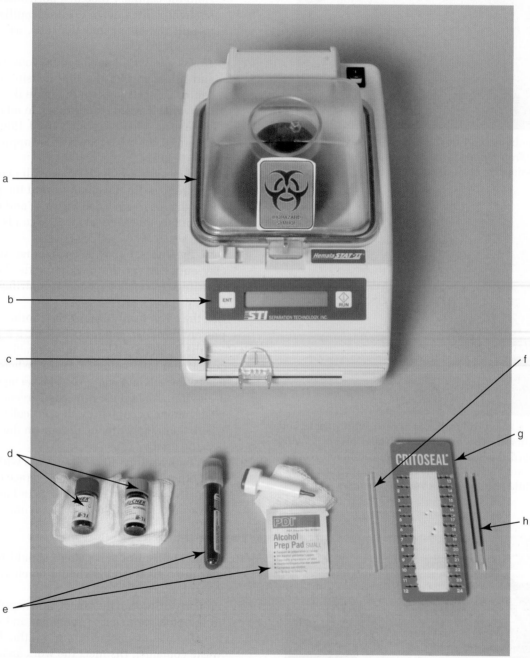

A, HemataSTAT instrument and supplies. *a,* HemataSTAT centrifuge area; *b,* HemataSTAT input controls; *c,* capillary tube reading tray with plastic slider; *d,* two liquid controls; *e,* blood specimens used in test; *f,* two plastic capillary tubes; *g,* Critoseal plastic sealant; *h,* two capillary tubes filled with blood and sealed before centrifuging.

PROCEDURE 5-4 Hematocrit: *HemataSTAT Method*—cont'd

B, HemataSTAT tube reading procedure. With both the capillary tube sealed end and the movable slider all the way to the left, press ENT to "read" according to the display.

C, Follow the display command to move the slider so the line is directly above the sealant/RBC interface, and press ENT.

D, Follow the display command to move the slider so the line is directly above the red blood cell–plasma interface, and press ENT.

E, Follow the display command to move the slider so the line is directly above the plasma-air interface, and press ENT.

F, Read the final result on the display, record, and press ENT for the next tube.

Equipment and Supplies (See Figure A, and Observe the Following)

- HemataSTAT centrifuge with locking cover for safety when spinning the specimens
- Input controls on each side of the digital screen
- Capillary tube reading tray with plastic slider
- Two liquid controls to check accuracy of high and low HCTs
- Blood specimens used in test—either venous blood collected in lavender EDTA tube or capillary blood
- Blood from finger using the lancet, alcohol, and sterile gauze
- Two plastic capillary tubes
- Critoseal plastic sealant for sealing one end of each capillary tube after collecting the blood specimen
- Two capillary tubes that have been filled with blood and sealed before centrifuging

(Continued)

PROCEDURE 5-4 Hematocrit: *HemataSTAT Method—*cont'd

Preparation—Preanalytical

1. Sanitize the hands, and put on a fluid-impermeable gown and gloves.
2. Check the expiration date and storage requirements of all supplies and controls.
3. All first-time operators should run and log results of the controls to check that their technique produces accurate results. Controls should then be run and logged periodically and whenever new supplies are used.

Procedure—Analytical

4. Collect two capillary tubes of anticoagulated blood; then seal and centrifuge them as directed.
5. Read the two tubes in the HemataSTAT instrument by following the digital screen instructions:
   - With the tube and slider all the way to the left, press ENT to "Read" (Figure B).
   - Move the slider so the line is directly above the sealant-RBC interface, and press ENT (Figure C).
   - Move the slider so the line is directly above the RBC-plasma interface, and press ENT (Figure D).
   - Move the slider so the line is directly above the plasma-air interface, and press ENT (Figure E).
   - Observe the final digital result, record, and press ENT to set the instrument for the next tube (Figure F).
6. Repeat the preceding procedure with the second tube. Check both readings to see if they are within 2% of each other, and then record the average of the two tubes.

Follow-Up—Postanalytical

7. Log and chart all results.
8. Properly dispose of biohazard waste materials, and disinfect the work area.
9. Remove personal protective equipment, and sanitize the hands.

✳ PROCEDURE 5-5 ESR: *Sediplast System Procedure*

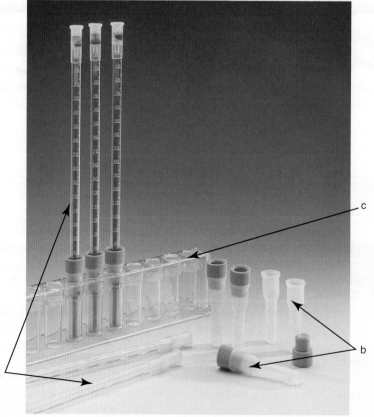

A, Sediplast system. *a,* 200-mm scaled pipette; *b,* citrate tubes; *c,* rack. *(From Rodak BF:* Hematology: clinical principles and applications, *ed 3, St Louis, 2007, Saunders. Courtesy Polymedco, Cortlandt Manor, NY.)*

PROCEDURE 5-5 ESR: *Sediplast System Procedure*—cont'd

B, Transfer whole blood from the EDTA Vacutainer tube to the indicated line on the citrate tube.

C, After replacing the citrate tube's pink top and mixing, place it in the rack. Press the pipette down fully into the citrate tube so that the blood rises up and over the top of the pipette. After 1 hour measure the red blood cell sedimentation (note the three readings in Figure *A*).

Equipment and Supplies (Figure A)

200-mm scaled Sediplast pipette; citrate tubes and rack; fresh venous blood specimen in EDTA (lavender top) Vacutainer tube

Procedure

1. Sanitize the hands, and don personal protective equipment.
2. Transfer the whole blood from the EDTA tube to the indicated line on the citrate tube (Figure B).
3. After replacing the citrate tube's pink top and mixing the specimen, place the tube in the rack.
4. Slowly press the Sediplast pipette down fully into the citrate tube so that the blood rises up and over the top of the pipette (Figure C).

5. After 1 hour, measure the number of millimeters the RBC fell in the pipette. This number is the RBC sedimentation rate (note the three different readings in Figure A).

Follow-Up

6. After recording the results as millimeters per hour (mm/hr) in the patient chart, dispose of the biohazardous pipettes properly and disinfect the work area.
7. Remove personal protective equipment, and sanitize hands.

✳ PROCEDURE 5-6 ESR: *Streck 30-Minute Procedure*

A, Streck 30-minute ESR system: *a,* liquid normal and high controls; *b,* black Streck citrate tubes; *c,* results of normal and high control tubes after 30 minutes; *d,* Streck rack with mm scale for reading the sed rates; *e,* bubble level indicator and adjustable legs for assuring rack is perfectly upright; *f,* magnifier for reading results; *g,* Vacutainer system for drawing EDTA tube and/or black citrate tube.

B, Collect the blood in a black-topped Streck citrate tube making sure to push and hold the tube stopper firmly against the holder. Position the tube in an angle that allows the bloodstream to hit the wall before mixing with the citrate solution to minimize the formation of blood foam. The blood will stop flowing near the indicated line on the bottom of the Streck tube's label. Immediately remove the tube and tilt 8 to 10 times.

C, Allow the liquid controls and the labeled blood specimen to come to room temperature while mixing thoroughly on a rotating blood mixer for 15 minutes.

PROCEDURE 5-6 ESR: *Streck 30-Minute Procedure*—cont'd

D, Place the ESR vacuum tube in any free position in the ESR-10 manual rack with the stopper in the upright position. Each tube position is marked with a red circle numbered 1 through 10. Align the tube so that the bottom of the liquid's curved meniscus is in line with the zero position on the measuring scale. (NOTE: Do not adjust the position of the tube by pulling on the stopper.)

E, After 30 minutes, record the numerical value at the top of the column of sedimented erythrocytes. Report the result as mm/hr Modified Westergren method. The tube on the left shows the RBCs settled to 4 mm/hr, and the tube on the right (the high control) shows a sedimentation rate of 84 mm/hr.

Equipment and Supplies (Figure A)

Streck equipment and supplies: black citrate tubes, normal and high liquid controls, balanced rack with built-in reading scale, magnifying reader, supplies for drawing the citrate tube or the EDTA tube to be transferred to the citrate tube

Procedure

1. Sanitize the hands, and don personal protective equipment.
2. Collect whole blood into the black ESR citrate tube to the exact volume. (NOTE: If using a butterfly needle, a waste tube will be needed to clear the air from the tubing [Figure B].) Blood from an EDTA tube may also be used. It will need to be transferred into the black tube. In both cases, the blood must be mixed immediately after drawing.
3. The ESR citrate tubes and liquid controls must be mixed on a rotating mixer for 15 minutes to come to room temperature (Figure C).
4. Place the ESR tubes in the ESR-10 manual rack with the stopper in the upright position. Align the tube so that the bottom of the liquid meniscus is in line with the zero position of the measuring scale. NOTE: Do not adjust the position of the tube in the rack by pulling on the stopper (Figure D).
5. Allow the tube to settle in an undisturbed, vertical position for 30 minutes. Then record the numerical value at the top of the column of sedimented erythrocytes (Figure E). Report the result as millimeters per hour using the Modified Westergren method.

Follow-Up

6. After recording the results as millimeters per hour (mm/hr) in the patient chart, dispose of the biohazardous tubes of blood properly and disinfect the work area.
7. Remove personal protective equipment, and sanitize hands.

5-6

✳ PROCEDURE 5-7 Prothrombin Time INRatio (HemoSense) Method

INRatio is a portable, precalibrated, battery-operated instrument that has its own built-in quality control testing method. Intended for use in quantitative prothrombin time (PT) testing in fresh capillary whole blood with the INRatio system. The INRatio system is intended for use by health care professionals or properly trained patients to monitor oral anticoagulation therapy.

A, INRatio—equipment and supplies. *a,* Gloves; *b,* lancet; *c,* alcohol and gauze; *d,* INRatio test strips; *e,* INRatio meter; *f,* biohazard sharps container.

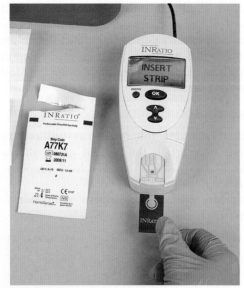

B, Insert the strip into the meter with "INRatio" readable at the bottom of the test strip.

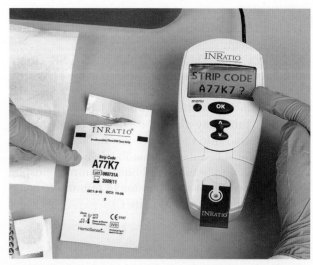

C, Check that the strip code on the meter matches the one on the test strip pouch when "STRIP CODE ####" appears in the display. If it does, press the "OK" key.

PROCEDURE 5-7 Prothrombin Time INRatio (HemoSense) Method—cont'd

D, The meter will then read "WARMING UP." Prepare the finger by warming, disinfecting, and drying thoroughly.

E, After the beep and the prompt "APPLY SAMPLE," incise the finger with the lancet and form a large hanging drop using gentle continuous pressure. Apply the hanging drop to the sample well on the test strip.

F, Alternatively the INRatio also provides plastic pipettes called "MICROSAFE Tubes" that are able to collect the exact amount of blood from the finger first, followed by transferring the specimen from the pipette to the test strip. The pipette should be held horizontally when collecting the blood by capillary action; and it should be held vertically when applying the drop to the sample well on the test strip.

G, The meter will beep, and the results will appear on the display when the test is complete. Read and record the INR and PT seconds from the digital screen.

Equipment and Supplies (Figure A)

- Gloves *(A)*
- Lancet with 21-gauge needle *(B)*
- Alcohol, gauze, and bandage for capillary puncture site care *(C)*
- INRatio test strips *(D)* (at room temperature and sealed in foil container until within 10 minutes of testing)
- INRatio meter *(E)* with digital readout screen that guides the operator through the procedure
- Biohazard sharps container *(F)*

Preparation—Preanalytical

1. Sanitize the hands, and don personal protective equipment.
2. Check to see that the test strip in the foil has warmed to room temperature and that the expiration date has not passed.
3. Prepare puncture site by warming and gently massaging.

(Continued)

PROCEDURE 5-7 Prothrombin Time INRatio (HemoSense) Method—cont'd

Procedure—Analytical

Below is a summary of the INRatio procedure. A more thorough explanation is found in the workbook skill sheet for Prothrombin Time—INRatio (HemoSense) Method.

4. Activate the INRatio meter by pressing any button. The meter should be on a level surface. Do not move during testing.
5. After the self-test, the meter will read "INSERT STRIP."
6. Open a test strip foil pouch, and remove the test strip. Insert the strip into the meter with "INRatio" readable at the bottom of the test strip (Figure B).
7. Check that the strip code matches the one on the test strip pouch when "STRIP CODE ####" appears in the display (Figure C). If it does, press the OK key. If it does not, press the UP/DOWN button to change the first digit. Press OK to enter the new digit. Repeat for each new digit until the instrument and the strip codes match; then press OK to finalize the code. The meter will then read "WARMING UP" (Figure D).
8. Prepare the finger by warming, disinfecting, and drying thoroughly. Then wait for the beep and the prompt **"APPLY SAMPLE."** The green sample light will also appear through the test strip sample well.
9. Incise the finger with the lancet. Wipe away the first drop, and form a large hanging drop using gentle continuous pressure.
10. Apply the hanging drop to the sample well on the test strip (Figure E).
11. Alternatively, the INRatio also provides plastic pipettes called "MICROSAFE Tubes" that are able to collect the exact amount of blood from the finger first, followed by transferring the specimen from the pipette to the test strip. The pipette should be held horizontally when collecting the blood by capillary action as seen in Figure F—Never squeeze the tube while sampling. The filled pipette is then held vertically when transferring the drop to the test slide by squeezing the bulb. NOTE: If the sample will not expel, there is a vent hole just above the blood sample in the pipette that may need to be covered while squeezing the bulb to deliver the specimen. In all these cases, it is important not to add any more blood to the sample well on the test strip after the blood has first been applied.

12. Wait while the meter performs the test and calculates the results. The message "TESTING SAMPLE" will display. The blood sample is traveling down the three channels. The center channel is the patient, and the outside channels are the controls.
13. The meter will beep, and the results will appear on the display when the test is complete. If an error message occurs, see the INRatio user's guide for proper action.
14. Read and record the INR and PT seconds from the digital screen (Figure G).

	INR	PT Seconds (NOTE: Ranges Vary Depending on Method)
Normal range	0.8 to 1.2	6.5 to 13 seconds
Therapeutic ranges	NOTE: Physician must determine therapeutic range for each patient	
Low anticoagulation	1.5 to 2.0	19.6 to 26.1 seconds
Moderate anticoagulation	2.0 to 3.0	26.1 to 39.2 seconds
High anticoagulation	2.5 to 4.0	32.6 to 52.2 seconds

Follow-up—Postanalytical

15. Discard the strip and any biohazard materials appropriately. The meter will turn off automatically after 10 minutes. Identify any critical values, and take appropriate steps to notify the physician.
16. Dispose of waste in the appropriate biohazard containers, and disinfect the work area.
17. Remove personal protective equipment, and sanitize the hands.

Photos A through G by Zack Bent.

Advanced Concepts

Complete Blood Count

Many physicians order a CBC because they want a more complete picture of the internal status of the blood cells. The CBC specimen usually requires a lavender-topped Vacutainer tube with EDTA. EDTA acts as a preservative that maintains the integrity of the blood cells and also works as an anticoagulant. Because the CBC consists of some moderately to highly complex tests, the blood specimen is usually sent to a reference laboratory to be tested with highly sophisticated instruments. See the laboratory requisition form in Figure 1-7 of Chapter 1 and locate the place on the form denoting where to order the CBC and determine the tube that should be used. Then look at a subsequent laboratory report form in Chapter 1 with the results of a CBC seen in Figure 1-1. Notice the elevated WBC count and the elevated neutrophils. This advanced section will help explain what these results may mean.

A CBC generally consists of seven or more laboratory tests that reflect the total count, analysis, and microscopic descriptions of the various cellular elements: RBCs, WBCs, and platelets (Table 5-3).

1. **RBCs** are counted and reported in millions per cubic millimeter or as a whole number times 10 to the ninth power per liter (International Units [SI]). Totals are then compared with reference ranges established for neonates (newborns), infants, children, men, and women.
2. **HCT** measures the percentage of packed RBCs compared with the total blood volume.
3. **Hgb** within the RBCs is measured. The value is expressed as grams per deciliter and is compared with the reference range.
4. **RBC indices** are mathematic ratios of the three aforementioned tests (Hgb, HCT, RBC count). These RBC tests are valuable for identifying various forms of anemia (a condition in which the RBC or Hgb levels are below normal) and polycythemia (abnormal condition of increased RBCs).

Table 5-3   Reference Ranges for Complete Blood Count (CBC)

Test	Neonates	Infants (6 mo)	Children	ADULTS Men	Women
1. Red blood cells	4.8-7.1 million/mm³	3.8-5.5 million/mm³	4.5-4.8 million/mm³	4.5-6.0 million/mm³	4.0-5.5 million/mm³
2. Hematocrit	44-64%	30-40%	35-41%	42-52%	36-45%
3. Hemoglobin	17-21 g/dL	10-15 g/dL	11-16 g/dL	15-18 g/dL	12-16 g/dL
4. Red blood cell indices					
MCV	96-108 µm	—	—	82-98 µm	
MCH	32-34 pg	—	—	26-34 pg	
MCHC	31-33 g/dL	—	—	31-37 g/dL	
5. White blood cells	9000-30,000/mm³	6000-16,000/mm³	5000-13,000/mm³	4000-11,000/mm³	
6. Differential white blood cell count					
Neutrophils	≥45% by 1 week of age	32%	60% of children 2 years and older	50-65%	
Bands	—	—	—	0-7%	
Eosinophils	—	—	0-3%	1-3%	
Basophils	—	—	1-3%	0-1%	
Monocytes	—	—	4-9%	3-9%	
Lymphocytes	≥41% by 1 week of age	61%	59% for children 2 years or older	25-40%	
7. Platelets	140,000-300,000/mm³	200,000-473,000/mm³	150,000-450,000/mm³	150,000-400,000/mm³	

From Stepp CA, Woods M: *Laboratory procedures for medical office personnel,* Philadelphia, 1998, Saunders.

MCH, Mean cell hemoglobin; *MCHC,* mean (average) cell hemoglobin concentration; *MCV,* mean cell volume.

- The mean (average) cell Hgb concentration (**MCHC**) is determined by the following formula:

$$MCHC = Hgb \times 100/HCT = g/dL \ or \ \%$$

This ratio is commonly calculated in the ambulatory care setting because Hgb and HCT are both CLIA-waived tests. The reference ranges for MCHC in Table 5-3 show a 1:3 ratio of Hgb to HCT, which is approximately 33%. If the patient's values fall below the reference range, the RBCs contain less Hgb than normal. This is often the case in iron deficiency anemia, chronic blood loss anemia, macrocytic anemia, and hypochromic anemia. All these conditions can be confirmed during the microscopic examination of a stained blood smear.

- The mean cell volume (**MCV**) and mean cell Hgb (**MCH**) indices compare the HCT volume and the Hgb value to the total RBC count, respectively. The formulas are as follows:

$$MCV = HCT \times 1000/RBC \ count = \mu mor \ fL \ (femtoliters)$$
$$MCH = Hgb \times 10/RBC \ count = pg \ (picograms)$$

By comparing the patient's MCV to the reference range, the general size of the RBCs can be determined. If the MCV is less than 80 μm, for example, the RBCs are microcytic (small); if the MCV is greater than 100 μm, the RBCs are macrocytic (large). The MCH indicates the concentration of Hgb compared with the average size of the RBCs.

5. **WBCs** are counted and reported in thousands per cubic millimeter or as a whole number multiplied by 10 to the ninth power per liter in SI units. The total WBC count is compared with reference ranges, such as those in Table 5-3 on the previous page.

6. **A differential count** that uses the stained blood smear is performed and the five types of leukocytes are counted and reported (Figure 5-34). The percentage of each WBC type is compared with the reference values shown in Table 5-3. The appearance of the RBCs and platelets is also observed and described in the report. The WBC tests are valuable in identifying **leukocytosis** (an abnormal increase in the number of WBCs), forms of **leukemia** (various cancers of the WBCs), and **leukopenia** (an abnormal decrease in the number of WBCs).

7. **Platelets** are counted by approximation on the stained slide or by an automated instrument; platelet counts are expressed in hundreds of thousands per cubic millimeter, or in SI units as a decimal fraction multiplied by 10 to the twelfth power per liter. The patient's results are compared with a reference range, such as that in Table 5-3. This information is useful in diagnosing various bleeding and clotting disorders.

Fig. 5-34 Examples of the seven peripheral blood cells seen in a differential: *1,* segmented neutrophil; *2,* banded neutrophil; *3,* eosinophil with large red granules; *4,* basophil with dark blue granules; *5,* small, mature lymphocytes; *6,* atypical lymphocyte (seen in mononucleosis and acute viral infections); *7,* large monocytes with large convoluted nuclei; *8,* small fragmented platelets; *9,* red blood cells. *(From Bonewit-West K: Clinical procedures for medical assistants, ed 9, St Louis, 2015, Saunders.)*

Abnormal Complete Blood Count Findings

The CBC gives a complete picture of the RBCs, WBCs, and platelets. High-quality medical care requires that laboratory values always be correlated with the clinical state. For example, if a patient exhibits signs and symptoms of fatigue and **hypoxemia** (lack of oxygen in the blood), the physician may suspect that a form of anemia is present. Remember, *anemia* is a condition in which the concentrations of RBCs and/or hemoglobin are less than normal. By ordering a CBC and observing all the RBC test results (RBC count, Hgb, HCT, and indices), the physician can then make a differential diagnosis.

Anemias

Table 5-4, on the next page, shows the effect of various forms of anemia on CBC test results. This information is confirmed by observing the stained blood smear during the differential. Figure 5-35 illustrates the way RBCs appear in the following forms of anemia:

- Folate (vitamin B_9) deficiency anemia: The macrocytic (enlarged) RBCs are caused by the poor formation of the RBCs in the bone marrow. (NOTE: Folate is the natural source of vitamin B_9, whereas folic acid is a synthetic form of B_9.)

- Iron deficiency anemia: The **hypochromic** (less than normal color) and microcytic (small) RBCs result from the inability to build healthy Hgb. This is the most common type of anemia and is caused by blood loss or inadequate iron in the diet.
- Hereditary spherocytosis: Because of a genetic abnormality, the RBCs have a spherical shape rather than the normal disk shape.
- Aplastic anemia: All the blood cell elements show a decrease in aplastic anemia as a result of the inability to produce cells in the bone marrow (see Table 5-4). Enlarged ovalocytes are the result of trauma to the stem cells in the bone marrow.
- Pernicious anemia: The cells appear enlarged, fragile, and abnormally shaped because the diet is deficient in vitamin B_{12} or because intrinsic factor (a chemical that allows B_{12} to be absorbed into the blood from the digestive tract) is lacking.
- Sickle cell disease: The RBCs collapse into a sickle shape under certain circumstances. This condition is caused by an inherited Hgb-S molecule.
- Thalassemia and hemolytic anemia produce an increase of reticulocytes (immature RBCs) in the peripheral blood attributable to RBC destruction (hemolysis) caused by the inherited thalassemia or other hemolytic causes.

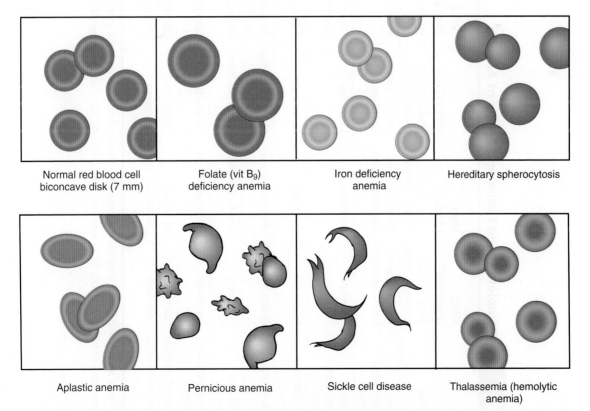

Normal red blood cell biconcave disk (7 mm) | Folate (vit B_9) deficiency anemia | Iron deficiency anemia | Hereditary spherocytosis

Aplastic anemia | Pernicious anemia | Sickle cell disease | Thalassemia (hemolytic anemia)

Fig. 5-35 Distinctive sizes, shapes, and colors of red blood cells associated with eight forms of anemia. *(From Stepp CA, Woods M: Laboratory procedures for medical office personnel, Philadelphia, 1998, Saunders.)*

Table 5-4   Complete Blood Count and Forms of Anemia

	RBC (per mm³)	Hgb (g/dL)	Hct (%)	MCV (per µm³)	MCH (pg)	MCHC (g/dL)	WBC (per mm³)	Reticulocyte Count (per mm³)	Platelet Count (per mm³)
Normal	Male, 4.7-6.1; female, 4.2-5.4	Male, 14-18; female, 12-16	Male, 42-52; female, 37-47	80-90	27-31	32-36	5000-10,000	0.5-2	150,000-400,000
Acute hemorrhagic anemia	Initial increase, latent decrease	Initial decrease, latent decrease	Normal initially, latent decrease	Increase	Decrease	Normal	Increase	Increase	Decrease
Chronic hemorrhagic anemia	Decrease	Decrease	Decrease	Slight decrease	Slight decrease	Slight decrease	Normal	Decrease	Normal
Iron deficiency anemia	Decrease	Decrease	Decrease	Decrease	Decrease	Decrease	Normal	Decrease	Normal to increase
Aplastic anemia	Gross decrease	Gross decrease	Gross decrease	Moderate decrease	Gross decrease	Gross decrease	Gross decrease	Decrease	Gross decrease
Pernicious anemia	Decrease	Gross decrease	Gross decrease	Increase	Increase	Increase	Slight decrease	Decrease	Slight decrease
Folate-deficiency anemia	Decrease	Gross decrease	Gross decrease	Increase	Increase	Increase	Slight decrease	Decrease	Slight decrease
Sickle-cell anemia	Decrease	Decrease	Decrease	Decrease	Normal	Normal	Increase	Increase	Normal
Hemolytic anemia	Decrease	Decrease	Decrease	Increase	Slight decrease	Normal	Normal	Increase	Normal to increase

From Frazier MS, Drzymkowski J: *Essentials of human disease and conditions*, ed 3, Philadelphia, 2004, Saunders.

HCT, Hematocrit; *Hgb*, hemoglobin; *MCH*, mean cell hemoglobin; *MCHC*, mean (average) cell hemoglobin concentration; *MCV*, mean cell volume; *RBC*, red blood cell; *WBC*, white blood cell.

White Blood Cell Disorders

The WBC count and differential can also be correlated to the patient's clinical state. For example, if a patient has an infection, the total WBC count may rise as the body fights the infection (leukocytosis). The type of infection can be determined by observing the percentage of each type of WBC in the differential. For example, an increase in the number of neutrophils would indicate a bacterial infection as opposed to an increase in the number of lymphocytes, which would indicate a viral infection. Also, the viral infection referred to as *mononucleosis* is known for the presence of atypical lymphocytes that appear larger than normal (Figure 5-36).

An abnormally low WBC count (leukocytopenia) may be a sign of malnutrition and/or patients undergoing chemotherapy. An extremely high abnormal WBC count with a decrease in the RBC and platelet counts may indicate leukemia. Again, the stained blood smear will shed more light on the disease process that is occurring. As previously stated, all the blood cells come from one stem cell or hemocytoblast. If the differentiation phase of the myeloblasts becomes uncontrollable, the number of bone marrow myelocytes increases and they begin to appear in the peripheral blood in increasingly greater numbers, to the detriment of RBCs and platelets. The patient would be diagnosed with acute myelocytic leukemia (**AML**) if this condition developed suddenly, or with chronic myelocytic leukemia (**CML**) if it is a long-term condition. If, on the other hand, the formation of the lymphocytes becomes uncontrollable, then immature lymphoblasts will appear in the peripheral blood. This form of leukemia can also be classified as acute (acute lymphocytic leukemia [**ALL**]) or chronic (chronic lymphocytic leukemia [**CLL**]). Monocytic leukemia, consisting of the overgrowth of monoblasts, is rare but can be either acute or chronic in nature.

CLIA-Nonwaived (Moderately Complex) Automated Hematology Systems

For offices that require more hematological information than just the waived Hgb and HCT measurements, semiautomated hematology instruments that are CLIA approved as moderately complex may be appropriate. When performing this level of diagnostic testing, the laboratory professional will need to complete the registration, accreditation, and certification process via the Centers for Medicare and Medicaid Services (CMS) and comply with more rigorous quality control and assurance standards, including the documented training of operators and additional quality assurance standards, to include documentation of the following:

- Daily instrument calibrations and standards
- Two levels of controls run routinely
- Maintenance checks of the instrument, temperature, and supplies
- Proficiency testing

To pass the required proficiency testing, the office must run a sample from an outside proficiency laboratory twice a year and submit its results to see if they are within the acceptable range established by the accreditation agency. If the results are not in the acceptable range, the office must take the appropriate steps to correct the problem.

QBC STAR Centrifugal Hematology System

The QBC STAR centrifugal hematology system (Becton Dickinson) provides the ambulatory care setting with more than just Hgb and HCT values. It also provides information regarding the WBC count, platelet count, and distribution of granulocytes (neutrophils, basophils, and eosinophils) versus nongranulocytes (lymphocytes and monocytes). This additional WBC information is helpful when dealing with infections. Neutrophils predominantly fight bacterial infections,

Fig. 5-36 Atypical reactive lymphocytes seen in mononucleosis. *(From Carr JH, Rodak BF: Clinical hematology atlas, ed 4, St. Louis, 2013, Saunders.)*

whereas lymphocytes fight viral infections. If the patient shows a high total WBC count (leukocytosis), the physician can determine which WBC demonstrates a higher percentage and act accordingly. This information is especially valuable to the pediatrician who needs to know whether a child should start taking antibiotics for a bacterial infection. Laboratory values must always be correlated with the clinical state.

The QBC system spins down a capillary sample of blood into its various layers (red cells, buffy coat, and plasma). A fluorescent dye and a miniature float within the tube can stain and disperse the buffy coat of WBCs and platelets into three additional layers (granulocytes, nongranulocytes, and platelets). Figure 5-37, *A* and *B,* shows the relative size of the centrifuged capillary specimen and the distribution of the centrifuged cell layers. A laser beam or a tungsten-halogen light beam is then directed at the separated layers of blood cells in the capillary tube to analyze each layer. The light beam strikes the cell layers at an angle, allowing sensors to detect the amount of light scattered and the amount absorbed by the cells. Each type of cell creates a different angle of scatter based on its volume, shape, and refractive index. After all the blood cell layers have been analyzed, the results are displayed and printed.

Quality Assurance

The QBC is a moderately complex instrument that requires regular monitoring with the high and low liquid controls. The control test results must be logged and plotted to detect any shifts, trends, or signs of inaccuracy. Proficiency testing with a specimen from an outside laboratory must also be done twice a year.

Coulter Counter System

The Coulter counter (Beckman Coulter, Fullerton, Calif) is a highly sophisticated hematology analyzer that performs an automated CBC. The test uses blood cells diluted with an electrolyte solution capable of conducting electricity. When the blood cells, which are poor conductors of electricity, pass through an opening (aperture) in the instrument, they cause a pulse or interruption (impedance) of the electrical circuit (Figure 5-38). The pulses are counted, analyzed, and calculated by the instrument, which produces a readout. Compare the normal and abnormal reports in Figure 5-39, *A* and *B.*

Fig. 5-37 **A,** QBC STAR tube after centrifugation. **B,** Identification of layers. (**B** *courtesy Becton Dickinson.*)

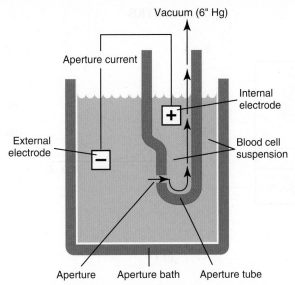

Fig. 5-38 The Coulter counter system, which uses electrical impedance technology. *(From Rodak BF:* Hematology: clinical principles and applications, *ed 4, St. Louis, 2012, Saunders. Courtesy Beckman Coulter.)*

Coulter STKS

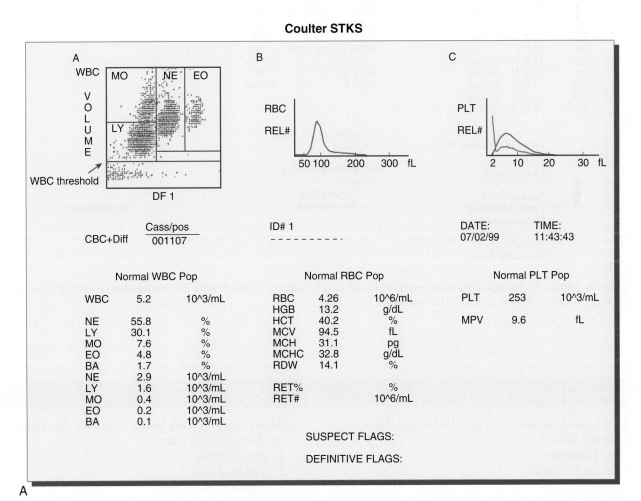

Fig. 5-39 A, Normal Coulter complete blood count readout.

(Continued)

Coulter STKS

	Abnormal WBC Pop	
WBC	18.0*RH 10^3/uL	
NE	63.0	%
LY	22.6	%
MO	6.9	%
EO	4.3	%
BA	3.2	%
NE	11.3 RH 10^3/uL	
LY	4.1 R 10^3/uL	
MO	1.2 R 10^3/uL	
EO	0.8 R 10^3/uL	
BA	0.6 RH 10^3/uL	

CBC+Diff   Cass/pos
            001104

ID 1 _ _ _ _ _ _ _ _

DATE: TIME:
07/02/99   11:41:03

	Abnormal RBC Pop		
RBC	1.98		10^6/uL
HGB	6.8	L	g/dL
HCT	20.0		%
MCV	101.1	H	fL
MCH	34.5		pg
MCHC	34.1		g/dL
RDW	18.5	H	%
RET %			%
RET #			10^6/uL

	Abnormal PLT Pop	
PLT	204	10^3/uL
MPV	13.0	fL

Imm Grans/Bands 2

Leukocytosis

Neutrophilia #
Lymphocytosis #
Monocytosis #
Eosinophilia #
Basophilia %
Basophilia #

SUSPECT FLAGS:
NRBCs

DEFINITIVE FLAGS:
Anemia
1+ Anisocytosis
1+ Macrocytosis

Large Platelets

B

Fig. 5-39, cont'd B, Abnormal Coulter complete blood count readout. *(From Rodak BF:* Hematology: clinical principles and applications, *ed 4, St. Louis, 2012, Saunders.)*

Review Questions

1. Which of the following is not a formed element in the blood?
   a. Platelets
   b. Prothrombin
   c. RBCs
   d. WBCs

2. Match the following terms with their description on the following page:
   a. granulocytes
   b. anticoagulant
   c. erythrocytes
   d. megakaryocyte
   e. plasma
   f. platelet
   g. EDTA

_____ complex liquid in which blood cells are suspended

_____ most numerous blood cells (occupying almost 50% of the blood)

_____ WBC group made up of neutrophils, eosinophils, and basophils

_____ agent that prevents clotting of whole blood

_____ cellular element important in hemostasis

_____ most common anticoagulant used in routine hematology procedures

_____ large bone marrow cell from which platelets are derived

3. Match the following terms with their definitions:

____ red cell	a. immature neutrophil
____ neutrophil	b. has coarse orange-red granules
____ eosinophil	
____ basophil	c. smallest WBC
____ lymphocyte	d. largest WBC
____ monocyte	e. has blue-black granules
____ platelet	f. made of fragments of cytoplasm
____ band cell	
	g. biconcave disk
	h. nucleus has two to five segments, and cytoplasm is pink/lavender with granules

4. Provide the missing terms found in the final steps of the common pathway of coagulation:

_____ → Thrombin

Fibrinogen → _____

5. Prothrombin (factor II) is a plasma protein dependent on vitamin _____.

6. Match each testing method with its appropriate test:

___ HemoCue	a. CBC
___ QBC	b. sedimentation rate
___ Westergren	c. coagulation test
___ HemataSTAT	d. Hgb
___ Protime	e. HCT

7. Match each RBC index with its ratio elements:

___ MCV	a. Hgb/RBC
___ MCHC	b. HCT/RBC
___ MCH	c. Hgb/HCT

8. Match each anemia with its cause:

__ iron deficiency anemia	a. destruction of circulating RBCs
__ hemolytic anemia	b. seen with blood loss (menses, ulcers, hemorrhaging)
__ aplastic anemia	c. inherited abnormal Hgb-S molecule
__ sickle cell anemia	d. destruction of stem cells in bone marrow from toxins
__ pernicious anemia	e. caused by decreased vitamin B_{12}

9. Match these leukocyte disorders with their descriptions:

_____ leukocytopenia	a. presence of atypical "reactive" lymphocytes
_____ ALL	b. increase in WBCs (usually from infection)
_____ mononucleosis	c. long-term cancer of granulocytes in bone marrow
_____ CML	d. sudden cancer of a nongranulocyte
_____ leukocytosis	e. abnormal decrease of WBCs

Websites

American Society of Hematology's image bank of slides of normal and abnormal blood cells:
www.ashimagebank.org/contents.asp

Dr. Joseph F. Smith Medical Library site offers information on ESRs:
www.chclibrary.org/micromed/00047230.html

Manufacturer information on INRatio (HemoSense):
www.hemosense.com/support/productlit.shtml

6

Chemistry

OBJECTIVES *After completing this chapter you should be able to do the following:*

1. Define and match key terms and abbreviations in this chapter.

Fundamental Concepts

2. Identify the plasma components in peripheral blood, and describe their function and significance.
3. Describe the proper specimen collection and processing for various chemistry tests.
4. Explain the basic principles of glucose and fat metabolism.

CLIA-Waived Chemistry Tests

5. Describe the Beer-Lambert law and the principle supporting the way in which chemical analytes are measured by photometry.
6. Explain the importance of performing instrument calibrations, optics checks, quality controls, and Westgard's rules of quality control monitoring.
7. Perform the following FDA-approved, CLIA-waived tests according to the most current OSHA safety guidelines and the test's objectives, conditions,

and standards that are listed in the Procedure Sheets found in the student workbook:
  a. glucose
  b. hemoglobin A_{1c}
  c. lipid panel
  d. i-STAT basic metabolic panel
  e. fecal occult blood

Advanced Concepts

8. Discuss the use of the hand-held i-STAT analyzer for point-of-care blood testing and list the eight critical chemistry tests performed during medical emergencies as seen on the i-STAT CHEM8+.
9. Match chemistry panels with the tests performed.
10. Identify when laboratory reports show chemistry values out of the expected range by comparing patient results with the laboratory's reference range, and then use the chart of basic blood chemistry tests to identify a possible disease condition related to high or low patient test results.

KEY TERMS

absorbance photometry indirect measurement of the amount of light that a solution absorbs

analyte substance being tested, such as glucose or cholesterol in a blood specimen

anion negatively charged ion

atherosclerosis formation of plaque along the inside walls of blood vessels

Beer-Lambert law law stating that the intensity of color change is directly proportional to the concentration of an analyte in a solution

carbohydrates sugars and starches

catalysts chemicals that produce specific changes in other substances without being changed themselves

cation positively charged ion

clinical diagnosis diagnosis based on the patient's initial signs and symptoms

clot activator chemical additive that accelerates the clotting of a blood specimen

definitive diagnosis final, confirmed diagnosis based on clinical signs and symptoms and the results of diagnostic tests

dyslipidemia abnormal amounts of fat and lipoproteins in the blood

endogenous cholesterol cholesterol manufactured in the liver

exogenous cholesterol cholesterol derived from the diet

galvanometer instrument capable of measuring the intensity of light

glucagon hormone produced by the pancreas to raise blood glucose levels by converting glycogen into glucose and noncarbohydrates into glucose

glycogen stored form of glucose found especially in muscles and the liver

glycosylated hemoglobin hemoglobin A molecule within red blood cells that becomes permanently bound to glucose

gout form of arthritis caused by accumulation of uric acid crystals in the synovial fluid

hyperglycemia elevated blood sugar levels

hyperinsulinemia excessively high blood insulin levels

hyperlipidemia excessive fat in blood, which gives plasma a milky appearance

hypoglycemia low blood sugar levels

insulin hormone produced by the pancreas to lower blood glucose level by moving it into body cells and converting glucose into glycogen for future use

insulin resistance condition in which insulin is not effective at moving the glucose from the blood into the cells (seen in type 2 diabetes)

ions electrolytes consisting of positively or negatively charged particles

ketoacidosis acidosis caused by an accumulation of ketones in the body, a result of the excessive breakdown of fats; occurs primarily as a complication of type 1 diabetes mellitus

lipoproteins protein-linked lipids

myoglobin iron-containing, oxygen-binding protein found in muscles

occult hidden or not visible to the naked eye

panels groups of tests that focus on blood cells, particular organs, or metabolic functions

reflectance photometry indirect measurement of the light that reflects off a solution

synovial fluid liquid found in joints

trans fats synthetic hydrogenated fats

transmittance photometry measurement of the amount of light passing through a solution

troponins I and T heart-specific indicators of a recent myocardial infarction (heart attack)

ABBREVIATIONS

2-hr PP	2-hour postprandial (after eating)	**Ig**	immunoglobulins (antibodies)
A_{1c}	hemoglobin A_{1c}, glycosylated hemoglobin, or glycated hemoglobin	**IGT**	impaired glucose tolerance
		K^+	potassium ion
ALP or AP	alkaline phosphatase (also abbreviated as alk phos)	**LD**	lactic acid dehydrogenase
		LDL	low-density lipoprotein(s), or "lousy" cholesterol
ALT (SGPT)	alanine aminotransferase		
AST (SGOT)	aspartate aminotransferase	**Na^+**	sodium ion
BUN	blood urea nitrogen	**NIDDM**	non–insulin-dependent diabetes mellitus (type 2)
Ca^{2+}	calcium ion		
Cl^-	chloride ion	**OGTT**	oral glucose tolerance test (2-hour post-prandial blood sugar)
CK or CPK	creatine kinase		
DM	diabetes mellitus	**SST**	serum separator tube
FBG	fasting blood glucose	**T_3**	triiodothyronine
FPG	fasting plasma glucose	**T_4**	thyroxine
GGT	gamma-glutamyltransferase	**TC/HDL ratio**	total cholesterol compared with high-density lipoprotein
GTT	glucose tolerance test		
HCO_3^-	bicarbonate ion	**TCO_2**	total carbon dioxide concentration
HDL	high-density lipoprotein(s), or "healthy" cholesterol	**TSH**	thyroid-stimulating hormone
		VLDL	very-low-density lipoprotein(s) (e.g., protein and triglyceride)
IDDM	insulin-dependent diabetes mellitus (type 1)		
iFOB	acronym for immunoassay for fecal occult blood		

👁 Fundamental Concepts

Clinical chemistry is the testing of the chemical **analytes** found in various liquid body specimens, such as urine, whole blood, serum, plasma, **synovial fluid** (from joints), pleural fluid (from the chest cavity), pericardial fluid (from the sac surrounding the heart), peritoneal fluid (from the abdominal cavity), and cerebrospinal fluid. The specimens most commonly tested in the ambulatory setting are urine and blood.

Chapter 5 detailed the various cellular elements found in blood (red blood cells [RBCs], white blood cells, and platelets) and the blood coagulation process. This chapter deals with the *liquid* portion of blood: plasma.

Blood Plasma

Plasma is a pale yellow, sweet-smelling, sticky fluid occupying slightly more than 50% of the total blood volume.

For a complete understanding of the numerous blood chemistry tests and their significance, the composition of plasma must be reviewed. Refer to the numbered flow chart (Figure 6-1) while reading about each component.

Approximately 90% of plasma *(1)* is water *(2)*, with hundreds of dissolved substances and gases, including the following:

- *Salts (3)*—electrolytes consisting of positively and negatively charged particles (**ions**) that maintain acid-base balance (e.g., sodium, chloride, potassium, and bicarbonate)
- *Nutrients (4)*—derived from the gastrointestinal tract after it digests and absorbs **carbohydrates** (sugars and starches) into glucose, fats into fatty acids, and proteins into amino acids, along with essential vitamins and minerals
- *Waste products (5)*—from cellular and molecular metabolism; carried in the plasma and excreted

Fig. 6-1 Plasma flow chart.

by the urinary system (e.g., urea, creatinine, uric acid)

- *Hormones (6)*—from various endocrine glands (e.g., thyroid, pancreas)
- *Enzymes (7)*—**catalysts** produced by living cells that cause specific changes in other substances without being changed themselves
- *Proteins (8)*—a major portion of plasma that can be divided into three categories: albumin, globulin, and clotting proteins
- *Albumins (9)*—hold the water within the blood vessels
- *Globulins (10)*—simple proteins further classified into *alpha (11)*, *beta (12)*, and *gamma (13)*; gamma globulins are also called immunoglobulins (**Ig** or antibodies)
- *Fibrinogen (14)* and *prothrombin (15)*—clotting proteins produced by the liver (when these clotting factors have been removed from plasma during the clotting process, the remaining fluid is referred to as *serum*)

Blood plasma is a dynamic, ever-changing liquid that reflects the inner workings of internal organs and tissues. In good health, each organ is constantly producing or removing its various chemical products within the plasma to maintain homeostasis. When disease strikes a particular organ or body system, homeostasis is interrupted and a change is seen in the blood chemistry. The measured change in blood chemistry allows a physician to detect or confirm the **clinical diagnosis** (diagnosis made on the basis of the patient's initial signs and symptoms). Follow-up chemistry

tests allow the physician and patient to monitor the progress of the disease.

Blood Chemistry Specimens
Reference Laboratory Specimens for Blood Chemistry Testing

Blood chemistry tests derived from a reference laboratory generally require a *serum specimen,* which is obtained from a coagulated (clotted) blood specimen. The vacuum tube of choice for serum specimens is usually the gold serum separator tube (**SST**) containing a gel and a **clot activator** (a chemical additive that accelerates the clotting of the blood specimen). To form a dense clot the SST containing the blood specimen must sit for 30 minutes after being drawn. The clotted specimen is then centrifuged for 20 minutes at a speed of 3000 revolutions per minute (rpm). NOTE: The specified time and rpm and/or the G-force *(g)* are dictated by your reference lab and your centrifuge. For example, Becton Dickinson's recommendations are the following: centrifuge at "Full Speed" (between 1100*g* and 1300*g*) for 10 minutes using swing-head centrifuges, or centrifuge for 15 minutes with fixed-angle centrifuges using balanced tubes in the centrifuge.

The centrifugation forces the clotted cells to the bottom of the tube. Also during centrifugation, the gel migrates up over the cells, separating the serum from the clot. Figure 6-2, *A* and *B,* shows the SST specimen (gold-topped tube) before and after centrifugation and Figure 6-2, *C,* shows the serum from a centrifuged red-topped "clot" tube.

Fig. 6-2 A, Gold SST before centrifugation. Note the position of the gel on the bottom. **B,** Gold SST after centrifugation. Note that the gel now separates the serum from the clotted cells. **C,** Centrifuged red-topped "clot" tube with no gel or clotting additive. *(Modified from Bonewit-West K:* Clinical procedures for medical assistants, *ed 9, St Louis, 2015, Saunders.)*

Some chemical analytes may be affected by the clot activator or gel in the SST tube, so the laboratory may request to collect the serum specimen in a plain red-topped tube that allows the blood to clot with no additives (see Figure 6-2, *C*).

Be sure to check the reference laboratory requisition (or the laboratory reference manual) to confirm the correct tube to draw for the ordered analyte(s). In the sample laboratory requisition illustrated in Figure 6-3, note the required tubes for individual chemistry tests and the tubes needed for the various "Testing by Alpha" based on their indicated color codes (seen in the bottom left of the requisition):

- G for gold or gel found in the SSTs—yields a serum specimen that is separated from the clot
- R for red-topped "clot" tubes—yields a serum specimen with no clot activators or gel
- P for purple ethylenediaminetetraacetic acid (EDTA) anticoagulant tubes—note the listed hematology tests that were performed in Chapter 5 that need an EDTA tube ("P")
- Light (Lt.) blue for sodium citrate anticoagulant—for coagulation testing (protime and APTT)

Also, notice the list of *panels* on the sample reference laboratory requisition. **Panels** are groups of tests that give results on either blood cells (such as complete blood count [CBC] panels), particular organs (e.g., Hepatic Panel), or metabolic functions (e.g., Met. Panel,

Basic, and Met. Panel, CMP). A panel of tests can usually be run on one analyzer with one serum specimen at a much lower cost than a series of individual tests. (The various panels of tests run in reference laboratories are discussed later in this chapter.) The listings of the panels, urine tests, and individual blood tests are each organized in alphabetical order on the requisition.

The required blood specimens for chemistry testing differ depending on which analyte is being tested and what testing method is used at the reference laboratory or ambulatory setting. See Figure 6-4 showing the proper specimen collection and handling requirements for a comprehensive metabolic profile as presented in a laboratory directory and/or an electronic medical record. It is critical that *all* the steps are followed in order to obtain accurate and reliable results. Also, note the causes for rejection of a specimen.

Physician's Office Laboratory Specimens for CLIA-Waived Chemistry Tests

The most common specimen in the physician's office laboratory (POL) for waived chemistry tests is the capillary puncture *whole blood* specimen. The blood is usually collected in a capillary tube containing an anticoagulant or directly into a testing device within a specified time frame. Testing devices may test the whole blood specimen directly, or they may separate the plasma from the whole blood before testing.

Patient Name:_____ DOB:_____ SS#:_____

Ordering Physician Signature:_____ Date:_____

Routine:_____ Standing Order:_____ Fasting:_____ Nonfasting:_____

Diagnosis Code: 1._____ 3._____
                       2._____ 4._____

Copy to:

_____

Panels
_____ CBC w/Diff   P
_____ CBC without Diff   P
_____ Electrolyte Panel   G
_____ Hepatic Panel   G
_____ Hgb and Hct   P
_____ Lipid Panel   G
_____ Met. Panel, Basic   G
_____ Met. Panel, CMP   G
_____ Renal Function Panel   G

Urine Testing
_____ U/A w/Micro
_____ Urinalysis-dip only

Individual Chemistry
_____ Alk Phos (ALP)   G
_____ BUN   G
_____ Calcium, Serum   G
_____ Cholesterol   G
_____ CK, Creat. Kinase Tot.   G
_____ FSH   G
_____ Glucose   G
_____ Hemoglobin, A1c   P
_____ *H. Pylori*   G
_____ Iron   G
_____ Iron Panel, incl. binding   G
_____ K (potassium)   G
_____ Magnesium   G
_____ Na (sodium)   G
_____ Phosphorus   G
_____ Prothrombin Time   Lt. Blue
_____ Rheumatoid Factor   G
_____ RA Titer   G
_____ Sed Rate   P
_____ SGOT (ALT)   G
_____ SGPT (AST)   G
_____ Uric Acid   G

Prostate Testing
_____ PSA Diag   G
_____ PSA M-Screening   G

Thyroid Specific Testing
_____ TSH   G
_____ T4 (Thyroxine)   G
_____ T3 Uptake   G
_____ Thyroid Panel w/TSH   G

Testing by Alpha
_____ 2 hr GTT   G
_____ 3 hr GTT   G
_____ 5 hr GTT   G
_____ Albumin   G
_____ Amylase   G
_____ APTT   Lt. Blue
_____ Bilirubin-Dorest   G
_____ Bilirubin-Total   G
_____ Chloride   G
_____ CO_2 G
_____ Digoxin   R
_____ HDL Cholesterol   G
_____ LD Lactate Dehyd.   G
_____ Mono Test   R
_____ Phenytoin   R
_____ Platelet Count   P
_____ Preg. Test   G
_____ RPR   G
_____ Protein, Total   G
_____ Tegretol   G
_____ TIBC   G
_____ Triglycerides   G
_____ Valproic Acid   R

G = Gold gel (SST tube)
R = Red (clot tube)
P = Purple (EDTA tube)
Lt. Blue = (sodium citrate)

Fig. 6-3 Sample lab requisition showing the required patient information at the top; two columns of tests divided into panels, individual tests, and Alpha tests; and the codes for the colored tubes at the bottom left.

Comprehensive Metabolic Profile

CPT Code:	80053

Tests included: albumin, albumin/globulin ratio (calculated), alkaline phosphatase, ALT, AST, BUN/creatinine ratio (calculated), calcium, carbon dioxide, chloride, creatinine, globulin, glucose, potassium, sodium, total bilirubin, total protein.

Type of specimen:	Serum
Amount:	4 ml
Collection supplies:	SST (send entire tube)
Collection techniques:	Let SST stand for 30 minutes. Centrifuge SST within 45 minutes of collection to separate serum from cells with gel barrier.
Patient preparation:	Patient should fast for 12 to 14 hours prior to collection.
Handling and storage:	Refrigerate or store at room temperature. Stable at room temperature for 24 hours and stable in the refrigerator for 72 hours.
***Causes for rejection:**	Nonfasting specimen, hemolysis, improper labeling of tube
Reference range:	Values given with report.

Use:
The CMP is used as a screening test to assess the overall health of an individual. It is used to detect any changes in the body's biologic processes that may be present, although the patient may not have had any symptoms to indicate these changes have occurred. Also see uses of individual tests.

Limitations:	See individual tests for limitations.
Methodology:	See individual tests for methodologies.

Fig. 6-4 Note all the criteria for collecting an acceptable blood specimen for a comprehensive metabolic profile dictated by the laboratory's directory. *Also, note the causes for rejecting a specimen. *(From Bonewit-West K:* Clinical procedures for medical assistants, *ed 9, St Louis, 2015, Saunders.)*

The manufacturer's instructions must be read and followed for each procedure to determine the exact type of specimen that should be used for each waived test.

Some waived tests may also use a venous anticoagulated whole blood specimen in place of the capillary blood specimen. Once again, only tubes designated by the manufacturer should be used. The following are examples of CLIA-waived specimens:

- **Glucose testing** may be run with the whole blood from a capillary puncture or venous blood specimen collected in a **gray-topped tube.** The gray tube contains an antiglycosylating additive that prevents the glucose from being metabolized by RBCs. NOTE: Some glucose monitors will not work with the gray-topped blood specimens.
- **Glycosylated hemoglobin** (hemoglobin A_{1c} molecule within RBCs that becomes permanently bound to glucose) can be performed with a capillary puncture specimen or a venous blood specimen collected in a **lavender-topped hematology tube.**
- **Cholestech** (Cholestech Corp., Hayward, Calif) lipid tests must be run with whole blood from either a capillary puncture specimen or a venous blood specimen collected in a **green-topped tube** containing the anticoagulant *lithium* heparin. (NOTE: Green-topped *sodium* heparin tubes should *not* be used because they will interfere with the Cholestech testing method.)
- The **i-STAT instrument** provides basic metabolic chemistry tests from whole blood drawn into a **green lithium heparin tube** that is then transferred to a syringe for loading the blood into the test cassette.

Glucose and Lipid Metabolism

In the ambulatory care setting, the most common CLIA-waived chemistry tests are designed to screen and monitor glucose and lipid metabolism. These in-office tests allow the physician to receive results immediately and counsel patients while they are still in the office. The physician may then order additional diagnostic tests from the reference laboratory to reach a **definitive diagnosis** (the final, confirmed diagnosis based on the initial clinical signs and symptoms of the patient compared with the results of the tests from the reference laboratory).

Glucose Metabolism

Glucose is a simple six-carbon sugar that all cells and tissues require for life-giving energy. Glucose enters the blood after the digestion of carbohydrates. Once glucose is in the blood, it is distributed, metabolized, and processed in the following cells, tissues, and organs:

- Body cells—all absorb blood glucose for energy
- Muscles—utilize glucose for energy and store excess glucose as **glycogen** (a stored form of glucose found especially in the muscles and liver) for future needs
- Adipose tissues (fat)—absorb fatty acids and glucose to produce triglycerides
- Liver—converts excess glucose into glycogen or combines glucose with fatty acids to produce triglycerides

Glucose levels in the blood must be maintained within a homeostatic range of 70 to 100 mg/dL. The monitoring and control of glucose levels within this range are regulated by two hormones: **insulin** and its antagonist, **glucagon** (Figure 6-5). Both hormones are produced by the islets of Langerhans within the pancreas to prevent **hyperglycemia** (abnormally high blood sugar levels) and **hypoglycemia** (abnormally low sugar levels).

When glucose levels rise, as seen after eating, the hormone insulin is secreted from the beta cells within the islets of Langerhans to lower the glucose levels and prevent hyperglycemia. *Insulin reduces the level of plasma glucose* by (1) promoting movement of glucose from the blood into body cells, (2) stimulating the conversion of glucose to glycogen in the liver and muscles, and (3) stimulating the conversion of glucose and fatty acids into triglycerides within the liver and adipose tissues.

When blood glucose levels decrease, as during fasting, the hormone glucagon is secreted from alpha cells within the islets of Langerhans to raise blood glucose levels and prevent hypoglycemia. *Glucagon increases plasma glucose* levels by stimulating the conversion of the stored glycogen in the liver and muscles back into glucose and then releasing the glucose into the blood.

Diabetes Mellitus

Diabetes mellitus (**DM**) is a disorder of carbohydrate metabolism characterized by hyperglycemia (elevated blood sugar levels) and glycosuria (sugar in the urine) resulting from the inadequate production or use of insulin. DM occurs when the pancreas is unable to

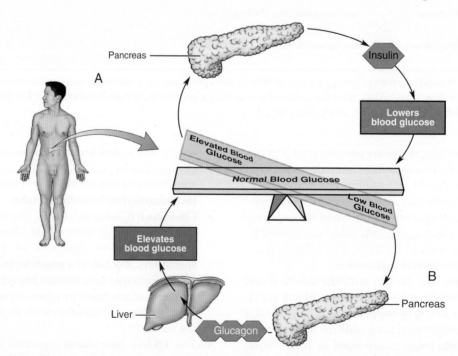

Fig. 6-5 Homeostatic balancing of glucose levels. **A,** When glucose level is too high, insulin lowers it to normal. **B,** When glucose level is too low, glucagon raises it to normal. *(From Herlihy M: The human body in health and illness, ed 5, St Louis, 2014, Saunders.)*

produce enough effective insulin to move the glucose from the blood into the body cells. There are several types of diabetes.

Insulin-Dependent Diabetes Mellitus (Type 1)

Insulin-dependent diabetes mellitus (**IDDM**) occurs in 5% to 10% of the diabetic population. It is the result of an autoimmune destruction of the pancreatic beta cells, which are then unable to produce insulin. Without insulin the body cannot move glucose out of the blood and into the tissues. Consequently, patients with IDDM must constantly monitor their blood sugar levels and inject the appropriate amount of insulin to prevent the harmful effects of hyperglycemia. If glucose levels remain high for long periods, the following severe complications may occur:

- *Microvascular problems,* caused by the abundance of sugar blocking the small blood vessels, may lead to kidney disease and renal failure; retinopathy and blindness; and poor circulation in the extremities (e.g., the feet), resulting in recurring infections that may result in gangrene and amputation.
- *Cardiovascular problems* caused by the subsequent formation of fatty plaque along the inside walls of the arteries may lead to atherosclerotic heart disease, hypertension, and stroke.
- **Ketoacidosis**, a dangerous blood condition, may lead to diabetic coma. Ketoacidosis occurs in IDDM when insulin is not present and the cells do not receive their glucose. It is the result of the body's effort to obtain its energy from fat rather than glucose. The by-products of the fat breakdown are ketones, which eventually make the blood dangerously acidic. When blood acidity and glucose levels are excessive, the patient becomes comatose.

By frequently monitoring glucose levels, the diabetic patient must administer insulin to keep any rising glucose levels suppressed, thus preventing the harmful effects of hyperglycemia and ketoacidosis. The insulin-dependent diabetic patient can also keep glucose levels in control by following a low-carbohydrate diet and exercising.

Non–Insulin-Dependent Diabetes Mellitus (Type 2)

Non–insulin-dependent, or type 2, diabetes mellitus (**NIDDM**) accounts for 90% to 95% of the diabetic population. It has become epidemic in the United States because of the increasing numbers of obese, sedentary individuals. These individuals generally produce insulin, but it cannot effectively move the glucose from the blood into the cells, a condition known as **insulin resistance**. This resistance creates high blood glucose levels (hyperglycemia). Scientific research has found that the beta cells of the pancreas become sluggish and cannot release the right amount of insulin at the right time, causing fluctuating periods of hypoglycemia (low blood sugar level) and hyperglycemia.

The ineffectiveness of insulin's response to glucose is referred to as *impaired glucose tolerance* (**IGT**). IGT may then lead to **hyperinsulinemia** (excessive blood insulin levels). Hyperinsulinemia causes abnormal amounts of fat levels in the blood (**dyslipidemia**) that lead to **atherosclerosis** (the formation of plaque along the inside walls of blood vessels) and hypertension. The cascade effect of NIDDM that begins with insulin resistance and hyperinsulinemia, which then leads to high blood pressure and heart disease, has been described as *metabolic syndrome* (Figure 6-6).

If individuals with NIDDM do not maintain control of their high glucose levels, they incur the same microvascular and cardiovascular complications as uncontrolled insulin-dependent patients with diabetes type 1 (IDDM). Research has shown that if individuals with NIDDM are diagnosed early, they can begin diet management, exercise, and the use of oral hypoglycemic medication to bring their sugar levels down. They may then avoid developing any of the negative complications caused by abnormally high blood sugar levels.

Table 6-1 summarizes the differences between type 1 and type 2 diabetes.

Prediabetes

Prediabetes is the state that occurs when blood glucose levels are higher than normal but not high enough for a diagnosis of diabetes. Studies have shown that type 2 diabetes develops in most people with prediabetes within 10 years. Studies have also shown that people with prediabetes can prevent or delay the development of type 2 diabetes by up to 58% through changes in lifestyle that include modest

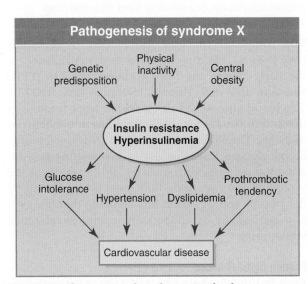

Fig. 6-6 Pathogenesis of syndrome X, also known as *metabolic syndrome. (From Belchetz P, Hammond P:* Mosby's color atlas and text of diabetes and endocrinology, *St Louis, 2003, Mosby.)*

Table 6-1	Comparison of Type 1 and Type 2 Diabetes Mellitus	
	Type 1	**Type 2**
Features	Usually occurs before age 30	Usually occurs after age 30
	Abrupt, rapid onset	Gradual onset; asymptomatic
	Little or no insulin production	Insulin usually present
	Thin or normal body weight at onset	85% are obese
	Ketoacidosis often occurs	Ketoacidosis seldom occurs
Symptoms	Polyuria (glycosuria promotes loss of water)	Polyuria sometimes seen
	Polydipsia (dehydration causes thirst)	Polydipsia sometimes seen
	Polyphagia (tissue breakdown causes hunger)	Polyphagia sometimes seen
Treatment	Insulin	Diet; oral hypoglycemic or insulin

From Chabner D: *The language of medicine,* ed 10, St Louis, 2014, Saunders.

weight loss with diets containing fewer refined carbohydrates (i.e., sugars and processed flour) and regular exercise.

Gestational Diabetes

Gestational diabetes occurs during pregnancy. The mother's IGT usually subsides after delivery of the baby. Signs and symptoms of gestational diabetes include glucosuria, hyperglycemia, excessive weight gain in the mother, and a baby weighing 9 pounds or more. Women who have gestational diabetes are also prone to developing type 2 diabetes later in life.

Transient Diabetes

Individuals may have diabetes during acute illness or when being administered steroid therapy. This form of diabetes usually lasts as long as the condition or treatment continues, and then subsides.

Blood Glucose Screening and Monitoring Tests

The American Diabetes Association recommends two tests to identify diabetes and prediabetes in the early stages: the fasting plasma glucose (**FPG**) test and the oral glucose tolerance test (**OGTT**). The blood glucose levels measured from these tests determine whether an individual has prediabetes or diabetes. The POL may perform CLIA-waived whole blood glucose tests that act as a screening test for potential patients with diabetes. If the results of the screening tests are high, they must be confirmed by the plasma test or serum test methods that are usually performed by moderately complex reference laboratories.

Fasting Blood Glucose

For a fasting blood glucose (**FBG**) test, a patient's fasting sample is usually taken in the morning after a fast of 10 to 14 hours. Patients cannot have any food from 10 PM on the night before until the test the next morning. Usually, they may drink only water, but check your institutional protocol for fasting preparations regarding proper timing and dietary restrictions. The patient's FBG level should be less than 100 mg/dL. If the FBG level is between 100 and 126 mg/dL on 2 different days, the patient is considered prediabetic. If the FBG level is greater than 126 mg/dL, the patient is considered diabetic (based on American Diabetes Association criteria). CLIA-waived glucose tests are for screening only and should be followed up with the more complex plasma tests for blood glucose measurements. A definitive diagnosis is usually made with a venous specimen that has been collected in a gray-topped tube.

Oral Glucose Tolerance Test or 2-Hour Postprandial Blood Sugar

Another method of screening for diabetes mellitus is the OGTT, also called a 2-hour postprandial blood sugar (**2-hr PP**). The OGTT begins with the measurement of FBG level. If the results are within an acceptable range after the initial test, the patient is given a glucose-rich drink or meal and retested after 2 hours. Normal blood glucose levels should be lowered to less than 140 mg/dL 2 hours after the drink or a meal. If the glucose level does not fall below 140 mg/dL but is not greater than 200 mg/dL, the patient is considered prediabetic. If the glucose level is greater than 200 mg/dL after 2 hours, the patient is considered diabetic.

Random Glucose Test

A blood specimen can also be collected at any time to see if the glucose level is within the normal range of less than 140 mg/dL. A random blood specimen with a glucose level greater than 200 mg/dL is indicative of diabetes.

Glucose Tolerance Test

A more thorough test for measuring an individual's glucose metabolism is the full glucose tolerance test

Fig. 6-7 Comparative patterns of GTT results. Compare the blood glucose levels for each condition during the initial fasting test, then the subsequent levels for each hourly test after consumption of the glucose drink.

(GTT), in which blood glucose levels are measured at fasting and then at 1-hour intervals for 2 to 6 hours. The test generally takes place at a reference laboratory or hospital outpatient laboratory.

The GTT begins the same way the OGTT does, in that the patient is fasting and is initially tested for blood glucose level. If the results of the fasting test show a high glucose level (greater than 126 mg/dL), no further testing is done. If the results are within an acceptable range, the patient is given a 100-gram dose of glucose to drink. Blood and urine specimens are collected and tested for glucose levels after the first half hour and then every hour for a specified period of time. The urine is tested to see if and when the blood glucose levels exceed the renal threshold level for glucose of 160 to 180 mg/dL. When the renal threshold level is exceeded, glucose is present in the urine.

During this test the patient should be monitored for signs of fainting or nausea. If these occur, or if the blood glucose levels exceed 300 mg/dL, the test should be terminated. If the physician suspects hyperglycemia (diabetes), it is typically a 3-hour GTT. If the physician suspects hypoglycemia, the test may continue for 5 or 6 hours. Figure 6-7 shows the patterns of faulty glucose metabolism during a GTT.

Glycosylated Hemoglobin/Glycated Hemoglobin (Hgb A$_{1c}$)

When hemoglobin A in the RBCs is exposed to high levels of glucose, the hemoglobin molecule is permanently glycosylated and changes into hemoglobin A$_{1c}$ (A$_{1c}$). Because the life span of an RBC is 80 to 120 days, the percentage of glycosylated hemoglobin molecules will be proportional to the overall concentration of glucose levels in the blood over the average life span of the RBCs (approximately 2 to 3 months). A normal percentage range of glycosylated hemoglobin in a whole blood specimen from adults is 2.2% to 4.8%.

The Hgb A$_{1c}$ test result is especially valuable to the person who is diagnosed with diabetes or prediabetes because it provides an accurate long-term index of the patient's average blood glucose level. Also, Hgb A$_{1c}$ test results are not subject to the daily fluctuations that occur in plasma glucose monitoring. Therefore the American Diabetes Association recommends the Hgb A$_{1c}$ as the best test to determine whether a patient's blood sugar level has been under control during the previous 2 to 3 months. For example, if an Hgb A$_{1c}$ test result of a diabetic person rises above the recommended 6% to 8%, the patient is at risk of developing the microvascular and cardiovascular complications previously discussed. This information can be used to encourage the patient to better understand and follow the treatment plan to prevent those complications.

Patients should be aware that the higher their Hgb A$_{1c}$ percentage rises, the less control they have in maintaining proper glucose levels. This information can be used to encourage the patient to better understand and follow the treatment plan to prevent those complications.

Lipid Metabolism and Testing

Lipids, or fats, are essential to the body. They are an alternate source of energy when blood glucose levels are low, and they are critical to cellular health. Research has shown that poor lipid metabolism and cardiovascular disease are directly linked. In an effort to help correct the growing problems of obesity and heart disease in the United States, annual lipid screening and monitoring tests are recommended. Lipid screening is approved as a CLIA-waived test.

Lipid Metabolism

Lipid metabolism begins with the ingestion of fats. Dietary fats and oils are digested into fatty acids, which are transported to the liver to be reassembled into lipids. These lipids, like glucose, are then transported by the blood to all the body tissues. The lipids are used in critical cellular metabolism or stored as body fat. Some of the essential functions and uses of lipids are the following:

- Production of steroidal hormones
- Transportation of fat-soluble vitamins (vitamins A, D, E, and K)
- Insulation against extreme temperatures
- Maintenance of healthy skin
- Protection of vital organs and nerves
- Potential source of energy when glucose is not available
- Reduction of feeling hungry

The two plasma lipids most routinely tested are cholesterol and triglycerides. These two lipids can be further categorized and tested according to the three ways they are transported in the blood in the form of **lipoproteins** (protein-linked lipids): high-density lipoproteins (**HDL**), low-density lipoproteins (**LDL**), and very-low-density lipoproteins (**VLDL**). Cholesterol, triglyceride, and lipoprotein levels are frequently ordered together in a lipid panel.

Cholesterol

Cholesterol is essential for the production of cell membranes, bile, myelin sheaths on nerves, and steroid hormones. Cholesterol is also required in the absorption of vitamin D. Cholesterol is found in the blood, bile, liver, brain, kidneys, and adrenal glands. Most of the cholesterol found in the blood is manufactured in the liver and is called **endogenous cholesterol**. In fact, the liver is able to produce all the cholesterol the body needs.

Another source of cholesterol, **exogenous cholesterol**, comes from what we eat. Foods high in saturated fats and **trans fats** tend to raise the blood level of cholesterol. Trans fats are synthetic hydrogenated fats found in partially hydrogenated margarines and oils used in cooking and baking. Saturated fats are found in meat, egg yolks, milk, and other dairy products that are usually hard or semisolid at room temperature. Both trans fats and saturated fats are known to elevate cholesterol levels, causing atherosclerosis (Figure 6-8).

Not all dietary fats have the adverse effects of saturated fats and trans fats. Research has found that mono*unsaturated* fats and poly*unsaturated* fats, which are naturally liquid at room temperature, actually lower the blood level of cholesterol. These fats can also reverse plaque buildup on blood vessel walls. Examples of "good" monounsaturated fats are canola oil, olive oil, and omega-3 oil from fish. Examples of good polyunsaturated fats are soybean, safflower, corn, and cottonseed oils.

Lipoproteins

Cholesterol and triglycerides are lipids that do not mix with the water in plasma. Consequently, the liver attaches a protein to these lipids, which then become

Normal arterial lumen   Atherosclerotic   Advanced arterial
                               plaque deposit   atherosclerotic disease

Fig. 6-8 Atherosclerosis is the buildup of fatty plaque in the arteries. *(From Stepp CA, Woods M: Laboratory procedures for medical office personnel, Philadelphia, 1998, Saunders.)*

lipoproteins. The following three types of lipoproteins are manufactured in the liver and are classified on the basis of their density:

- HDL (high-density lipoprotein) is referred to as the "healthy" cholesterol because it has the lowest fat content and appears to protect against the accumulation of fatty deposits in blood vessels. In fact, HDL is capable of removing excess cholesterol from the interior walls of the blood vessels and carrying it back to the liver to be excreted.
- LDL (low-density lipoprotein) is referred to as the "lousy" cholesterol because it forms plaque on the interior walls of the blood vessels (atherosclerosis) as a result of its higher fat content. LDL becomes elevated in the blood after saturated fats and trans fats are ingested. Some individuals are also genetically predisposed to producing LDL endogenously within the liver.
- VLDL (very-low-density lipoprotein) is made predominantly of proteins linked to triglycerides. VLDL is also directly linked to the formation of plaque and atherosclerosis.

Total Cholesterol/High-Density Lipoprotein Ratio

The total blood cholesterol level (TC) is compared with the HDL level in the form of a ratio. This ratio provides an important index for determining the cardiac risk a patient faces because of atherosclerosis. The **TC/HDL ratio** is more valuable than TC level alone because it takes into account whether a high level of TC is made up of the HDL "healthy" cholesterol or the undesirable LDL cholesterol. A ratio greater than 4.5 indicates that the person either is not producing enough good HDL or is producing too much bad LDL. In either case, the individual will need to do the following to lower cardiovascular risk:

- Exercise routinely, which will cause the HDL level to rise and the triglyceride level to decrease.
- Change eating habits in favor of foods that are low in refined carbohydrates and high in fiber (e.g., whole grains, vegetables, fruits), which will lower glucose and triglyceride levels.
- Lower the dietary intake of trans fats and saturated fats found in baked goods, dairy products, and fatty meats. This will lower the LDL levels.
- Change to a diet containing natural monounsaturated fats and polyunsaturated fats found in olive, canola, soybean, safflower, and other oils. This will raise HDL levels.
- Take cholesterol-lowering medications (e.g., statins) as prescribed by the physician.

Triglycerides

Triglycerides are a direct result of diets rich in carbohydrates. Triglycerides account for 95% of the fat stored in adipose tissue. High levels of triglycerides are also associated with atherosclerotic risk. Like cholesterol, triglycerides are transported in the plasma bound to proteins as either LDL (15%) or VLDL (85%). When elevated, triglycerides produce a milky-white appearance in the plasma, a condition called **hyperlipidemia**. Triglyceride levels rise significantly in the blood after sweets or alcohol are ingested and when blood insulin levels are high (hyperinsulinemia). Therefore, when testing for triglyceride levels in the blood, laboratories require the patient to fast 12 to 14 hours before testing and to refrain from alcohol 2 days before testing. Triglyceride levels can be lowered by exercising and decreasing dietary intake of sweets and alcohol.

The Lipid Panel

The lipid panel of tests consists of TC, HDL, LDL, VLDL, triglycerides, and the TC/HDL ratio. Medical research has established a direct link between blood lipid levels and coronary artery disease that may lead to subsequent myocardial infarcts (heart attacks). Myocardial infarction is the leading cause of death in the United States. An individual's cardiovascular risk can be determined by comparing the results of the tests in the lipid panel with the individual's age, weight, height, blood pressure, and smoking habits. Early detection of an at-risk individual can reduce the risk of cardiovascular disease and heart attack if the individual begins an appropriate preventive treatment plan consisting of exercise, diet, and medication therapy.

Also, a high triglyceride result in the panel may indicate metabolic syndrome in patients with central obesity. It is important to remember that the patient must not have alcohol for 48 hours before being tested for triglycerides because alcohol raises the triglyceride levels.

CLIA-Waived Chemistry Tests

Most of the CLIA-waived blood chemistry tests that are performed or observed in ambulatory settings are *quantitative* analyses. The numerical blood levels of glucose, lipids, glycosylated hemoglobin, electrolytes, blood urea nitrogen (BUN), and creatinine are all quantified by electronic photometers. The CLIA-waived fecal **occult** blood (hidden or not visible to the naked eye) test is a *qualitative* analysis that simply detects the presence or absence of blood in a fecal specimen.

Principle of Photometers and Spectrophotometers

Each blood chemistry testing method in this section involves collecting a capillary puncture whole blood specimen into a testing device containing premeasured reagents that react with the analyte being tested. The reagents change color as they react to the analyte in question (similarly to the color changes occurring in

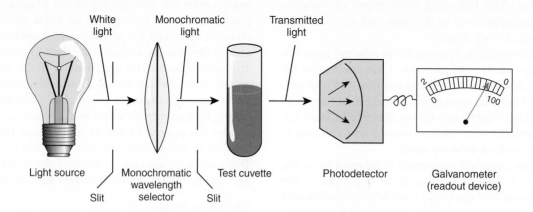

White light   Monochromatic light   Transmitted light

Light source   Monochromatic wavelength selector   Test cuvette   Photodetector   Galvanometer (readout device)

Slit   Slit

Fig. 6-9 Principles of photometry: A spectrum of light passes through the specimen and strikes a photodetector. The intensity of light received by the photodetector is then sent to a readout device that is able to convert the light intensity to a quantitative concentration of the analyte being tested. The intensity of the color changed by the specimen is directly proportional to the concentration of the analyte within the specimen based on the Beer-Lambert law. *(From Stepp CA, Woods M:* Laboratory procedures for medical office personnel, *Philadelphia, 1998, Saunders.)*

urine dipsticks). The testing devices are inserted into an electronic analyzer that sends a spectrum of light through the specimen. A photometer located within the analyzer measures the amount of light that passed through the specimen or reflected off the specimen. The intensity of the color changed by the specimen is directly proportional to the concentration of the analyte within the specimen. This equation is known as the **Beer-Lambert law**.

The chemical analyzers used in blood chemistry testing are highly sensitive photometers and spectrophotometers that directly measure the amount of light passing through the solution (**transmittance photometry**), indirectly measure the amount of light that the solution absorbs (**absorbance photometry**), or indirectly measure the amount of light the solution reflects (**reflectance photometry**). Once the light passes through the solution (or reflects off the specimen), it activates a photodetector that activates a **galvanometer** (an instrument capable of measuring the intensity of light). The galvanometer sends the information to an electronic program that converts the information into a quantitative digital readout (Figure 6-9).

Quality Assurance When Using Optical Instruments

Optical tests depend on all the elements in the light path functioning correctly to receive accurate and reliable results. To accomplish this, each analyzer provides an "optics check" or calibration device or setting that ensures the instrument's optics are working correctly.

Be sure to observe and document all the quality assurance and quality control steps in the instruction manuals for the chemical analyzer being used to. The skill check sheets and corresponding logs for the tests covered in this text are located in the workbook and on-line in Evolve. They all have the following preanalytical requirements:

- Instruments must be calibrated *daily*, and the calibration results must be documented in the calibration log. Newer analyzers may self-calibrate with each specimen and will not require documentation.
- Run liquid controls for each test method according to the manufacturer's recommendations to check the technique and accuracy of the various testing devices, such as the glucose strip, the Hgb A_{1c} cartridge, and the Cholestech cassette. Document the results of the controls on their control logs. If they do not fall within the manufacturer's acceptable range, check the following:
  1. Was the control specimen processed poorly, or was the testing technique poor?
  2. Were the reagents or liquid controls stored at the wrong temperature? Had they expired?
  3. Was the instrument dirty or faulty?
- Always check the expiration date of the testing device, and do not use it to run the test if the expiration date has passed.
- Because the testing device kits for each test must be stored and tested within a specific temperature range, record and monitor the daily room temperature and refrigerator temperature on a log sheet, as found in the workbook appendix. Also pay strict attention to the length of time it is necessary to wait for a testing device that has been stored in the refrigerator to come to room temperature.
- Always retain the most current package inserts that come with the liquid controls and the testing kits and attach them to the procedure sheets for each test method.

Westgard's Rules for Monitoring Quality Control Results

In Chapter 2 the weekly documentations of the liquid control results were placed onto a Levey-Jennings graph and analyzed for excessive scatter, trends, and shifts (see Figures 2-4 through 2-7). The control's mean (average) value and its reference range (±2 standard deviations) were compared with a target that would show if the daily results were consistently accurate and precise (see Figure 2-8). In this chapter each of the chemical analyzers requires the periodic running of one to three liquid controls to determine whether the testing procedure is able to consistently detect both the normal values and the abnormal values of the analytes being measured.

Westgard has set up four additional rules to help evaluate the reliability of a test method when the controls have been run over time. By plotting the monthly documented logged control results onto a Levey-Jennings graph, one can see if any of the following rules have been broken, which indicates a faulty testing system. Do not run patient tests, and contact the manufacturer if any of the following patterns appear on the Levey-Jennings chart:

1. Both levels of control results are outside the manufacturer's reference range.
2. The same control level falls outside of the reference range in two successive runs.
3. One of the controls falls outside of the ±1 standard deviation in four successive runs.
4. One of the controls consistently falls above the mean value or consistently falls below the mean value for 10 consecutive runs.

A monthly Levey-Jennings graph and exercise are provided in Chapter 6 of the workbook. Also, when running the tests in the lab class, plot the results of the controls for all the students and analyze their accuracy and precision to see if the plotted results pass the criteria for reliability.

CLIA-Waived Glucose Tests

Present blood glucose levels can be readily screened and monitored with simple hand-held glucometers. Blood glucose levels over time can also be monitored by testing the percentage of glycosylated hemoglobin (A_{1c}) in a whole blood specimen.

Glucose Monitoring Devices

Numerous brands of glucose meters have been approved for home use and for point-of-care monitoring and screening. Technology continues to make it easier to collect blood specimens and obtain the glucose results in seconds. For example, multiple-site lancets can now be used to collect a very small amount of blood from sites other than the finger, such as the forearm. NOTE: Although forearm testing can give sensitive fingertips a break from testing, forearm testing is not recommended whenever the blood sugar levels may be running low, such as before meals, after exercising, and after administering insulin. It has been proved that fingerstick blood samples will show hypoglycemia more quickly than forearm testing, thus alerting the patient to possible insulin shock.

Noninvasive infrared absorption technology has also made it possible to measure the blood glucose levels with no stick at all.

Glucose meters are also becoming more and more sophisticated, with computerized readouts that graph the patient's glucose readings throughout each day of the week. The computerized visual data help the patient and physician see exactly when glucose levels become unmanageable during the week. The patient may then take the appropriate steps to prevent those problems. The Contour (Bayer, Pittsburgh, PA) procedure check sheet is provided in the workbook and is demonstrated in Procedure 6-1, located at the end of this section. This monitor is similar to the OneTouch Ultra (LifeScan, Milpitas, Calif). Both devices can be viewed on the Internet (along with many other glucose monitoring methods) by accessing the various manufacturers' websites. (NOTE: Never run the supplies or controls from one manufacturer on a different manufacturer's analyzer.)

Glycosylated Hemoglobin A_{1c}

The Hgb A_{1c} test is generally used for monitoring patients with diagnosed diabetes or prediabetes at 3- and 6-month intervals to ensure they are keeping their long-term glucose levels under control. Several brands of analyzers measure Hgb A_{1c} levels. The Bayer A1CNOW+ procedure check sheet is provided in the workbook and is demonstrated in Procedure 6-2, located at the end of this section. It uses a dedicated testing meter that is packaged with 20 test cartridges and 20 sampling packets that all share the same code as the meter. When the 20 tests are completed, the meter is deactivated. Another kit with a new dedicated meter and its 20 coded cartridges and sampling packets is then purchased for the next 20 A_{1c} tests.

Cholesterol and Lipid Profiles with the Cholestech LDX

Total blood cholesterol testing and lipid profiles have become standard screening tests in POLs. The Cholestech LDX is a popular analyzer capable of measuring either single blood cholesterol levels or the full panel of lipids plus glucose. Its procedure check sheet is provided in the workbook and demonstrated in Procedure 6-3, located at the end of this section.

Liver Enzyme Testing with the Cholestech LDX

The Cholestech is also approved for CLIA-waived testing for two liver enzymes: alanine aminotransferase (**ALT**) and aspartate aminotransferase (**AST**). Levels of these enzymes may become elevated if a person is taking statin drugs (i.e., cholesterol-lowering drugs such as Zocor or Lipitor) and is experiencing liver damage. If enzyme results are elevated, the physician may consider a different therapeutic drug. NOTE: Because levels of these enzymes are also elevated during muscle damage, the physician must interpret the significance of the results on the basis of an entire clinical evaluation of the patient. See Figure 6-10 showing the supplies and equipment for measuring the two liver enzymes: ALT and AST.

i-STAT CHEM8+

The i-STAT system consists of a hand-held analyzer and single-use disposable cartridges. The analyzer automatically controls all functions of the testing cycle including fluid movement within the cartridge, calibration, and continuous quality monitoring. (NOTE: A pictorial Procedure 6-4 i-STAT has been placed at the end of this section and a complete procedure skill sheet is provided in the workbook.)

The CLIA-waived i-STAT CHEM8+ cartridge can be used to test all the following blood chemistries and provide the results in minutes:

- Sodium (Na^+)
- Potassium (K^+)
- Chloride (Cl^-)
- Ionized calcium (Ca^{2+})
- TCO_2
- Glucose (Glu)
- Blood urea nitrogen (BUN)
- Creatinine (Crea)
- Hematocrit (Hct)
- Hemoglobin (Hgb)

Fecal Occult Blood Testing—Three Methods

Fecal occult blood testing is a simple, inexpensive test to detect blood that may be hidden or not visible to the naked eye (occult) on or in a stool specimen. It is a useful aid in the diagnosis of a number of gastrointestinal disorders and is typically part of a routine physical examination or a mass screening clinic of the population for colorectal cancer.

The presence of blood in fecal matter may be the result of bleeding from hemorrhoids, polyps, diverticulitis, dysentery, parasites, fissures, colitis, stomach ulcers, or colorectal cancer. If a positive result is obtained, additional follow-up diagnostic tests are performed, such as proctosigmoidoscopy, colonoscopy, barium enema x-ray studies, or endoscopy to determine the cause of the bleeding.

Fig. 6-10 Cholestech system with supplies and results showing elevated liver enzymes: ALT (SGPT) = 59 units/L; AST (SGOT) = 43 units/L.

Cancer of the colon is one of the leading causes of death in the United States. The early stages of colon cancer are usually painless and asymptomatic. By the time an individual becomes aware of the condition, the cancer is typically at the metastasizing phase. Therefore early detection is especially critical while it is still localized and curable. The American Cancer Society recommends that a fecal occult blood test be a routine part of the physical examination of adults. Some patients are embarrassed about the collection of a fecal specimen, and must be encouraged to collect such a specimen and submit it for testing.

Occult Blood Testing with the Guaiac Slide Method

The principle of the test is to apply samples from various fecal specimens to paper slides coated with guaiac (a wood resin that reacts with blood). The paper slides are contained within cardboard testing devices that are then mailed or returned to the testing site. If blood is present, the hemoglobin will react with the guaiac and turn blue when a developing solution (hydrogen peroxide) is applied. False-positive test results can occur if the patient's diet is high in red meat, turnips, horseradish, or bananas. Certain therapeutic drugs, such as nonsteroidal anti-inflammatory drugs, aspirin, iron preparations, and anticoagulants, may also cause positive findings because of their effects on the gastrointestinal tract. The procedure for fecal occult blood check sheet is provided in the workbook and is demonstrated in Procedure 6-5, located at the end of this section.

ColoCARE Method Using Test Pads

An alternative patient-friendly method of testing for occult blood consists of simply floating a test pad in the toilet after a bowel movement. The test pad is

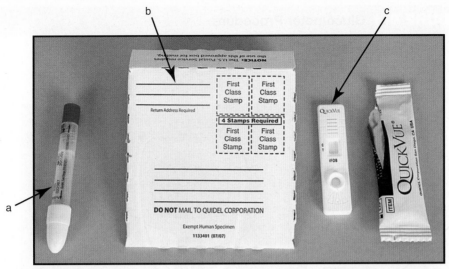

Fig. 6-11 The QuickVue iFOB test is a rapid immunochemical diagnostic tool intended to detect the presence of blood in stool specimens. *a,* Fecal specimen collection tube; *b,* mailer to send specimen to office; *c,* in office test kit.

checked for a change in color that is produced when blood is in the toilet water. When blood is present, the test pad will show areas of blue or green. See Procedure 6-6 for this ColoCARE method of testing for fecal occult blood.

NOTE: Results are dependent on the patient's interpretation. This method may be less sensitive than the guaiac slide method but may be more acceptable to patients who tend to be noncompliant in submitting a fecal specimen.

iFOB (Immunoassay Fecal Occult Blood) Method

The QuickVue **iFOB** test is a rapid immunochemical diagnostic tool intended to detect the presence of blood in stool specimens. iFOB is the acronym for immunoassay fecal occult blood (see Figure 6-11). This highly sensitive qualitative test uses an antibody-antigen reaction (rather than the guaiac methods described earlier) and utilizes a test kit similar to the lateral flow tests covered in Chapter 7: Immunology. This new method of testing occult blood is demonstrated in Procedure 6-7 at the end of this section and a check sheet is available in the workbook. A video demonstration of the entire procedure is also available at the following website: www.quidel.com/assets/swf/iFOBTrainingvideoHQ.htm.

Summary of CLIA-Waived Tests

All the CLIA-waived tests covered in the preceding sections are *screening* tests to detect possible risks to a patient's health. The glucose test detects possible diabetes, the lipid profile detects possible cardiovascular disease, the i-STAT detects possible chemical

imbalances related to the body's homeostatic state, and the occult blood test detects possible colon cancer.

Diabetes and cardiovascular diseases have become so prevalent in the United States that in 2005 the Centers for Medicare and Medicaid Services approved coverage of glucose screening and preventive cardiovascular screening for all Medicare beneficiaries. The new coverage went into effect as part of the larger Medicare Prescription Drug, Improvement, and Modernization Act of 2003. The approved cardiovascular screening includes three tests to detect early risk for cardiovascular disease: TC, HDL, and triglycerides. The TC/HDL ratio can also be determined by these tests, which can be ordered individually or as part of a lipid panel.

Becoming Proficient at CLIA-Waived Chemistry Testing

Now that you have learned about the significance of glucose, hemoglobin A_{1c}, lipid panels, basic chemical homeostasis, and occult blood tests, take time to complete the following:

1. Answer the CLIA-waived portion in Chapter 6 of the workbook using your structured notes and text.
2. View the videos on-line to see glucose quality controls and fecal occult instructions and testing.
3. Perform the Chapter 6 on-line exercises, which are designed to reinforce your terminology and CLIA-waived test knowledge.
4. Study Procedures 6-1 through 6-7 at the end of this section before performing your lab procedures.

✳ PROCEDURE 6-1 Glucometer Procedure

A, Equipment and supplies. *a,* Gauze; *b,* alcohol; *c,* lancet; *d,* test strip; *e,* liquid control; *f,* test strip container with control reference range; *g,* Contour glucometer.

B, Glucometer procedure showing the specimen being pulled into the tip of the strip as it is held in the drop of blood.

C, When a beep sounds, remove the strip from the drop of blood.

PROCEDURE 6-1 Glucometer Procedure—cont'd

D, The glucometer will display the glucose result after 5 to 30 seconds depending on the model (e.g., The glucometer *Elite* in the picture displays the result in 30 seconds, and the newer Bayer *Contour* displays the result in 5 seconds.)

Equipment and Supplies (Figure A)

- Gauze and personal protective equipment (gloves and gown)
- Alcohol
- Lancet
- Test strips
- Liquid control
- Strip container with liquid control reference range
- Contour glucose monitor

Patient Specimen

Note if the patient's capillary specimen is random, fasting, or 2-hr PP. Each of these specimens will have a different reference range.

NOTE: The Contour pictured in Figure A is an upgraded version of the glucometer Elite seen in these pictures; the procedure steps remain the same.

Procedure

1. Sanitize the hands, and put on gloves.
2. Turn on the meter by inserting the end of the strip that contains the metallic contact bars.
3. Perform a capillary puncture, and wipe away the first drop. Then touch and hold the exposed end of the strip into the base of the second drop of blood. This allows the strip to "sip," or draw the blood in without interruption (Figure B). Do not smear or place blood on the top or bottom of the strip.

4. When a beep sounds, quickly remove the strip from the blood to keep it from overfilling (Figure C).
5. After 5 to 30 seconds the result on the Contour meter is displayed on the screen (Figure D).
6. Discard all the test materials in the appropriate biohazard containers.
7. Remove and discard gloves into the biohazard container. Sanitize hands.

The expected results for this test are as follows:

	Fasting	2-hr PP (After Drinking Glucose-Rich Beverage)
Normal	<100 mg/dL	<140 mg/dL
Prediabetes	100-125 mg/dL	140-199 mg/dL
Diabetes	≥126 mg/dL	≥200 mg/dL

Quality Control Procedures

The "coding" or calibration of the glucometer Elite and Contour glucose monitors is set when each strip is inserted into the glucometer. Liquid controls are provided by the glucose meter manufacturer and should be run the same way patient specimens are run to ensure that your technique and the system are providing reliable results.

The glucose liquid controls must be run with each new shipment of glucose strips, with each new operator, and on the days when glucose testing is performed. Patient samples cannot be run if the control results are not acceptable. If the controls are run again and they are still not acceptable, there are three areas to investigate: (1) the *technique* used to process the specimen and run the test, (2) the liquid control and/or the *reagent* expiration dates and their temperature and time requirements, and (3) the *monitor's* optics and maintenance requirements. If all these areas are acceptable and a new set of controls still does not work, call the manufacturer.

A control log has also been provided in the workbook to track the results of multiple glucose control readings. The results can then be plotted on a Levey-Jenning's graph as seen in Chapter 1 in order to observe trends, shifts, randomized errors, and excessive scatter. An extra control log and a control graph are provided in the workbook appendix and on the Evolve website to plot the results of multiple control readings. Check the plotted control graph for signs that show when the multiple results are out of the control limits based on Westgard's four rules.

Photo A by Zack Bent.

6-1

A, Supplies and equipment for the Test Kit Method for A_{1c}. *a,* Gauze; *b,* bandage; *c,* heparin tube for venous blood sample; *d,* alcohol swab; *e,* lancet for capillary blood sample; *f,* sample dilution kit containing capillary tube collector and sampler body; *g,* test cartridge; *h,* A_{1c} monitor programmed to work only with the 20 cartridges in the kit; *i,* box containing 1 monitor and 20 sample dilution kits and 20 cartridges.

B, After lancing the finger and wiping away the first drop, gently touch the blood drop and fill the capillary blood collector from the #1 packet, as seen above.

C, After wiping any blood from the outside of the capillary tube, firmly insert the blood collector into the top of the dilution sampler body, as seen above.

D, The <u>fully</u> inserted sample is then mixed with the dilution by tilting 6 to 8 times. Then stand the sampler on the table.

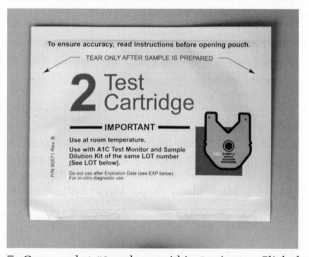

E, Open packet #2 and use within 2 minutes. Click the cartridge into the monitor from the same kit.

PROCEDURE 6-2 A1CNOW+ Glycosylated Hemoglobin Procedure—cont'd

F, The inserted cartridge will start the monitor, which indicates a "WAIT" message.

G, Wait for the "SMPL" to appear before proceeding with the next step.

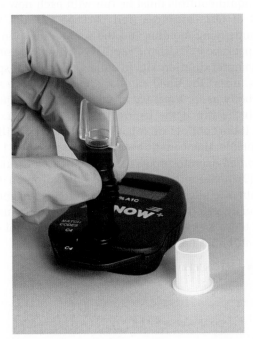

H, Remove the sampler from its base, and push it down onto the white well of the cartridge. The monitor must be on a level surface and cannot be moved until the test is complete.

I, Next, the A$_{1c}$ result will appear along with an intermittent "QCOK" indicating that the test controls were within their normal limits and then a number indicating how many more tests are available in the kit.

(Continued)

6-2

PROCEDURE 6-2 A1CNOW+ Glycosylated Hemoglobin Procedure—cont'd

Equipment and Supplies

See Figure A.

Patient Specimen

Use only **fresh capillary blood** or venous whole blood collected in a **green heparin tube.** Venous blood may be used only if the tube is less than 1 week old and has been under refrigeration during that time. The blood being tested should fill the small glass capillary tube located on the capillary holder provided in the kit (Figure B). Do not allow blood to touch the holder. If using the venous tube of blood, dispense the well-mixed blood onto a slide, and obtain the blood by dipping the capillary tube into the drop at a 45-degree angle. Once the glass capillary tube has been filled with the specimen, the analysis must begin within 5 minutes.

Procedure

1. Sanitize the hands, and put on personal protective equipment (gown and gloves).
2. Remove the blood collector from the foil #1 sampler dilution kit. Touch the tip of the capillary tube that is attached to the holder into the small drop of blood from the finger stick or the venous blood drop on the slide until the capillary is filled (Figure B).
3. Wipe the outer sides of the capillary tube with tissue, being careful not to draw out any of the blood sample within the tube.
4. Insert the capillary holder into the sampler body that also came from the #1 sampler dilution kit (Figure C). Push together and twist until the holder and sampler body snap into place.
5. The fully inserted sample is then mixed with the dilution by tilting 6 to 8 times (Figure D). Then, stand the sampler on the table.
6. Open the #2 test cartridge (Figure E) foil package, and perform the following within 2 minutes: click the cartridge into the monitor that came in the same kit box; check code numbers, which must match.
7. While the monitor indicates "WAIT" (Figure F), prepare the sample by removing the base.

8. Do not add the sample until the monitor indicates "SMPL" (Figure G).
9. Push sampler down onto the white well of the cartridge (Figure H). The monitor must be on a level surface and cannot be moved until the test is complete.
10. After several minutes, the monitor will indicate "QCOK" followed by the test result (Figure I), which in this case shows a result of 5.2 followed by the number of tests left in the kit.
11. Record the results from the display, and report to the physician.
12. Properly dispose of all biohazard supplies, disinfect the area, remove gloves, and sanitize hands.

The expected results of an A_{1c} test are the following:

Nondiabetics	3-6%
Controlled diabetics	6-8%
Poorly controlled diabetics	As much as 20% or higher

NOTE: Because A_{1c} is also affected by hemoglobin concentration, the patient's hemoglobin level should be tested to ensure that it is in the normal range.

Quality Control Procedures

The liquid controls must be run with each new shipment of test cartridges (foil package #2) and their accompanying monitor and the sample dilution kits (foil package #1). Use the capillary holder from one of the sampler dilution kits to collect the control specimens. Insert the filled capillary holder into the sampler body as for a patient specimen. Patient samples cannot be run if the control results are not acceptable. If the controls are run again and they are still not acceptable, there are three areas to investigate: (1) the *technique* used to process the specimen and run the test, (2) the liquid control and *reagent* expiration dates and their temperature and time requirements, and (3) the *analyzer's* optics and maintenance requirements. If all these areas are acceptable and a new set of controls still does not work, call the manufacturer.

Photos A through I by Zack Bent.

PROCEDURE 6-3 Cholestech Method of Measuring Lipids and Glucose

A, Cholestech analyzer and supplies. *a,* Cholestech LDX analyzer; *b,* printer with self-adhesive individual reports; *c,* liquid control box with insert reference sheet of values for level 1 and level 2 controls; *d,* optics check container and cassette for daily optics checks; *e,* foil wrap and testing cassette; *f,* capillary tubes and plungers for collecting and dispensing capillary blood samples.

6-3

PROCEDURE 6-3 Cholestech Method of Measuring Lipids and Glucose—cont'd

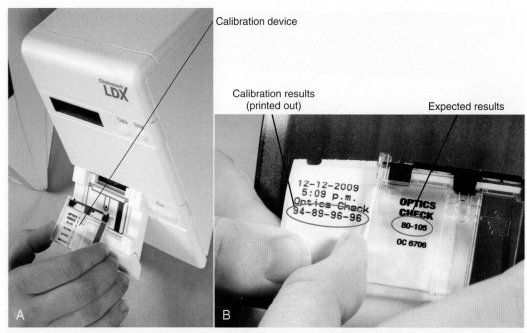

Calibration device

Calibration results
(printed out)

Expected results

B, Calibration check. *(A)* Place the "Optics Check" calibration cassette in the drawer of the Cholestech. *(B)* The results of the optical reading in all four testing areas will be displayed and printed.

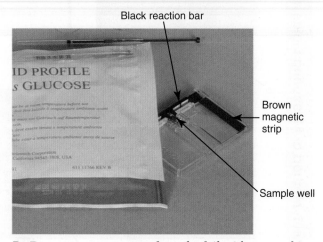

Black reaction bar

Brown
magnetic
strip

Sample well

D, Remove a new cassette from the foil without touching the brown magnetic strip or black reaction bar.

C, Micropipetter for obtaining and dispensing liquid controls and venous blood collected in a green lithium heparin tube. (1) First, press thumb down on plunger to dispense out the air before entering sample. (2) Release thumb while in sample, causing the pipette to fill. (3) Clean outside of pipette with gauze. (4) Press thumb down again to deliver the sample into the cassette, and then remove the pipette from the device before releasing thumb to avoid pulling the specimen back into the pipette. *(From Proctor D, Adams A: The medical assistant: an applied learning approach, ed 12, St Louis, 2014, Saunders.)*

PROCEDURE 6-3 **Cholestech Method of Measuring Lipids and Glucose—cont'd**

E, Collect blood into the capillary tube with the black plunger inserted into the red end of the capillary tube. Collection should be completed within 10 seconds.

F, Transfer the blood into the cassette test well using the plunger as seen above within the next 5 minutes (this avoids clotting of the specimen). Also, observe the positioning of the cassette with the testing bars to the left of the well and the hand on the cassette pointing down toward the well.

(Continued)

6-3

PROCEDURE 6-3 Cholestech Method of Measuring Lipids and Glucose—cont'd

G, Immediately place the cassette with the specimen in the opened drawer, and press RUN. Results will be printed after 5 minutes.

Equipment and Supplies (Figure A)

- Cholestech LDX analyzer
- Printer that provides individual self-adhesive patient readouts
- Control box with level 1 and level 2 liquid controls (stored in refrigerator)
- Optics check container and optics check cassette (stored at room temperature)
- Individual foil wrap and test cassette for running a test on a patient or a liquid control (stored in refrigerator)
- Cholestech capillary tubes and black plungers for collecting and transferring capillary blood samples (stored at room temperature)

Patient Sample

If a lipid panel including triglycerides is ordered, the patient should not drink alcohol for 48 hours before testing and should have fasted for 10 to 12 hours. The test can be run with whole blood from a finger stick that is collected in the appropriate capillary tube with its black plunger inserted. Whole blood from a green-topped lithium heparin tube can also be used. (NOTE: Green-topped *sodium* heparin tubes are not acceptable.) Cholestech provides an automatic micropipetter that consists of a disposable plastic-tipped pipette placed on the end of a plunger (Figure C). The plunger is pushed in before entering the tube of blood. Once in the blood, the plunger is released, causing the correct amount of blood to flow into the plastic tip. The

blood can then be transferred to the Cholestech testing device by pushing down on the plunger.

Procedure

1. Allow the refrigerated cassette to come to room temperature (at least 10 minutes before opening).
2. Make sure the analyzer is plugged in and warmed up.
3. Remove the cassette from its foil pouch, and place it on a flat surface. Do not touch the black bar or the brown magnetic strip (Figure D). Hold the cassette by the short sides only.
4. Press RUN. The analyzer will perform a self-test, and the screen will display "Self-Test Running," then "Self-Test OK."
5. The cassette drawer will open, and the screen will display "Load Cassette and Press Run." The drawer will remain open for 4 minutes, after which it will close with the message "System timeout. Run to continue." If the RUN button is not pushed within 15 seconds of the message, the drawer will close and the screen will go blank. If this happens, simply press RUN and allow the analyzer to go through the self-test again; then proceed.
6. Collect a blood sample from a finger stick into the Cholestech LDX capillary tube with its plunger in place (Figure E). (Or use the Mini-Pet pipette provided by Cholestech to collect the Vacutainer blood and the control samples.)

PROCEDURE 6-3 Cholestech Method of Measuring Lipids and Glucose—cont'd

7. The blood or control sample must then be plunged into the cassette well within 5 minutes after collection, or the blood may clot (Figure F).
8. Immediately place the filled cassette into the drawer of the analyzer (Figure G).
   a. Keep the cassette level after the sample is applied.
   b. The black reaction bar faces toward the analyzer.
   c. The brown magnetic strip is on the right.
9. Press RUN. The drawer will close and the screen will display "(Test names) Running."
10. When the test is complete, the analyzer will beep and the screen will display results. At the same time, the printer will provide the results. (NOTE: Pressing the DATA button will display the calculated results of all tests on the screen if you are running a panel of tests. The DATA button will also display questions that must be answered to determine the cardiac risk factor.)

The interpretation of the lipid panel as it relates to cardiovascular risk is as follows (based on American Heart Association recommendations):

Total Cholesterol Levels	What It Means
<200 mg/dL	Desirable
200-239 mg/dL	Borderline high risk for heart disease
≥240 mg/dL	High risk for heart disease

LDL Cholesterol Levels	What It Means
<100 mg/dL	Optimal
100-129 mg/dL	Near-optimal
130-159 mg/dL	Borderline high
160-189 mg/dL	High
≥190 mg/dL	Very high

HDL Cholesterol Levels	What It Means
<40 mg/dL	High risk for heart disease
40-59 mg/dL	Less risk for heart disease
≥60 mg/dL	Desirable

TC/HDL ratio ≤4.5 is desirable.

Triglycerides	What It Means
<150 mg/dL	Desirable
150-199 mg/dL	Borderline high
200-499 mg/dL	High
≥500 mg/dL	Very high

Cholestech results when testing ALT (SGPT) and AST (SGOT) enzymes: ALT and AST are enzymes that are measured to help assess liver damage. ALT and AST levels are monitored in patients who are taking certain medications to lower cholesterol level, control diabetes, or treat other diseases. A normal ALT range is 10 to 40 units/L. A normal AST range is 10 to 30 units/L.

Quality Control Procedures

The calibration "optics check" cassette should be run daily. It does not require any specimen in its well. Simply place the cassette in the drawer of the Cholestech. The results of the optical reading in all four testing areas will be displayed and printed (see Figure B). Document the results on the calibration log and compare the numbers with the required range designated on the cassette. If any number falls out of range, patient tests cannot be run until the cause is determined and corrected.

The two levels of liquid controls should be run at least monthly, or with a new user, or whenever a new set of cassettes is opened. Use the Mini-Pet pipette to transfer the control solution into the cassette well, and run the control as you would a patient sample. Document the results on the control log and compare them with the control's package insert. If the results do not fall in the required range, patient samples cannot be run until the cause is determined and corrected.

6-3

✳ PROCEDURE 6-4 i-STAT Chemistry Analyzer Procedure

Preanalytical supplies: *(a)* Venipuncture items using a 4-mL lithium heparin tube, and *(b)* the safety transfer device that will be used to transfer the blood from the Vacutainer tube to the 1-mL syringe.

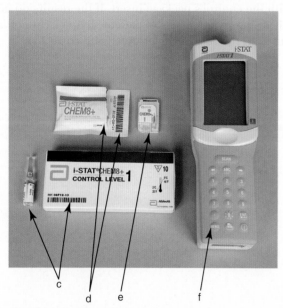

Analytical supplies and analyzer: *(c)* Liquid control ampule and package, *(d)* foil cartridge CHEM8+ package with bar code, *(e)* cartridge, and *(f)* the hand-held analyzer.

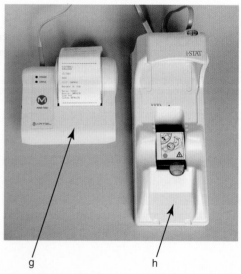

Postanalytical supplies: *(g)* Printer and *(h)* recharging dock for analyzer.

PROCEDURE 6-4 i-STAT Chemistry Analyzer Procedure—cont'd

A, Collect blood, making sure the 4-mL heparin tube fills completely and that the blood is mixed by tilting 10 times. The specimen should be tested within 10 minutes. NOTE: During this time, enter in the operator and patient information followed by scanning the cartridge's bar code.

B, Using the safety transfer device, pull well-mixed blood from the tube into about half of a 1-mL syringe. If air enters the syringe, do not push it back into the blood tube.

C, Remove any air at the tip of the syringe along with three drops of blood onto a gauze pad. Then carefully push the blood into the cartridge well until the blood reaches the arrow and there is still blood remaining in the well but not overflowing.

D, Swing the cover tab over the well from left to right using one finger. Do not press on the beige circle area directly over the well. Push down on the tab until it snaps into place.

(Continued)

PROCEDURE 6-4 i-STAT Chemistry Analyzer Procedure—cont'd

E, Use the grooved area to the left of the well, or the sides of the cartridge, to slowly insert it into the analyzer.

F, After 2 to 3 minutes the results will appear on the screen. Note the "→ Page" command on the bottom of the screen indicating more results will appear on a second screen. Press the print button to send the results to the printer via wireless transmission or via the docking device USB connection.

Equipment and Supplies

Specimen Collection—Preanalytical

- 4-mL lithium heparin tube
- Safety transfer device and 1-mL syringe

Testing Supplies and Analyzer—Analytical

- Liquid controls
- Foil cartridge package with bar code
- CHEM8+ cartridge
- Hand-held analyzer

Print Equipment—Postanalytical

- Printer
- Recharging dock for analyzer

Patient Sample

The FDA-approved CLIA-waived i-STAT test requires a whole blood sample from a completely filled green-topped *lithium* heparin tube. (NOTE: Green-topped *sodium* heparin tubes are not acceptable.) The well-mixed blood is then transferred to a 1-mL syringe using the safety transfer device, and then it must be inserted into the test cassette within 10 minutes.

Procedure

1. Allow cassette to come to room temperature (at least 10 minutes before opening).
2. Key in operator and patient information into the hand-held analyzer, followed by scanning the cartridge bar code until a beep is heard.

3. *Within 10 minutes* of drawing a 4-mL specimen of blood into a vacuum tube, perform the following (Figure A):
   - Mix the specimen by tilting 10 times.
   - Connect a safety tip or safety transfer device to a 1-mL syringe.
   - Invert the green top tube with the specimen and pierce the green stopper with the syringe safety tip or the transfer device.
   - *Slowly* pull back on the syringe plunger until it is about one-half full; note any air bubbles that enter syringe while transferring and do not push them back into specimen (Figure B).
   - Disconnect syringe from vacuum tube and continue to hold it with tip pointed upward; then hold a gauze pad at the tip of the syringe to absorb blood while syringe plunger is slowly pushing out the air and approximately three drops of blood.
   - Tear open the foiled cartridge pouch and remove the cartridge by holding the sides and placing it on a flat surface.
   - Hold the syringe tip directly over and into the sample well and carefully push the blood into the cartridge until the blood reaches the blue arrow indicator and there is still blood remaining in the well but not overflowing (Figure C).

PROCEDURE 6-4 i-STAT Chemistry Analyzer Procedure—cont'd

4. Move the tab over the well from left to right using one finger; do not press on the beige circle area directly over the well; push down on the tab until it snaps into place (Figure D).
5. Use the grooved area to the left of the well or hold the sides of the cartridge to slowly insert it into the analyzer (Figure E).
   - The hand-held analyzer first displays "Identifying Cartridge" and then a "time-to-result" bar appears.
   - *Do not* **remove cartridge until the "Cartridge Locked" message on the hand-held analyzer is removed and results are displayed on screen.**

6. Review results
   - After 2 to 3 minutes, the results will appear on the screen (Figure F). The "→ Page" command on the bottom of the screen indicates more results will appear on a second screen. Press the print button to send the results to the printer by wireless transmission or by the docking device USB connection.
   - The hand-held device shows the numerical values and units with the results. It also shows bar graphs with tic marks for reference ranges.

Test	Test Symbol	Units	Reportable Range	Reference Range	Results	Critical Low/High
Sodium	Na^+	mmol/L	100-180	138-146		
Potassium	K^+	mmol/L	2.0-9.0	3.5-4.9		
Chloride	Cl^-	mmol/L	65-140	98-109		
Total carbon dioxide	TCO_2	mmol/L	5-50	24-29		
Ionized calcium	iCa^{2+}	mmol/L	0.25-2.50	1.12-1.32		
Glucose	Glu	mg/dL	20-700	70-105		
Urea nitrogen	BUN	mg/dL	3-140	8-26		
Creatinine	Crea	mg/dL	0.2-20.0	0.6-1.3		
Hematocrit	Hct	% PCV	10-75	38-51		
Hemoglobin*	Hgb	g/dL	3.4-25.5	12-17		
Anion gap*	AnGap	mmol/L	10-99	10-20		

*These results are figured mathematically from the other results (not directly).

Quality Control Procedures

The calibration "optics check" is performed using the simulator provided by i-STAT. Simply place the simulator into the same port as the patient cassette. The results of the optical reading will be displayed and printed. If the result falls out of range, patient tests cannot be run until the cause is determined and corrected.

The two levels of liquid controls should be run at least monthly, or whenever a new set of cassettes is opened. Use the syringe to transfer the well-mixed control solution into the cassette well, and run the control as you would a patient sample. Document control results and compare them with the control package insert. If the results do not fall in the required range, patient samples cannot be run until the cause is determined and corrected.

Photos by Zack Bent.

6-4

✳ **PROCEDURE 6-5** Occult Blood: *ColoScreen III Method*

A, Fecal occult blood kit and supplies. *a,* ColoScreen III box with supplies and directions; *b,* three specimen slides; *c,* three wooden applicators; *d,* hydrogen peroxide developer.

B, The patient applies a thin fecal smear to each box after lifting the *front flap* of the specimen slide. *(From Stepp CA, Woods M:* Laboratory procedures for medical office personnel, *Philadelphia, 1998, Saunders.)*

C, The patient enters all the information on the front flap of each slide *after* applying three different specimens to each of the three slides. The three slides of labeled specimens are then mailed or carried to the laboratory. *(From Stepp CA, Woods M:* Laboratory procedures for medical office personnel, *Philadelphia, 1998, Saunders.)*

D, In the lab, two drops of developer are applied to each test area after lifting the *flap on the back* of the specimen slide. *(From Stepp CA, Woods M:* Laboratory procedures for medical office personnel, *Philadelphia, 1998, Saunders.)*

PROCEDURE 6-5 Occult Blood: *ColoScreen III Method*—cont'd

E, Apply developer to the monitoring section of the slide to confirm that the positive turns blue and the negative does not. *(From Stepp CA, Woods M: Laboratory procedures for medical office personnel, Philadelphia, 1998, Saunders.)*

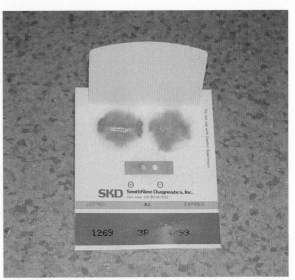

F, Observe the blue positive occult blood test results in the upper patient areas of the slide and confirm the control results at the bottom: positive blue *(left)* and negative white *(right)*. *(From Stepp CA, Woods M: Laboratory procedures for medical office personnel, Philadelphia, 1998, Saunders.)*

Equipment and Supplies for ColoScreen III Method (Figure A)

- ColoScreen III
- Three specimen slides
- Three wooden applicators
- Hydrogen peroxide developer

   Check for proper storage (e.g., temperature, light). Check the expiration date. Locate the package insert and patient instructions.

Patient Preparation and Pretest Instruction

Two days before the test and during the specimen-collecting day, the patient should eat a high-fiber diet, including well-cooked poultry or fish, cooked fruits and vegetables, bran cereals, raw lettuce, carrots, and celery, and moderate amounts of peanuts and popcorn. The patient should refrain from ingesting the following items, which may interfere with the test results: red and partially cooked meats, turnips, cauliflower, broccoli, parsnips, melons (especially cantaloupe), alcohol, aspirin, and vitamin C.

   When collecting specimens, the patient should use the slides, applicators, and the take-home instructions as follows:

1. After a bowel movement, use the wooden applicator to collect a small sample by scraping the surface of the feces and spread a thin layer in box A of the slide (Figure B). Using the same applicator, collect

a second sample from a different part of the feces and spread it in box B.
2. Discard the wooden applicator, reseal the cover of the slide, and complete the information requested on the outside of the cover (Figure C).
3. Repeat the preceding steps with the next two consecutive bowel movements and the two remaining slides.

Test Procedure

4. Apply gloves, and observe Universal Precautions. Confirm that all necessary information was written on slide covers.
5. Open the back sides of all three slides, and place two drops of developer on each specimen (Figure D). Any blue reaction in the specimen area indicates a positive result. A positive result may be read in as early as 30 seconds to 2 minutes, but do not record a negative (no blue) until at least 2 minutes have passed.
6. Perform the monitor test (internal control) by placing one or two drops between the monitor boxes and waiting 30 seconds to 2 minutes to read the results and confirm that the positive turned blue and the negative did not (Figure E).
7. Observe if there are positive blue specimen reactions and validate the results of the control monitors showing blue on the positive dot and nothing on the negative dot (Figure F).

6-5

✳ PROCEDURE 6-6 Occult Blood: *ColoCARE Method*

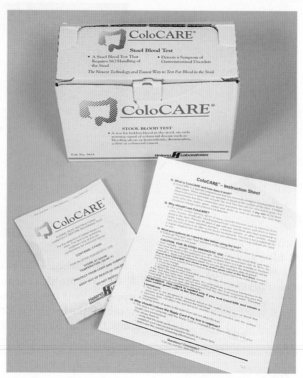

A, ColoCARE method for fecal occult blood. Patient receives foil packet with three test pads, a reply card, and an instruction sheet.

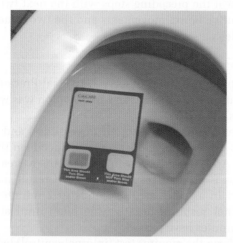

B, Negative occult blood test result with no color in the large test box. The controls show blue in the positive left lower corner and no color in the negative control box in the lower right corner.

C, Positive occult blood test showing blue color in the large test box. The controls once again show blue in the positive left lower corner and no color in the negative control box in the lower right corner.

PROCEDURE 6-6 Occult Blood: *ColoCARE Method* —cont'd

First Bowel Movement	Second Bowel Movement	Third Bowel Movement
Date _____	Date _____	Date _____
ColoCARE Test area	**ColoCARE** Test area	**ColoCARE** Test area
This area should turn blue and/or green · This area should NOT turn blue and/or green	This area should turn blue and/or green · This area should NOT turn blue and/or green	This area should turn blue and/or green · This area should NOT turn blue and/or green

D, Patient marks the diagram on the reply card labeled "first bowel movement" with an **"x" in each area of the pad that turned a blue and/or green color.** The areas include the large test area and the two smaller areas at the bottom (the positive and negative control areas). The same directions apply to the second and third bowel movements.

Equipment and Supplies for ColoCARE Method

Patient receives foil packet containing three test pads and a reply card, along with an instruction sheet (Figure A).

Patient Preparation and Pretest Instruction

Two days before the test and during the specimen-collecting day, the patient should eat a high-fiber diet, including well-cooked poultry or fish, cooked fruits and vegetables, bran cereals, raw lettuce, carrots, celery, and moderate amounts of peanuts and popcorn. The patient should refrain from ingesting the following items, which may interfere with the test results: red and partially cooked meats, turnips, cauliflower, broccoli, parsnips, melons (especially cantaloupe), alcohol, aspirin, and vitamin C.

At-Home Test Procedure

1. After a bowel movement, do not flush or put toilet paper in the toilet. **Perform the following steps within 5 minutes after bowel movement.**
2. Open foil pouch by tearing along the dotted line at the bottom of the pouch, being careful not to tear the pad inside and remove one ColoCARE pad from the pouch. Tape the pouch closed to protect the remaining pads from light and moisture.
3. Hold the ColoCARE pad with the printed side up. Carefully release the pad, allowing it to float on the water in the center of the toilet bowl.
4. Observe the ColoCARE pad for 30 seconds, and note any blue or green appearance on the pad (see Figures B and C for possible negative and positive results).
5. After testing the first bowel movement, mark the diagram on the reply card (Figure D) labeled "First Bowel Movement" with an **"x" in each area of the pad that turned a blue or green color.** The areas include the large TEST AREA and the two smaller areas at the bottom of the pad (the positive and negative control areas). After recording the results on the reply card, flush the floating test pad down the toilet.
6. Repeat step 5 for the next two consecutive bowel movements, and mark the second and third diagrams on the reply card according to the same instructions.
7. Fill out all the patient information required on the reply card, and either mail it to the office or bring the card back to the office for interpretation.

Photos A, B, and C by Zack Bent.

6-6

✳ PROCEDURE 6-7 Occult Blood: *iFOB Method*

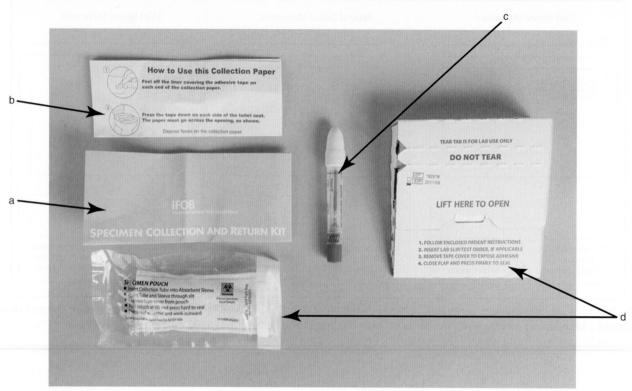

A, Patient supplies for collecting fecal specimen at home for iFOB method: *a,* step-by-step illustrated instruction sheet; *b,* specimen collection paper to place across toilet seat; *c,* specimen collection tube with internal sampling probe to pierce the specimen; *d,* plastic biohazard bag and mailer to send specimen to the lab or office.

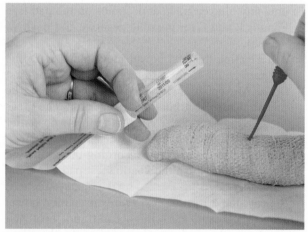

B, Demonstrating how to pierce the specimen using the collection tube's blue probe. The patient is then instructed to recap the blue sampler into the collection tube (on the left), firmly tighten, and shake well. The specimen is then inserted into the provided absorbent sleeve, and then into the biohazard plastic bag. The bagged specimen is then placed into the cardboard mailer and returned to the office or laboratory within 24 hours.

C, After receiving the patient's specimen, the medical assistant or lab tech shakes the specimen thoroughly, and then unscrews the pale blue–capped end of the collection tube. Using the absorbent sleeve or a gauze pad, quickly snap away the plastic tip of the collection tube as seen above.

PROCEDURE 6-7 Occult Blood: *iFOB Method*—cont'd

D, Next, holding the sampler collection tube vertically, squeeze six (6) drops into the sampling well. Allow the sample to remain undisturbed for 5 to 10 minutes. (This allows the sample to flow laterally across the test area ["T"] and the control area ["C"].)

E, After 5 to 10 minutes, inspect the "T" area for a line indicating a positive result for fecal occult blood, or no line indicating a negative result for fecal blood. In both cases the "C" (control) must show a line indicating the test kit results are "valid." This patient's results show a valid negative result for fecal occult blood.

Patient Supplies for iFOB Method (Figure A)

- Instruction sheet
- Specimen collection paper to place across toilet seat
- Specimen collection tube with internal sampling probe to pierce the stool specimen
- Absorbent pouch, plastic biohazard bag, and mailer to send specimen to the lab or office

Patient Preparation and Pretest Instruction

The QuickVue iFOB test is specific to human hemoglobin. Therefore, the patient does not need to follow the food restrictions in the previous fecal occult tests. Patients with the following conditions, however, should not be considered for testing, because these conditions may interfere with test results:

- Menstrual bleeding
- Bleeding hemorrhoids
- Constipation bleeding
- Urinary bleeding

The patients with the aforementioned conditions may be considered for testing after such bleeding ceases.

Alcohol and certain medications such as aspirin, indomethacin, reserpine, phenylbutazone, corticosteroids, and nonsteroidal anti-inflammatory drugs may also cause gastrointestinal irritation and subsequent bleeding in some patients.

Enter the Patient Identification Information on the Collection Tube Label

1. When collecting specimens, the patient should use the take-home instructions as follows:
   - Do not collect specimen if bleeding is present from hemorrhoids, constipation, urination, or menstruation.
   - Urinate before positioning collection paper (or a paper plate).
   - Do not urinate on fecal specimen or collection paper.
   - Position paper on rear half of toilet seat and press the tape down on each side.
   - Deposit fecal specimen on the collection paper.
2. Unscrew the dark blue sampler probe from the collection tube that contains a liquid buffer solution:
   - Using the probe, pierce the specimen in at least five different sites (Figure B).
   - Insert the sampler back into the collection tube, firmly tighten the tube, and then shake the tube well.
   - Flush remaining specimen and collection paper.

(Continued)

PROCEDURE 6-7 Occult Blood: *iFOB Method*—cont'd

3. Make sure the patient's identification line has the patient's name on the label. Then, in the following order, insert the collection tube that has the well-mixed specimen and solution into the:
   - Absorbent sleeve
   - Plastic specimen pouch
   - Cardboard mailer
   - Mail or bring to the medical office or laboratory

Test Procedure After Receiving Specimen

4. Apply gloves, and observe Universal Precautions. Confirm that all necessary information was written on the collection tube.
5. Shake tube well and unscrew pale blue cap.

6. Cover the tip with the absorbent sleeve or gauze and snap the tip away (Figure C).
7. Squeeze 6 drops into the test well (Figure D).
8. Read results as positive, negative, or invalid after 5 to 10 minutes (Figure E) based on the following criteria:
   - Positive result: A pink line appears next to the letter T and next to the letter C.
   - Negative result: Only one pink line forms next to the letter C.
   - Invalid test: If there is no pink line next to the letter C, the test results are invalid and should not be reported.

 # Advanced Concepts

i-STAT

Additional CLIA-waived point-of-care chemistry analyzers, such as the i-STAT, have been approved for POLs. Originally, this hand-held i-STAT device was designed for critical care situations in which blood chemistry test results were needed immediately *(stat).* The technology was designed to ensure that a non–laboratory-trained health professional could run the chemistry tests at the patient's bedside and obtain reliable results. Table 6-2 shows the critical test values that are typically monitored during a patient's "crisis" situation. The reasons that these values are needed are discussed in the following paragraphs.

Almost all metabolic processes in the body are dependent on or affected by pH, blood gas, and electrolyte levels. The pH is critical for maintaining proper physiological molecular structure and chemical reactions. The electrolytes (Na^+, K^+, Cl^-, and ionized Ca^{2+}) are involved with pH regulation, water distribution, proper muscle and nerve function, oxidation-reduction reactions, and enzymatic reactions. Proper concentrations of blood gases (oxygen and carbon dioxide) are also critical for maintaining correct tissue oxygenation and pH balance.

Glucose level determinations help in evaluating disorders of carbohydrate metabolism; evaluating acidosis and ketoacidosis; evaluating dehydration, coma, hypoglycemia, and neuroglycopenia; and establishing a diagnosis of diabetes.

Blood urea nitrogen (BUN) and creatinine measurements are commonly used to evaluate renal function. An abnormally high level of urea nitrogen in the blood is an indication of kidney impairment, or kidney failure due to the kidney's inability to remove urea from the blood. Other causes of increased values for urea nitrogen include gastrointestinal bleeding and a high-protein diet. Causes of decreased urea values include pregnancy, severe liver insufficiency, overhydration, and malnutrition.

The whole blood hematocrit and hemoglobin measurements are useful for determining if RBC quantity is sufficient to maintain a proper oxygen level during a surgical procedure. It is a key indicator of the body's state of hydration, anemia, or severe blood loss, as well as the blood's ability to transport oxygen.

Piccolo Xpress

Demands for improved patient care and greater cost control are driving profound changes in the structure of health care delivery. Within and outside of traditional hospital environments, evolving technology is permitting some types of diagnostic testing and patient monitoring to move from the clinical laboratory to the near-patient environment. Many health care professionals whose roles have traditionally involved hands-on patient care are now being asked to take a role in clinical chemistry testing as well.

Laboratorians, with their training and experience, know that rigorous quality control (QC) is an absolute necessity for accurate test results on which treatment decisions can confidently be based. The Piccolo Xpress point-of-care chemistry analyzer incorporates a process called iQC ("intelligent Quality Control") that meets established QC standards independently of the operator's skill level. iQC is a series of sophisticated automatic checks that verify the chemistry, optics, and electronic functions of the analyzer during each run and ensure that operators in a wide range of environments report only accurate and reliable results.

Table 6-2 Normal and Critical Blood Chemistry Results (on i-STAT Analyzer)

		Arterial	Venous	Critical Ranges
Reference Ranges	pH	7.35-7.45	7.32-7.42	<7.200 or >7.55
	P_{CO_2}	35-45 mm Hg	41-51 mm Hg	<20 or >65 mm Hg
	P_{O_2}	80-100 mm Hg		<50 mm Hg
	Sodium	136-146 mmol/L		<120 or >160 mmol/L
	Potassium	3.5-5.0 mmol/L		<2.5 or >6.0 mmol/L
	Chloride	101-114 mmol/L		<80 or >130 mmol/L
	Glucose	Fasting: 73-115 mg/dL		Adult: <40 or >500 mg/dL
				Newborn (birth to 3 months): <40 or >200 mg/dL
	BUN (UN)	Adults (>12 years): 8-20 mg/dL		
	Hct	Male subjects: 42-52% Female subjects: 37-47%		<15%
	Hgb	12-17 g/dL		<7 g/dL

The Piccolo Xpress point-of-care chemistry analyzer is a lightweight portable instrument that processes whole blood, serum, or plasma samples in self-contained, single-use reagent disks. Transparent to the operator, iQC checks the analyzer, the reagent disk, and the sample during each run to verify correct electronic and chemistry performance. If it detects uncharacteristic performance, iQC automatically suppresses a single chemistry test result or the entire panel of results and immediately alerts the operator to any problems. From the self-test at power-up to the recording and printing of patient results, the Piccolo Xpress conducts multiple QC checks automatically with each run; iQC ensures that the operator reports only accurate and reliable results.

Metabolic Panels: Basic and Comprehensive

Not all offices can afford the previously described chemistry analyzers. When physicians need to know blood chemistry values to arrive at a definitive diagnosis, they will have either the medical assistant or the phlebotomist draw a blood sample (usually a gold SST) and send it to a reference laboratory for testing, or they will send the patient to the reference laboratory. Depending on what the physician needs to know, a metabolic panel, which typically consists of 6 to 12 or more chemistry tests, will be ordered. The panels are usually ordered as part of an annual physical exam, when a patient is being prepared for surgery, or when a patient is exhibiting specific symptoms. Metabolic panels provide the physician with a comprehensive picture of the patient's carbohydrate and lipid metabolism. They also provide information regarding the liver, kidney, heart, and thyroid functions. Typical tests in a metabolic panel include electrolytes, lipids, glucose, BUN, bilirubin, enzymes, and hormones. The report in Figure 6-12 shows each analyte's result along with the lab's reference range. Note that when an analyte is out of range, it is noted in a column next to the reported value. Laboratories are now required to indicate when analytes are outside of their particular reference range because ranges may vary between different methods of testing. The physician must interpret these chemistry results along with the rest of the patient's examination to make a definitive diagnosis.

Renal Panel

The renal, or kidney, panel consists of tests that portray how the kidney is functioning. The kidney is responsible for excreting the following chemical wastes: urea, creatinine, and uric acid. By observing increases in BUN, blood creatinine, and uric acid levels, the physician can determine when the kidney has become impaired as well as the degree of impairment. This panel of tests is helpful in monitoring the diabetic patient who is at risk for kidney failure. Elevated uric acid levels alone are associated with gout (a form of arthritis caused by the accumulation of uric acid crystals in the synovial fluid of joints). The kidneys and lungs maintain the body's water and pH balance by releasing or retaining charged electrolyte ions—chloride (Cl^-), potassium (K^+), sodium (Na^+), and bicarbonate (HCO_3^-). Therefore testing the levels of these electrolytes may also be included in the renal panel.

Electrolyte Panel

The electrolyte panels give a picture of the patient's water-salt balance and the ability to maintain proper

TEST		RESULTS	REFERENCE RANGE	UNITS
		DATE & TIME RECEIVED	ACCESSION NUMBER	
		10/20/2010 20:45		
		LOCATION	DATE REPORTED	
			10/21/2010	
PHYSICIAN			PATIENT'S INFORMATION	

TEST		RESULTS	REFERENCE RANGE	UNITS
CHEMISTRY 23 - PANEL B				
CALCIUM, TOTAL, SERUM	LO	7.4	8.5-10.5	mg/dL
PHOSPHORUS	LO	2.8	3.0-4.6	mg/dL
URIC ACID	LO	3.2	3.5-7.2	mg/dL
CHOLESTEROL	LO	123	151-240	mg/dL
TRIGLYCERIDE		121	58-258	mg/dL
LDH		217	118-242	IU/L
SGOT (AST)	HI	41	10-37	IU/L
SGPT (ALT)	HI	45	10-40	IU/L
GGTP	LO	8	11-51	IU/L
ALKALINE PHOSPHATASE		63	39-117	IU/L
BILIRUBIN, TOTAL		0.3	0.1-1.5	mg/dL
ALBUMIN	LO	2.4	3.7-5.2	g/dL
TOTAL PROTEIN	LO	3.6	6.0-8.5	g/dL
ALBUMIN/GLOBULIN RATIO		2.0	1.0-2.2	RATIO

Fig. 6-12 Example of an abnormal metabolic panel report. Notice the second column indicating if an analyte is *"HI"* or *"LO"* as compared to its reference range. *(From Zakus SM:* Mosby's clinical skills for medical assistants, *ed 4, St Louis, 2001, Mosby.)*

pH. The most common electrolytes measured in the serum are the following:

- K+ and Na+, two positively charged ions, or **cations**
- Cl− and HCO$_3$−, two negatively charged ions, or **anions**

Hepatic Panel

The hepatic panel is a series of tests to determine liver function and damage. The liver is involved in the following metabolic functions:

- It metabolizes glucose from the gastrointestinal tract into stored glycogen.
- It metabolizes amino acids from the gastrointestinal tract into plasma proteins—albumin, some globulins, and the clotting proteins (fibrinogen and prothrombin).

- It metabolizes fatty acids from the gastrointestinal tract into the various blood lipids.
- It processes bilirubin, a waste product from the breakdown of hemoglobin, and excretes it in the bile.
- When the liver is impaired, the blood chemistry will reflect *increases* in bilirubin levels and *decreased* levels of albumins and clotting proteins owing to the impairment of protein production. However, significant impaired liver function must be present for these analytes to show abnormality. Therefore a liver panel will also include a series of enzyme tests to help determine whether the liver is damaged.
- Enzymes are usually located within the cells of organs and tissues. Enzymes are catalysts that assist in the particular metabolic changes required of the

Fig. 6-13 Myocardial infarction enzyme patterns seen in the blood during the 9 days after a heart attack. *(From Stepp CA, Woods M:* Laboratory procedures for medical office personnel, *Philadelphia, 1998, Saunders.)*

cells. An enzyme's name always ends with the suffix *-ase*. The word root preceding the *-ase* explains the chemical reaction in which the enzyme is involved. When a tissue or organ is damaged, it releases its specific enzymes into the blood. Because the liver is involved in so many intracellular metabolic reactions, levels of all the following enzymes may become elevated in the blood when it is damaged:

- Alkaline phosphatase (alk phos, **ALP**, or **AP**)
- Gamma-glutamyltransferase (**GGT**)
- Aspartate aminotransferase (AST)
- Alanine aminotransferase (ALT)
- Lactic acid dehydrogenase (**LD**)

Patients who are taking medications (e.g., statin drugs that lower blood cholesterol) may have their ALT or AST levels tested to see if the liver is being damaged by the medication. Other damaged organs may release some of these enzymes as well. Once again, the physician must interpret the chemical results along with the complete clinical picture of the patient before making a definitive diagnosis.

Cardiac Panel

When the heart is injured, as in a myocardial infarction (heart attack), it releases the following into the blood:

- **Troponins I and T**—muscle proteins that, when elevated, are excellent heart-specific indicators of a recent myocardial infarction.
- Creatine kinase (**CK or CPK**)—an enzyme found in muscle and brain tissue that is elevated soon after the heart is damaged. Two other heart enzymes, LD (LDH) and AST (SGOT), are also elevated. Figure 6-13 illustrates the cardiac enzyme pattern typical of patients with myocardial infarction.
- **Myoglobin** is an iron-containing, oxygen-binding protein found in muscles (similar to hemoglobin in

RBCs) that is also elevated in blood after a myocardial infarction.

Thyroid Panel

The thyroid gland plays a critical role in body metabolism by producing two hormones: thyroxine (T_4) and triiodothyronine (T_3). Their production is regulated by the pituitary gland, which releases thyroid-stimulating hormone (**TSH**). A panel of these analytes—TSH, T_4, and T_3 uptake—would be ordered to help in the diagnosis of an overactive or underactive thyroid gland. The T_3 uptake is a test that measures the amount of iodine that is "taken up" to synthesize the T_3 hormone.

Individual Analytes and Their Disease Associations

The laboratory requisition, as previously seen in Figure 6-3 at the beginning of the chapter, listed many individual tests that can be ordered, as well as the panels of tests. Individual tests are preferred over panels once the diagnosis is made and the condition requires frequent monitoring. Table 6-3 lists the most common chemistry tests categorically, their expected ranges, and the possible disease associations if the test results are high or low.

Summary

Because blood chemistry is so crucial to diagnosis and patient care, technology will continue to provide POLs with new and improved, user-friendly chemical testing analyzers. Be sure to stay informed through local diagnostic test suppliers and the Internet for the latest in chemistry testing. The websites for each of the CLIA-waived testing methods presented in this chapter are also listed. Review the latest news at each site, as well as their educational departments and their demonstration videos.

Table 6-3   Common Chemistry Panels and Possible Disease Associations

Test	Expected Range (Note: The exact ranges will vary due to testing method, population, location, etc.)	POSSIBLE DISEASE ASSOCIATIONS	
		High Levels	Low Levels
Renal Panel—Kidney			
BUN (blood urea nitrogen)	8-26 mg/dL	Impaired kidney function Acute renal failure Cardiovascular failure Obstruction of urine flow	No clinical significance
BUN/creatinine ratio	10-20	Prerenal impairment Dehydration Congestive heart failure Gastrointestinal bleed	Renal tubular necrosis
Creatinine	0.7-1.4 mg/dL	Impaired kidney function Acute glomerulonephritis Obstruction of urine flow	No clinical significance
Uric acid	3.6-8 mg/dL (male subjects) 2.5-6.78 mg/dL (female subjects)	Gout Decreased renal function Emotional stress Total fasting	Use of some drugs
Electrolytes			
Chloride	98-108 mmol/L	Congestive heart failure Dehydration Cushing's disease Diabetes insipidus Severe hyperaldosteronism	Nephritis Diuretic administration Starvation Severe vomiting Severe hypoaldosteronism
Potassium	3.5-5.3 mmol/L	Urinary obstruction Renal failure Ketoacidosis Hypoaldosteronism	Diarrhea Diuretic administration Starvation Hyperaldosteronism Renal tubular defects
Sodium	135-146 mmol/L	Severe dehydration Brain injuries Diabetic coma Cushing's disease Hyperaldosteronism Lack of ADH Renal failure	Metabolic acidosis Diarrhea Renal tubular disease Polyuria Addison's disease Overhydration Hypoaldosteronism Renal SIADH
Hepatic—Liver			
Bilirubin	0.1-1.2 mg/dL	Massive hemolysis Obstructive jaundice Cirrhosis Carcinoma Renal calculi	No clinical significance

Table 6-3 **Common Chemistry Panels and Possible Disease Associations—cont'd**

Test	Expected Range (Note: The exact ranges will vary due to testing method, population, location, etc.)	POSSIBLE DISEASE ASSOCIATIONS	
		High Levels	Low Levels
Hepatic—Liver—cont'd			
A/G ratio (albumin/globulin ratio)	1.1-2.5	No clinical significance	Viral hepatitis
			Ulcerative colitis
			Burns
			Multiple myeloma
			Sarcoidosis
			Metastatic carcinoma
			Nephrotic syndrome
			Diabetic ketosis
			Congestive heart failure
Albumin	3.5-5.0 g/dL	Dehydration	Impaired synthesis (cirrhosis, hepatitis)
			Hemorrhage
			Acute nephritis
			Protein-losing gastroenteropathies
			Inadequate protein intake
			Excessive protein breakdown
			Burns
Globulin	1.7-3.5 g/dL	Chronic active hepatitis	No clinical significance
		Multiple myeloma	
		Hodgkin's disease	
		Collagen disease	
		Tuberculosis	
		Brucellosis	
		Sarcoidosis	
Protein	6-8.5 g/dL	Multiple myeloma	Impaired kidney function
		Dehydration	
		Vomiting	
		Diarrhea	
Blood Enzymes			
ALP (alkaline phosphatase)	117-390 units/L (child)	Obstructive jaundice	Scurvy
	39-117 units/L (adult)	Paget's disease	
		Rickets	
		Osteomalacia	
		Hepatocellular disease	
		Biliary obstruction	
		Cirrhosis	
AST (SGOT) aspartate transaminase	0-37 units/L (male)	Myocardial dysfunction	No clinical significance
	0-31 units/L (female)	Acute hepatitis	
		Cirrhosis	
		Mononucleosis	

(Continued)

Table 6-3   Common Chemistry Panels and Possible Disease Associations—cont'd

Test	Expected Range (Note: The exact ranges will vary due to testing method, population, location, etc.)	POSSIBLE DISEASE ASSOCIATIONS	
		High Levels	Low Levels
Blood Enzymes—cont'd			
ALT (SGPT) alanine transaminase	0-40 units/L (male) 0-31 units/L (female)	Viral hepatitis Biliary obstruction	No clinical significance
CK (creatine kinase)	10-90 units/L (depending on method of testing)	Myocardial infarction Duchenne's muscular dystrophy	No clinical significance
GGT (gamma-glutamyltransferase)	11-50 units/L (male) 7-32 units/L (female)	Cirrhosis Congestive heart failure Alcoholism Obstructive jaundice Hepatocellular disease	No clinical significance
LD or LDH (lactic acid dehydrogenase)	118-242 units/L (male) 122-220 units/L (female)	Myocardial infarction Hemolytic anemia Acute leukemia Hepatic disease Pulmonary infarction	No clinical significance
Minerals			
Calcium	8.5-10.5 mg/dL	Dehydration Myeloma Hyperparathyroiditis Sarcoidosis Bone metastases Leukemia Lymphoma Paget's disease Acute renal failure Hypervitaminosis D Addison's disease	Regional enteritis Ulcerative colitis Diarrhea Hypoparathyroidism Cushing's disease Pancreatitis Malabsorption Malnutrition Rickets Tetany (neonates) Vitamin D deficiency Some renal and intestinal disorders
Phosphorus	2.5-4.5 mg/dL	Addison's disease Hypervitaminosis D Acromegaly Hypoparathyroidism Chronic renal failure	Hyperparathyroidism Vitamin D deficiency Rickets Malabsorption IDDM
Iron	40-160 mcg/dL	Hemolytic anemia Hemochromatosis Increased release from body stores Decreased use of iron (e.g., lead poisoning) Sideroblastic anemia	Iron deficiency anemia Pregnancy Insufficient dietary intake of iron

Table 6-3 Common Chemistry Panels and Possible Disease Associations—cont'd

Test	Expected Range (Note: The exact ranges will vary due to testing method, population, location, etc.)	POSSIBLE DISEASE ASSOCIATIONS	
		High Levels	Low Levels
Blood Gases			
Carbon dioxide	Dependent on method and if blood is arterial or venous	Aldosteronism Respiratory acidosis Metabolic alkalosis	Diarrhea Metabolic acidosis Respiratory alkalosis
Metabolism			
Cholesterol	140-200 mg/dL LDL <100 mg/dL HDL >50 mg/dL	Atherosclerotic disease Alcoholism Defects in lipoprotein metabolism Hypothyroidism Diabetes mellitus	Malnutrition
Glucose	65-100 mg/dL	Diabetes mellitus (hyperglycemia) Cushing's disease	Hypoglycemia Addison's disease
Triglycerides	30-150 mg/dL	Atherosclerotic disease Alcoholism Hyperlipidemia Hypothyroidism Pancreatic disorders Diabetes mellitus (poorly controlled)	Malnutrition

ADH, Antidiuretic hormone; *IDDM*, insulin-dependent diabetes mellitus; *SIADH*, syndrome of inappropriate secretion of antidiuretic hormone.

Review Questions

1. What type of specimen is required for most blood chemistry tests in the POL (hint: think of the waived tests)? When collecting blood for a reference laboratory?

2. When plasma glucose level is high, what hormone is secreted?

3. What percentage of diabetes mellitus cases in the United States are type 2, or non–insulin-dependent cases?

4. The presence of sugar in the urine is called

   _____.

5. A type of blood glucose test that requires no special fasting or other preparation is the
   a. GTT.
   b. fasting glucose.
   c. 2-hour postprandial glucose.
   d. random glucose test.

6. Explain the reason for testing Hgb A_{1c}.

7. List the two main sources of cholesterol in the blood.

8. Why is LDL cholesterol referred to as "lousy" cholesterol and HDL referred to as "healthy" cholesterol?

9. What is the purpose of calibrating a blood chemistry analyzer?

10. List three reasons that a control would not fall within its designated range.

11. List the ranges for each of the following total cholesterol categories:
    a. desirable cholesterol level:
    b. low-risk cholesterol level:
    c. high cholesterol level:

12. Match the following:
    _____ LDL
    _____ HDL
    _____ glycogen
    _____ hypoglycemia
    _____ hyperglycemia
    _____ lipoprotein

    a. an abnormal increase in the glucose level in the blood
    b. a complex molecule consisting of protein and a fat such as cholesterol
    c. the form in which carbohydrate is stored in the body
    d. a lipoprotein consisting of protein and cholesterol that removes excess cholesterol from blood vessel walls
    e. an abnormally low level of glucose in the blood
    f. a lipoprotein consisting of protein and cholesterol that adheres to blood vessel walls, forming plaque

13. What is the main reason for performing the fecal occult blood test? List the three methods for testing fecal occult blood.

14. Match the blood chemistry profiles for the various body organs or diseases with their corresponding chemistry tests:
    ___ renal profile
    ___ liver profile
    ___ cardiac profile
    ___ lipid profile
    ___ gout

    a. uric acid
    b. BUN, creatinine, uric acid, electrolytes
    c. CK, LDL, AST (SGOT), and lipids
    d. bilirubin, alkaline phosphatase, albumin, globulin, ALT (SGPT)
    e. cholesterol, LDL, HDL, triglycerides

Websites

American Diabetes Association:
www.diabetes.org/home

Bayer Contour information:
www.bayercontour.com/Blood-Glucose-Monitoring/Product-Portfolio

Demonstration video on how to use the LifeScan OneTouch Ultra glucose monitor from Johnson & Johnson:
www.lifescan.com

Training video on how to run the Cholestech LDX:
www.cholestech.com/support/ldx_training.htm

i-STAT information:
www.abbottpointofcare.com/istat/www/products/Cartridge_Brochure.pdf
www.codemap.com/abbott

Information on iFOB testing:
www.quidel.com/assets/swf/iFOBTrainingvideoHQ.htm

Piccolo Xpress information:
www.abaxis.com/medical/

Excellent physician office resource for lab equipment and supplies:
www.physiciansofficeresource.com/physicians/physician-office-lab.asp

7

Immunology

OBJECTIVES   *After completing this chapter you should be able to do the following:*

1. Define and match key terms in this chapter.

Fundamental Concepts

2. Explain the following concepts related to the immune process:
   - List the three lines of defense against harmful invaders.
   - Differentiate between cell-mediated immunity and humoral immunity.
   - Match the classes of immunoglobulins (antibodies) with their locations and/or functions.
   - List the four ways to acquire adaptive (acquired) immunity.
3. Discuss the principles of in vivo and in vitro immunology tests as they relate to allergy testing.

CLIA-Waived Immunology Tests

4. Give examples of direct and indirect immunology tests based on the detection of antigens or antibodies.
5. Describe mononucleosis, *H. pylori, and HIV infections,* and explain how they are diagnosed.
6. Perform the following CLIA-waived immunology tests according to the stated task, conditions, and standards listed in the Learning Outcome Procedure Sheets in the student workbook:
   - Pregnancy test
   - Infectious mononucleosis test
   - *Helicobacter pylori* test
   - HIV blood and/or oral test

Advanced Concepts

7. Discuss advanced immunological techniques such as agglutination, enzyme-linked immunosorbent assay, and chromatographic immunoassay.
8. Explain the basic principles of ABO and Rh blood typing, and discuss the relationship between hemolytic disease of the newborn and the Rh negative status of the mother.
9. Explain how antibody titers are used by physicians in the diagnosis and prognosis of disease conditions.
10. Identify common immunology tests within three categories: bacterial infections, viral infections, and detection of other antigens such as hormones and cancer-related substances.

KEY TERMS

active immunity long-term protection against future infections resulting from the production of antibodies that were formed naturally during a specific infection or artificially by vaccination

agglutination clumping of blood cells or latex beads caused by antibodies adhering to their antigens

allergen an antigen that causes an allergic reaction

antibodies immunoglobulins produced specifically to destroy foreign invaders (antigens)

antigens substances that are perceived as foreign to the body and elicit an antibody response

autoimmune diseases destructive tissue diseases caused by antibody/self-antigen reactions

cell-mediated immunity T lymphocytic cell response to antigens

chromatographic pertaining to a visual color change that appears when an enzyme-linked antibody/antigen reaction takes place

complement proteins proteins that stimulate phagocytosis and inflammation and are capable of destroying bacteria

erythroblastosis fetalis a hemolytic anemia in newborns resulting from maternal-fetal blood group incompatibility

helper T cells (TH4 or CD4) antigen-activated lymphocytes that stimulate other T cells and help B cells produce their antibodies

heterophile antibody antibody that appears during an Epstein-Barr viral infection (mononucleosis) and has an unusual affinity to antigens on sheep red cells

histamine compound released by injured cells that causes the dilation of blood vessels

humoral immunity B lymphocytic cell response to antigens resulting in the production of specific antibodies to destroy a foreign invader; also called antibody-mediated immunity

iFOB (immunoassay Fecal Occult Blood) new method for testing fecal occult blood

immunosorbent pertaining to the attachment of an antigen or antibody to a solid surface such as latex beads, wells in plastic dishes, or plastic cartridges

inflammation overall reaction of the body to tissue injury or invasion by an infectious agent, characterized by redness, heat, swelling, and pain

interferons proteins secreted by infected cells to prevent the further replication and spread of an infection into neighboring cells

in vitro within a laboratory apparatus

in vivo within a host or living organism

killer T cells antigen-activated lymphocytes that attack foreign antigens directly and destroy cells that bear the antigens; also called cytotoxic cells

memory B cells antigen-activated B lymphocytes that remember an identified antigen for future encounters

memory T cells antigen-activated T lymphocytes that remember an antigen for future encounters

mucous membrane thin sheets of tissue that line the internal cavities and canals of the body and serve as a barrier against the entry of pathogens into the body

natural killer cells special type of lymphocyte that attacks and destroys infected cells and cancer cells in a nonspecific way

normal flora nonpathogenic microorganisms that normally inhabit the skin and mucous membranes

passive immunity short-term acquired immunity created by antibodies received naturally through the placenta and the colostrum (first breast milk) to an infant, or received artificially by injection

phagocytes cells capable of engulfing, ingesting, and destroying microorganisms and cellular debris

phagocytosis process of engulfing, digesting, and destroying microorganisms and cellular debris

plasma cells a subgroup of B lymphocytes that produce the antibodies that travel through the blood specifically targeting and reacting with antigens

self-antigens substances within the body that induce the production of antibodies that attack an individual's own body tissues; also called autoantigens; they may result in an autoimmune disease

serology branch of laboratory medicine that performs antibody/antigen testing with serum

suppressor T cells antigen-activated lymphocytes that inhibit T and B cells after a sufficient number of cells have been activated

titer a quantitative test that measures the amount of antibody that reacts with a specific antigen

vaccination process of injecting harmless or killed microorganisms into the body to induce immunity against a potential pathogen (also called immunization)

wheal raised induration (hardened tissue), such as a hive caused by an antibody/antigen reaction

👁 Fundamental Concepts

Overview of Immunology

The immune system is a remarkable defense system that protects the human body against invading pathogens, toxins, allergens, and cancer cells. When the body is under attack by any of these invaders, it has a full arsenal of defenses to destroy the invader, as well as protect itself from future attacks. A key ingredient in this defense mechanism is the body's production of **antibodies** (immunoglobulins produced specifically to destroy foreign invaders). These antibodies are produced after the body detects the presence of specific **antigens** (substances that are perceived as foreign to the body). Once antibodies are produced, they attack the antigens, forming an antibody/antigen complex that destroys or renders the invader harmless.

Biotechnology research has made it possible to detect and measure specific antibodies and their specific antigens in blood and body fluids. Antibody/antigen testing is a rapidly expanding laboratory science called *immunology*. Because antibodies are usually found in serum, the laboratory department performing antibody/antigen testing may also be referred to as the **serology** *department*.

The science of immunology dates to the 1500s, when it was recorded that China had developed a technique of exposing individuals to a powder made from smallpox scabs to produce protection against the disease. The thought was that if children or young adults were exposed in a healthy state, the disease would not be as devastating; unfortunately, that did not always occur. In the late 1700s, Edward Jenner, an English country doctor, found that injecting individuals with material from cowpox provided effective protection against smallpox. This preventive process of injecting harmless or killed microorganisms into the body to induce immunity against a potential pathogen was known as **vaccination** or immunization.

The field of immunology has benefited from a tremendous amount of new research and subsequent knowledge over the past 100 years. In fact, the cells responsible for the body's immune response were not discovered until the 1960s. Another recent finding is that the body may respond to **self-antigens** (substances within the body that induce the production of antibodies that attack an individual's own body tissues; also called *autoantigens*). Antibody/self-antigen reactions may cause a variety of destructive tissue diseases referred to as **autoimmune diseases**.

The Immune Process

The overall immune process that occurs as the body protects itself against foreign invaders can be viewed as three lines (or battlefields) of defensive mechanisms. Figure 7-1 is a simplified picture of these lines of defense. The foreign invaders are portrayed at the top of the flow chart. Their goal is to enter the body and cause destruction. The first two lines of defense are considered "nonspecific immunity"—nonspecific because they fight all invaders in the same way. The third line of defense, at the bottom of the illustration, is referred to as "specific immunity" because it intelligently identifies each invader on the basis of its specific antigens. The B cells are then able to produce a specific antibody capable of destroying the invader.

First Line of Defense: Natural Barriers

The first line of defense stops invaders from entering or growing on the body. The skin and **mucous membrane** (thin sheets of tissue lining the internal cavities and canals) serve as anatomical barriers that prevent the entry of pathogens into the body. They also secrete chemicals that discourage the growth of pathogenic bacteria. These secretions maintain a skin pH of 5.6, which allows the growth of **normal flora** (nonpathogenic microorganisms that normally inhabit the skin and mucous membranes) while inhibiting the growth of pathogens. In the respiratory tract the mucous membranes contain mucus, which entraps foreign organisms. Coughing and sneezing help move foreign organisms out of the body.

Second Line of Defense: Nonspecific Internal Response

The second line of defense is the internal nonspecific response to all invaders that have passed the natural barriers and entered the body. When invaders break through the barriers, the body quickly responds by sending **phagocytes** (cells capable of engulfing, ingesting, and destroying pathogens and cellular debris) to the site of invasion. Two white blood cells—neutrophils and monocytes (which become macrophages in the tissue)—engulf, ingest, and destroy the invaders by the process of **phagocytosis**.

Natural killer cells are a special type of lymphocyte sent to the scene of invasion to attack and destroy the body's infected cells and cancer cells in a nonspecific way. Protective proteins such as interferons and complement proteins also play an important role at

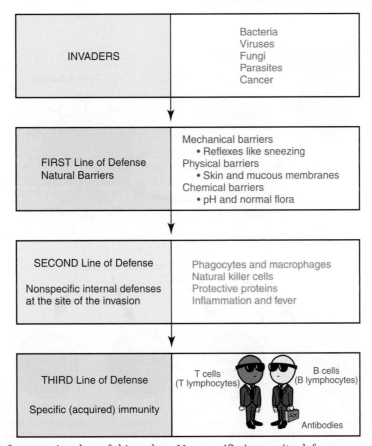

Fig. 7-1 Three lines of defense against harmful invaders. Nonspecific immunity defenses are external barriers, and then internal responses to the invaders. Specific immunity (the third line of defense) involves "intelligent" T cells, B cells, and the production of antibodies. *(Modified from Herlihy M: The human body in health and illness, ed 5, St Louis, 2014, Saunders.)*

the site of invasion. **Interferons** are proteins secreted by infected cells to prevent the further replication and spread of the infection into neighboring cells. **Complement proteins** are proteins that further stimulate phagocytosis and **inflammation** (reaction of the body to tissue injury or invasion by an infectious agent) and are capable of destroying bacteria. Complement proteins swarm over a bacterium and punch holes in its membrane, causing it to fill with fluid and explode.

At the same time that these defenders are doing their jobs to destroy the invader, the injured tissues are initiating a nonspecific *inflammatory* response. The clinical signs of inflammation are heat, redness, swelling, and pain. Inflammation begins when **histamine** is released by the injured cells, causing the dilation of blood vessels. The increased blood flow to the affected areas results in redness and heat. Fluids in the plasma leak into the tissue because of the increased permeability of the vessels, causing the swelling and pain.

The second line of defense is generally seen within the first 12 hours of an infection. For example, the first signs and symptoms of influenza start with swollen glands, sore throat, chills, and fever. These symptoms are the result of an active nonspecific battle against the invaders consisting of the phagocytes, natural killer cells, and protective proteins and the subsequent inflammatory response.

Third Line of Defense: Acquired (Adaptive) Immunity

The third line of defense is activated when the first two lines have failed to bring the invasion under control. It is the "intelligent" identification of the invader based on its antigenic properties. The T cells and B cells work together to produce the specific antibodies that will destroy the invader or render it harmless. This adaptive process takes 6 to 10 days to accomplish. The T and B cells are also capable of developing immunological memory so that a second encounter with the same organism will induce a heightened immune reaction.

Both these intelligent lymphocytes provide different immunological functions, as described in the following sections.

Cell-Mediated Immunity. T cells, small lymphocytes associated with the thymus gland, are involved in **cell-mediated immunity**. They become involved at the site of the invasion, where they become activated after they receive an antigen presentation from the macrophages (Figure 7-2).

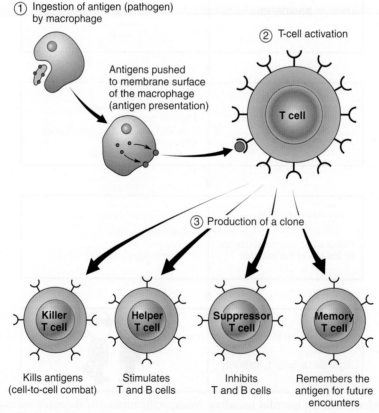

① Ingestion of antigen (pathogen) by macrophage

② T-cell activation

Antigens pushed to membrane surface of the macrophage (antigen presentation)

T cell

③ Production of a clone

Killer T cell

Helper T cell

Suppressor T cell

Memory T cell

Kills antigens (cell-to-cell combat)

Stimulates T and B cells

Inhibits T and B cells

Remembers the antigen for future encounters

Fig. 7-2 Activation of T cells from the antigens provided by the macrophage resulting in cell-mediated immunity. The three-step process results in four subsets of T cells. *(From Herlihy M: The human body in health and illness, ed 5, St Louis, 2014, Saunders.)*

Once activated, T cells rapidly duplicate themselves into clones that differentiate into the following four subgroups:

1. **Killer T cells**, or cytotoxic cells (TC), are antigen-activated lymphocytes that attack foreign antigens directly and destroy cells that bear the antigens.
2. **Helper T cells** (TH4 or CD4) stimulate other T cells and help B cells produce their antibodies. (These are the cells infected by the human immunodeficiency virus [HIV].)
3. **Suppressor T cells** (TS) inhibit the T and B cells after a sufficient number of cells have been activated.
4. **Memory T cells** remember the antigen for future encounters. They are ready to respond to subsequent exposure to the specific antigens with increased speed and intensity.

Of the lymphocytes circulating in the blood, 70% to 80% are T cells.

Humoral Immunity (Antibody-Mediated Immunity). B cells are involved in **humoral immunity**. Humoral immunity begins with the interaction of a B cell with a specific antigen and the lymphokine (chemicals) from the T helper cell (Figure 7-3).

Once it is activated, it rapidly duplicates into a clone and differentiates into the following two subgroups:

1. **Plasma cells** produce the antibodies (immunoglobulins) that travel through the blood specifically targeting and reacting with the antigens, resulting in the destruction of the invader.
2. **Memory B cells** remember the antigen for future encounters. They also are ready to respond to subsequent exposure to the specific antigens with increased speed and intensity.

Classes of Antibodies (Immunoglobulins). Biomedical researchers have found that antibodies are part of the globulin group of proteins that circulate in the blood. Because of their globulin properties, antibodies are referred to as *immunoglobulins (Ig)*. The researchers have classified immunoglobulins into the following groups, based on their shapes, locations, and functions:

- IgE are the immunoglobulins involved in acute allergic reactions.
- IgM are the primary responders in the first encounter with an invading antigen.
- IgG respond to the antigens and allergens in subsequent invading or allergic encounters.
- IgA protect mucous membranes from bacterial and viral infections.
- IgD are involved in lymphocyte activation and suppression.

Ways to Acquire Specific Immunity. Once a specific antibody is present in the blood, the individual is said to be immune to its particular disease, pathogen,

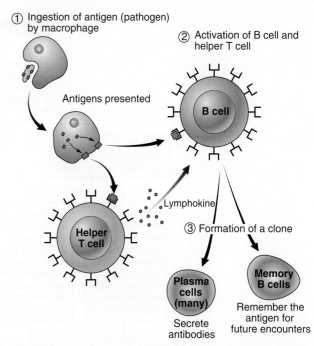

① Ingestion of antigen (pathogen) by macrophage

② Activation of B cell and helper T cell

Antigens presented

B cell

Helper T cell

Lymphokine

③ Formation of a clone

Plasma cells (many)
Secrete antibodies

Memory B cells
Remember the antigen for future encounters

Fig. 7-3 Activation of B cells by antigens and T helper cells resulting in humoral (antibody) immunity. The three-step process results in the production of antibodies by the plasma cells. *(From Herlihy M: The human body in health and illness, ed 5, St Louis, 2014, Saunders.)*

or antigen. There are four ways to acquire specific immunity: (1) active immunity acquired naturally, (2) active immunity acquired artificially, (3) passive immunity acquired naturally, and (4) passive immunity acquired artificially (Figure 7-4).

Active immunity is long-term protection against future infections that results from the production of antibodies that were formed naturally during an infection or artificially by vaccination. In both cases the antibody is remembered in the memory B cells, making the individual immune to future encounters with the pathogen.

Passive immunity is short-term protection against infections created by antibodies received naturally through the placenta (or the colostrum to an infant) or artificially by the injection of antiserum or gamma globulins. Passive immunity is only temporary.

Two Types of Allergy Testing

In Vivo Testing

The body is capable of overreacting to antigens by producing too many antibodies (immunoglobulins), resulting in allergic or autoimmune conditions such as asthma, hives, breathing difficulties, and gastrointestinal inflammation. Allergy tests have been performed to visualize the specific reaction between an **allergen** (an antigen that causes an allergic reaction) and its specific antibody. Tests are done **in vivo** (within a host or living organism) by injecting or pricking an antigen

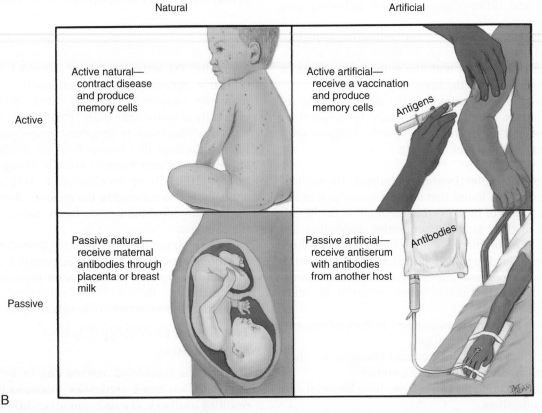

Fig. 7-4 **A,** Forms of acquired humoral (antibody) immunity and their ability to provide permanent or temporary immunity. **B,** Examples of the four combinations of active/passive immunity and natural/artificial immunity. (**A** *from Stepp CA, Woods M:* Laboratory procedures for medical office personnel, *Philadelphia, 1998, Saunders;* **B** *from Applegate EJ:* The anatomy and physiology learning system, *ed 4, St Louis, 2011, Saunders.)*

| NEG | ±1 | +1 | +2 | +3 | +4 |

Fig. 7-5 In vivo antibody/antigen test, with negative and positive skin reactions to an antigen. If the patient has the specific antibodies that react with the injected antigen, a wheal (raised induration) forms. *(From Bonewit-West K:* Clinical procedures for medical assistants, *ed 9, St Louis, 2015, Saunders.)*

into the skin and seeing whether a **wheal** (raised induration or hardened tissue, such as a hive) forms in response to the antibody/antigen reaction. Figure 7-5 shows a negative reaction and various positive reactions to skin tests. Tuberculosis screening tests and allergy skin tests are examples of in vivo immunology tests.

In Vitro Testing

Laboratory immunology tests (also referred to as *serology tests*) are now being performed **in vitro** (within the laboratory test tube) outside of the body. It is now possible to test the antigen/antibody reaction using only the serum from a tube of blood. Through this testing method, a multiwell plate is coated with various food proteins and/or inhalants that are possible allergens capable of causing allergic reactions. The patient's serum is then added to each well. If the patient's serum contains IgE or IgG antibodies to any of the specific food or inhalant proteins, a binding reaction occurs. The degree of antibody-antigen binding depends on the concentration of antibodies present in the patient's serum. The reaction is then detected through a color change and assessed spectrophotometrically. The wells showing a strong reaction and high level of IgG immunoglobulins will indicate an allergic response to the items in the wells. A typical serological food panel test will indicate possible allergies in the following food groups: gluten, peanuts, dairy, meat/fowl, fruits, fish/crustacea/mollusk, grains, vegetables, spices, and herbs.

CLIA-Waived Immunology Tests

CLIA-Waived Enzyme-Linked Immunoassays

Manufacturers produce a large variety of immunology testing devices. In most of these rapid screening tests, a liquid specimen is absorbed and travels across a testing area that enzymatically changes color if an antibody/antigen reaction takes place. The tests typically include an internal control that must also change color to prove the testing device is working. The control area is usually located just beyond the test area to make sure the solution has traveled all the way through the test area. This method is often referred to as a *lateral flow immunochromatographic assay*. Figure 7-6 shows the before and after reactions of a positive and a negative urine pregnancy test.

The presence of specific antibodies and/or antigens associated with a specific disease can be detected in the blood or other body specimens by mixing them with their specific antigen or antibody and observing a reaction. The test kits usually provide a visual reaction when the antibody/antigen complex is formed. Biotechnology continues to develop numerous CLIA-waived test kits designed to rapidly detect the presence of an antigen (direct test) or an antibody (indirect test) associated with a particular disease or infection. These screening tests are usually displayed and interpreted **chromatographically** (pertaining to a visual color change that appears when the enzyme-linked antibody/antigen reaction takes place).

Table 7-1 lists the common CLIA-waived tests that use the lateral flow method to detect the presence of an antigen or antibody associated with a specific disease or condition. Some test kits provide the antibody and test for its antigen in the specimen (direct tests). Other test kits provide the antigen and test for its specific antibody in the specimen (indirect tests). In both cases a color reaction occurs if both antibody and antigen are present, and the results are recorded as positive. If the color reaction does not occur in the test area, the result is recorded as negative. Also note that if a color does not develop in the internal control area, the patient's result is invalid, and the test must be repeated.

A variety of test kits are available for CLIA-waived screening tests for pregnancy, mononucleosis, *Helicobacter pylori* infections, HIV, and the new **iFOB** (immunoassay fecal occult blood) method for testing fecal occult blood (as seen in Chapter 6). NOTE: This

Fig. 7-6 In vitro pregnancy test showing the lateral flow immunochromatographic test method. **A,** Test device before adding specimen (*S,*= specimen is placed in well; *T,*= specimen travels through test area; *C,*= control must turn color to prove device is functioning correctly). **B, Positive** result in test area and control area (two pink bands). **C, Negative** result in test area and positive reaction in control area.

Table 7-1	Common CLIA-Waived Tests That Use the Lateral Flow Method	
WHEN BOTH ANTIGEN AND ANTIBODY ARE PRESENT → POSITIVE RESULT		
Screening Tests	**Antigens (When Testing for Antigen in Specimen = Direct Test)**	**Antibodies (When Testing for Antibody in Specimen = Indirect Test)**
Pregnancy	HCG from mother's placenta in urine specimen (Direct)	Anti-HCG antibodies in test kit
Bladder tumor–associated antigen (BTA)	BTA from bladder cancer in urine specimen (Direct)	Monoclonal antibodies in test kit react with BTA
Mononucleosis	Heterophile antigens in test kit	IgM heterophile antibody produced against EBV found in blood specimen (Indirect)
Helicobacter pylori	*H. pylori* antigens in test kit	IgG antibodies specific against *H. pylori* found in blood specimen (Indirect)
HIV	HIV-1 antigens in test kit	Antibodies against HIV-1 found in blood or cheek cells (Indirect)
Immunoassay for fecal occult blood (iFOB)*	Blood from fecal matter (Direct)	Immunochemical color reaction occurs if positive
Influenza A and B†	Viral antigens from nasal swab specimen (Direct)	Antiviral antibodies in test kit
Streptococcus A infection†	Streptococcal antigen extracted from throat swab (Direct)	Antistreptococcal antibodies in test kit
Drug testing in urine‡	Drug will inhibit immune reaction	Reaction does *not* appear in test area if positive

EBV, Epstein-Barr virus; *HCG,* human chorionic gonadotropin; *HIV,* human immunodeficiency virus.
*iFOB was covered in Chapter 6.
†Antigenic direct testing for the presence of influenza A and B infection and streptococcus A infection is covered in Chapter 8.
‡Drug testing in urine is covered in Chapter 9.

text provides the directions that apply to the specific manufacturer's kits portrayed in the procedures. Never assume that the instructions from a new kit or a kit from another manufacturer are the same. The instructions packaged with each box of testing kits should be read thoroughly, followed, and saved as a reference for as long as there are kits to be tested with the box's lot number.

Pregnancy Testing

Pregnancy testing is based on the detection of a hormone called *human chorionic gonadotropin (HCG)*, which is found in urine or blood. HCG levels in blood and urine may detect pregnancy 1 to 5 days after conception. HCG is produced by the chorionic villi of the developing placenta, with levels peaking between the fiftieth and eightieth days of pregnancy. After this time the levels decline and remain at a lower level, and then disappear a few days after the birth.

The CLIA-waived immunoassay provides a qualitative detection of HCG. The test takes approximately 5 minutes to perform and is easy to read. The following points are important to remember:

- The urine specimen container must be free of detergents; a clean, disposable urine container is best for collection.
- A first morning urine specimen is recommended because it will contain the highest concentration of HCG. Specific gravity testing should be performed to determine if the urine specific gravity is more than 1.010. An overly diluted specimen with a specific gravity less than 1.010 could cause a false-negative result.
- The urine should be refrigerated if testing cannot be performed within an hour. The urine must be brought back to room temperature before testing.
- Follow the manufacturer's recommendations for storage of the kit. If the kit is refrigerated, it also must be brought to room temperature before testing.
- Do not use expired kits.
- Do not use the supplies or reagents from one kit with another kit.
- Test results will show "negative" or "positive," but be sure to chart "negative for pregnancy" or "positive for pregnancy."
- Observe Health Insurance Portability and Accountability Act (HIPAA) guidelines regarding patient confidentiality.
- Observe Occupational Safety and Health Administration (OSHA) guidelines when dealing with specimens.

The **SureStep Pregnancy Test** procedure check sheet is provided in the workbook and is demonstrated in Procedure 7-1, located at the end of this section.

Automated urine pregnancy testing is also available on the Clinitek instrument that was presented in

Fig. 7-7, A & B Automated pregnancy test. **A,** *(a)* Urinalysis normal liquid control (containing hCG pregnancy hormone); *(b)* Clinitek pregnancy test packet containing *(c)* a urine pipette; and *(d)* a test cartridge. **B,** Pregnancy cartridge placed on Clinitek instrument that will electronically test and record the results.

Chapter 3: Urinalysis. Figure 7-7, *A,* shows the urine liquid controls containing the HCG hormone; and the testing supplies that are used to prepare the pregnancy cartridge for testing on the Clinitek instrument seen in Figure 7-7, *B*.

Mononucleosis Testing

The causative agent of mononucleosis is the Epstein-Barr virus (EBV). The infection is often called the "kissing disease" because it is transmitted by direct oral contact through saliva. Mononucleosis is an acute infectious disease most frequently seen in children and young adults. *Clinical signs* and symptoms are mental and physical fatigue, severe weakness, headache, fever, sore throat, and swollen lymph nodes. *Hematological findings* may show an increase in the number of reactive lymphocytes. *Immunologically,* the antibody that is produced during EBV infection is called a **heterophile antibody**. This heterophile antibody has an unusual affinity for antigens on the red blood cells (RBCs) of sheep.

The heterophile antibody is produced by patients infected with mononucleosis usually by the fifth to eighth day after infection. Within 3 weeks of infection, 80% of the patients have a detectable level of heterophile antibodies. In the 20% of patients who do not produce the antibody, the diagnosis depends solely on the clinical and hematological findings. In the outpatient laboratory, rapid mononucleosis tests that detect heterophile antibodies are easy to perform and provide reliable results.

The **QuickVue+ Mononucleosis Test** Procedure check sheet is provided in the workbook and is demonstrated in Procedure 7-2 at the end of this section.

Helicobacter pylori Testing

H. pylori are spiral-shaped bacteria believed to be the cause of most peptic ulcers (90% of duodenal and 80% of gastric ulcers). This organism weakens the mucous lining of the stomach and duodenum. Stomach acids and bacteria are able to penetrate the sensitive lining beneath the mucous layer and cause an ulcer. Symptoms of an ulcer include a gnawing pain in the abdominal area a few hours after eating and during the night. These symptoms are relieved by eating and taking antacids. Ulcers are now being treated with antibiotic drugs that kill the *H. pylori* bacteria along with drugs that reduce the amount of stomach acid.

The **QuickVue+ *Helicobacter pylori* gII Test** procedure check sheet is provided in the workbook and is demonstrated in Procedure 7-3, located at the end of this section.

Human Immunodeficiency Virus

HIV attacks and destroys the T helper (CD4) lymphocytes. As previously stated in this chapter, the T helper cells play a critical role in protecting the body against infection by cell-mediated immunity. They also help the B cells produce their specific antibodies during humoral immunity. As more and more T helper cells are destroyed by the HIV infection, the body becomes less able to fight infections and becomes more susceptible to opportunistic infections. Acquired immunodeficiency syndrome (AIDS) is the condition that eventually occurs and is characterized by the presence of life-threatening infections and cancers (see Chapter 1 for more information on AIDS and this bloodborne pathogen).

At this time, there is no known cure once someone has an HIV infection. Therefore, in 2013 the CDC (Centers for Disease Control and Prevention) and WHO (World Health Organization) have both advised prevention measures to control the disease.

This requires early detection and early treatment of HIV-infected individuals. The sooner the virus is detected via immunological testing, the sooner treatment with antiretroviral (ARV) medications may begin. The current recommended treatment of just one tablet daily is able to keep the virus from duplicating and destroying the T cells, thereby halting the progression to AIDS and reducing the possibility of infecting others.

CLIA-waived HIV tests are now readily available to detect the presence of the HIV antibodies in blood and in oral specimens. The immunological tests for HIV are able to detect HIV infection 3 months after a risk event. A risk event is defined by any of the following list of activities:
- Sex (vaginal and/or oral) with multiple sex partners
- Sex with someone who is HIV positive or whose HIV status is unknown
- Sex between a man and another man
- Use of illegal injected drugs or steroids
- Use of shared needles or syringes
- Participation in exchanged sex for money
- Diagnosis or treatment for hepatitis, tuberculosis, or a sexually transmitted disease like syphilis

Patients who are "at risk" of HIV infection are now encouraged to take a 10- to 20-minute blood test in outpatient clinics and/or perform an oral self-test from a kit that is available at pharmacies.

Remember, HIV is a bloodborne pathogen. Therefore, it is critical that health care workers testing for HIV adhere to the OSHA Bloodborne Pathogens Standard to avoid exposure during the testing process. The CLIA-waived HIV blood and oral testing procedure check sheets are provided in the workbook and are demonstrated in Procedures 7-4 and 7-5 located at the end of this section.

In both testing methods, it is very important to provide the patient with information and/or counseling regarding HIV infection and its relationship to AIDS. They also need to understand the five possible test results (i.e., positive, negative, false positive, false negative, and invalid). Be aware that the patients being tested may be very fearful and that proper knowledge presented in a therapeutic way will help them dispel the fear and take positive action toward preventive behavior and treatment. Positive HIV tests will need to be verified at the hospital or reference laboratory using the enzyme-linked immunosorbent assay (ELISA) test, with a confirmatory test called the Western immunoblot method.

PROCEDURE 7-1 SureStep Pregnancy Test Procedure

A, SureStep pregnancy test. *a,* Test device; *b,* pipette; *c,* urine specimen.

B, SureStep pregnancy test results. *1,* Test device before adding specimen (*C,* control; *T,* specimen travels through test area; well: holds specimen); *2,* positive reactions in test area and control area (two pink bands); *3,* negative reaction in test area and positive reaction in control area.

(Continued)

PROCEDURE 7-1 SureStep Pregnancy Test Procedure—cont'd

Equipment and Supplies (Figure A)—Preanalytical

- Test device from foil package stored in SureStep box
- Pipette from foil-wrapped package
- Urine specimen
- Gloves *(not pictured)*

Procedure—Analytical

1. Sanitize the hands, and apply gloves.
2. Remove the test device from its protective pouch, and label it with the patient's identification. Bring it to room temperature before opening to prevent condensation.
3. Draw the urine sample to the line marked on the pipette, approximately 0.2 mL. Use separate pipettes and test devices for each specimen and control.
4. Dispense the entire contents of the pipette into the sample well.
5. Wait for the pink bands to appear.
   - High concentrations of HCG can be observed as soon as 40 seconds.
   - Low concentrations may need 5 minutes of reaction time.
   - Do not interpret results after 10 minutes.
6. At 5 minutes, read and record the results (Figure B).
   - Positive test result: Two distinct pink bands appear, one in the patient test region *(T)* and one in the control region *(C)*.
   - Negative test result: Only one pink band appears in the control region *(C)*. No pink band is apparent in the patient test region *(T)*.
   - Invalid: Pink band is absent from the control region. Repeat the test with a new device. If the problem persists, call for technical assistance.

Follow-Up—Postanalytical

7. Properly dispose of biohazard waste material, and disinfect the work area.
8. Remove personal protective equipment, and sanitize the hands.
9. Document patient and control results on lab log.

Quality Control Procedure

In addition to the internal control region built into the test device, external positive and negative liquid controls should be performed when a new kit is used. Also, each operator of the test should perform a positive and negative control once with each testing method to confirm that his or her testing technique is correct. The results of the control tests should be documented on the HCG control log.

The positive liquid control procedure is performed in the same way as the patient procedure, with a new pipette and testing device. Observe and record the results in 5 minutes. Repeat the procedure with a drop of well-mixed negative control.

✳ PROCEDURE 7-2 QuickVue+ Mononucleosis Test Procedure

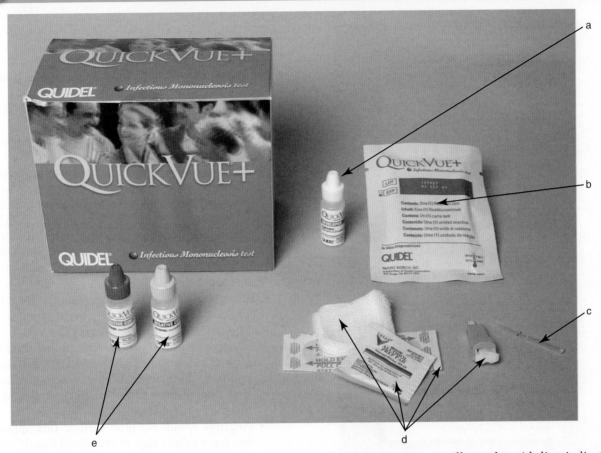

A, QuickVue+ infectious mononucleosis test kit. *a,* Developer; *b,* reaction unit; *c,* capillary tube with line indicating volume of blood; *d,* capillary puncture supplies; *e,* positive and negative external liquid controls.

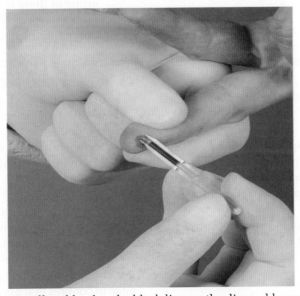

B, Collecting capillary blood to the black line on the disposable capillary tube.

(Continued)

PROCEDURE 7-2 QuickVue+ Mononucleosis Test Procedure—cont'd

C, Results of mononucleosis test. *1*, Reaction unit before testing; *2*, positive result and "test complete" result; *3*, negative result and "test complete" result.

Equipment and Supplies (Figures A and D)—Preanalytical

QuickVue+ mononucleosis test kit containing the following:

- Developer
- Individually wrapped reaction units
- Capillary tubes (for capillary specimens) and pipettes (for venous specimens)
- Capillary puncture supplies or venipuncture supplies
- Positive and negative liquid external control
- NOTE: the package insert is seen in Figure D

Procedure—Analytical

1. Sanitize the hands, and apply gloves.
2. Remove the test device from its protective pouch, and label it with the patient's identification.
3. Draw a capillary sample to the line marked on the capillary tube (Figure B).
   - If using whole blood from a venous specimen, use the pipette provided in the kit.
   - Use separate pipettes and devices for each specimen and the controls.
4. Dispense all the blood from the capillary tube into the "Add" well, or transfer a large drop from the venous whole blood specimen with the pipette.
5. Add 5 drops of developer to the "Add" well. Hold the bottle vertically above the well, and allow drops to fall freely.
6. Read the results at 5 minutes (Figure C). The "Test Complete" line must be visible by 10 minutes.
7. Interpretation of results; see Figure D:
   - Positive result: A vertical line in any shade of blue forms a plus sign in the "Read Result" window along with a blue "Test Complete" line. Even a faint blue vertical line should be reported as a positive.
   - Negative result: No blue vertical line appears, leaving a minus sign in the "Read Result" window along with a blue "Test Complete" line.
   - Invalid result: After 10 minutes, no line is observed in the "Test Complete" window, or a blue color fills the "Read Result" window. If either of these occurs, the test must be repeated with a new reaction unit. If the problem continues, request technical support.

Follow-Up—Postanalytical

8. Properly dispose of biohazard waste material, and disinfect the work area.
9. Remove personal protective equipment, and sanitize the hands.
10. Document patient and control results on the lab logs and the patient's chart.

Quality Control Procedures

The internal control occurs in the "Test Complete" window built into each reaction unit. External positive and negative liquid controls are provided with each new kit. Each new operator of the test should perform liquid positive and negative external controls once to confirm that his or her testing technique is correct. Chart the control results in the control log with the operator's initials. Also, external controls should be tested and charted when a new kit is used.

PROCEDURE 7-2 QuickVue+ Mononucleosis Test Procedure—cont'd

QuickVue + Mononucleosis Test

FOR INFORMATIONAL USE ONLY ■ FOR INFORMATIONAL USE ONLY ■ FOR INFORMATIONAL USE ONLY

Not to be used for performing assay. Refer to most current package insert accompanying your test kit.

TEST PROCEDURE – WHOLE BLOOD

Read all of the procedural instructions before running patient samples.

Remove the Reaction Unit from the pouch and place it on a well lit and level surface.
The "Read Result" window contains a horizontal blue line pre-printed on the membrane.

Capillary Tube Procedure

For fingertip blood, fill the capillary tube (50 μL) to line.
Dispense all blood into the "Add" well.

Venipuncture Procedure

For whole blood samples in tubes, use the sample pipette provided.
Place one drop of sample in the "Add" well.

Hold the Developer bottle vertically.
Add 5 drops of Developer to the "Add" well.

Read results at 5 minutes.

"Test Complete" line must be visible by 10 minutes.

INTERPRETATION OF RESULTS
FOR PATIENT SAMPLES, POSITIVE AND NEGATIVE CONTROLS

Positive Result

Any shade of a blue vertical line forming a (+) sign in the "Read Result" window along with the blue "Test Complete" line, is a positive result. **Even a faint blue vertical line should be reported as a positive.**

Negative Result

No blue vertical line in the "Read Result" window along with the blue "Test Complete" line, is a negative result.

Invalid Result

Test results are invalid:
■ If after 10 minutes no signal is observed in the "Test Complete" window. (View #1.)
■ If after 10 minutes a blue color fills the "Read Result" window. (View #2.)

An invalid result indicates either the test was not performed correctly or the reagents are not working properly.

Should an invalid result occur, re-test the sample using a new Reaction Unit.

If the problem continues, contact Technical Support toll-free in the U.S. at (800) 874-1517. Outside the USA, contact your local representative.

LIMITATIONS

1. As is the case of any other diagnostic procedure, the results obtained by this kit yield data that must be used in addition to other information available to the physician.
2. QuickVue+ Infectious Mononucleosis test is a qualitative test for the detection of IM heterophile antibodies.
3. A negative result may be obtained from patients at the onset of the disease due to antibody concentration below the sensitivity of this test kit. If symptoms persist or increase in intensity, the test should be repeated.
4. Some segments of the population who contract Infectious Mononucleosis do not produce measurable levels of heterophile antibodies. Approximately 50% of children under 4 years of age who have IM may test as IM heterophile antibody negative.[4]

B

D, Package insert showing instructions for QuickVue+ test and how to interpret results. *(From Bonewit-West K: Clinical procedures for medical assistants, ed 9, St Louis, 2015, Saunders.)*

✳ PROCEDURE 7-3 QuickVue *Helicobacter pylori* gII Test (CLIA-Waived) Procedure

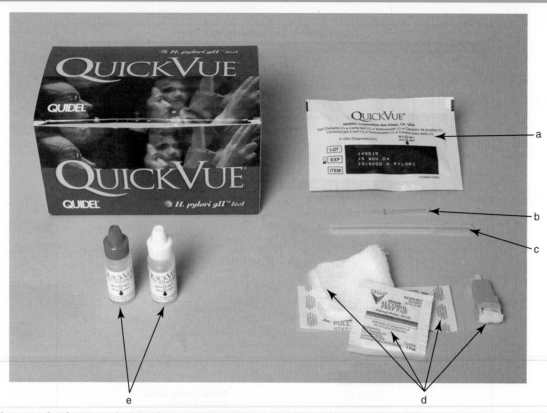

A, QuickVue *Helicobacter pylori* test kit. *a,* Test cassette; *b,* capillary tube for obtaining capillary puncture blood specimen; *c,* transfer pipette for venous blood specimens; *d,* capillary puncture supplies; *e,* positive and negative external liquid controls.

B, *Helicobacter pylori* test results. *1,* Test cassette before adding specimen; *2,* positive result: pink band in test area and blue internal control band; *3,* negative result: no band in test area and blue internal control band.

PROCEDURE 7-3 QuickVue *Helicobacter pylori* gII Test (CLIA-Waived) Procedure—cont'd

Equipment and Supplies (Figure A)—Preanalytical

- Foil-wrapped test cassette
- Capillary tube for capillary puncture blood
- Transfer pipette for venous blood
- Capillary puncture supplies
- Positive and negative external liquid controls
- Gloves and OSHA disposal equipment (*not pictured*)

Procedure—Analytical

1. Sanitize the hands, and apply gloves.
2. Add 1 drop of venous whole blood (using disposable dropper in the kit), 1 capillary tube (from kit) of whole blood from a capillary puncture (see Procedure 7-2), or 2 hanging drops of whole blood from a finger stick to the round sample well on the test cassette.
3. Do not move the test cassette until the assay is complete. Read and record the results of the test after 10 minutes or less (Figure B).
   - Positive result: A pink line appears next to the letter *T* and a blue line next to the letter *C*.
   - Negative result: Only a blue line forms next to the letter *C*. The blue line is the internal control indicating that the capillary flow occurred and the functional integrity of the strip was maintained. If the blue line does not show, the test results are invalid and should not be reported.
4. Discard all the test materials in the appropriate biohazard containers.
5. Remove and discard gloves in the biohazard container and sanitize the hands.

Follow-Up—Postanalytical

6. Disinfect the work area.
7. Chart the patient and control results on the lab logs and the patient chart.

Quality Control Procedure

The external positive and negative controls should be performed when a new kit is used and with each new operator of the test method. The procedure is done by adding 2 drops of the positive control to a test well and reading and recording the results after 5 minutes. The same procedure is done with the negative control.

✳ PROCEDURE 7-4 Uni-Gold Recombigen HIV Blood Test

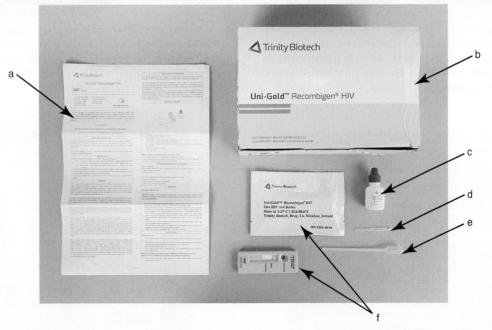

A, Uni-Gold Recombigen HIV supplies: *(a)* package insert and patient information sheets; *(b)* box with 20 test devices; *(c)* wash solution; *(d)* fingerstick sample collector and transfer pipette; *(e)* disposable pipette to use with venipuncture whole blood; *(f)* foil pouch and its test device.

(Continued)

B, Using standard phlebotomy procedures, collect a venipuncture whole blood specimen using a blood collection tube containing EDTA, or acid citrate dextran (ACD), or heparin anticoagulant.

C, Alternatively, collect the whole blood sample from a finger stick using the smaller sample transfer pipette. NOTE: It is important to hold the pipette gently in a horizontal position and allow the blood to fill to the mark on the pipette without squeezing the bulb.

D, Using appropriate personal protective equipment (PPE) including a face shield, deliver one drop of venipuncture blood from its pipette as it is held vertically over the test port. Then carefully dispose the pipette into a biohazard container.

E, Alternatively, after collecting the blood from a finger stick, immediately squeeze the bulb on the pipette until the blood is fully discharged into the sample port while using PPE including a face shield. Discard the empty pipette into a biohazard container.

F, After the blood is in the port, hold the wash bottle vertically over the port and deliver four (4) drops. Then set the timer for 10 minutes. Read results after 10 minutes but not more than 12 minutes of incubation time.

G, Valid test results after 10 minutes: *(a)* negative HIV test result showing no line in the test area and a line in the control area; *(b)* preliminary positive HIV test result showing lines in both the test and control areas.

PROCEDURE 7-4 Uni-Gold Recombigen HIV Blood Test—cont'd

H, Invalid test results that cannot be reported because of the following: *(a)* these two tests do not show a reaction in the control area; *(b)* these three tests do not show a full red area in the sample port.

Equipment and Supplies Preanalytical

Uni-Gold Recombigen HIV supplies (Figure A):
- Package insert and patient information sheets (NOTE: read these thoroughly before testing)
- Box with 20 test devices
- Wash solution
- Fingerstick pipette for sample collection and transfer
- Disposable pipette to transfer venipuncture whole blood
- Foil pouch and test device
- Other supplies *(not pictured)*
- Positive and negative external liquid controls
- PPE to include gloves, face protection, gown, and OSHA disposal equipment
- Blood collection supplies for capillary or venipuncture samples (e.g., lancets, gauze, alcohol swab, appropriate Vacutainer tube, bandages)

Procedure—Analytical

1. Sanitize the hands, and apply PPE.
2. Document that information sheet has been given to the patient, and that patient has read it.
3. Allow the unopened foil packet and wash solution to come to room temperature. **Only perform one test at a time.**
4. Open kit and lay the testing device on a clean, flat surface.
5. Label the device with the appropriate patient information.
6. Collect the sample via venipuncture using EDTA (lavender-top tube) or heparin (green-top tube) (see Figure B). Alternatively, collect the sample from a finger stick using the appropriate transfer pipette until the blood reaches the mark as seen in Figure C. Note that it is important to hold the

pipette gently in a horizontal position and allow the blood to fill to the mark on the pipette.

7. Add one (1) free-flowing drop of the venous whole blood to the sample port (using the proper disposable transfer pipette in the kit; see Figure D. Alternatively, immediately dispense all the blood in the capillary pipette from the finger stick into the sample port as seen in Figure E. NOTE: Both of the aforementioned procedures should be done with a barrier shield or a full face mask to protect the operator from possible blood exposure to the mucous membranes.
8. Discard the pipette in biohazard waste.
9. Next, hold the dropper bottle of wash solution above the sample port in a vertical position, and add four (4) free-flowing drops of the wash solution to the sample port as seen in Figure F.
10. Do not move the test cassette until the assay is complete. Read and record the results of the test after 10 minutes but not more than 12 minutes (see Figure G).
    a. Negative result: Only one red line forms next to the letter *C*. The pink/red line is the internal control indicating that the capillary flow occurred and the functional integrity of the test was maintained. Report as "Negative."
    b. Positive result: A pink/red line appears next to the letter *T* and next to the letter *C*. Report as "Preliminary Positive."
    c. Invalid results: For a test to be valid, a pink/red control line must be present, and the sample port must show a full red color. See Figure H for examples of five possible invalid results. If any of these results appear, do not report the patient result. The test must be repeated with a new testing device.

(Continued)

PROCEDURE 7-4 Uni-Gold Recombigen HIV Blood Test—cont'd

11. Discard all the test materials in the appropriate biohazard containers.
12. Remove and discard gloves in the biohazard container, and sanitize the hands.

Follow-Up—Postanalytical

13. Properly dispose of biohazard waste material, and disinfect the work area with 10% bleach or proper decontaminant.
14. Document the results on the lab log and the patient's chart.

Quality Control Procedure

The external positive and negative controls should be performed when a new kit is used and with each new operator of the test method. The procedure is done by adding one (1) drop of the positive control to the test device using the venipuncture pipette, followed by four (4) drops of the wash solution, and reading and recording the results after 10 minutes. The same procedure is done with the negative control.

✳ PROCEDURE 7-5 HIV OraQuick Test

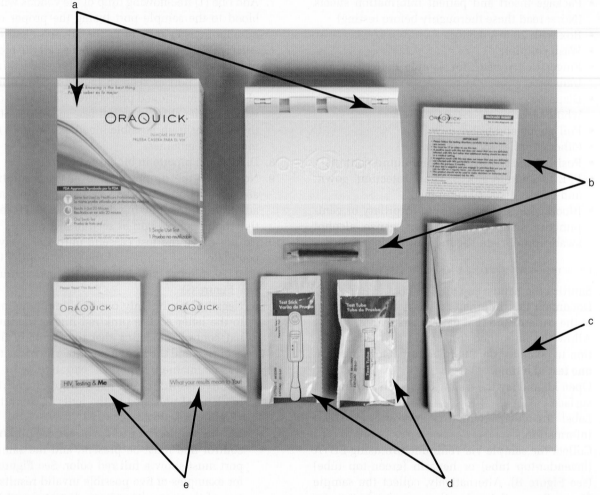

A, OraQuick HIV self-test kit contents. *(a)* Box and plastic test kit containing the flip chart directions and the following displayed items; *(b)* required manufacturer's insert and pencil for writing start and finish times; *(c)* plastic bag for disposal of the test supplies when finished; *(d)* foil-wrapped test stick and test tube; *(e)* two booklets labeled as follows: *Please Read This Book First—HIV, Testing, and Me* and *What Your Results Mean to You!*

PROCEDURE 7-5 HIV OraQuick Test—cont'd

B, Test instructions: Steps 1 and 2—Gently pop off the test tube's cap. Then hold the test tube upright and place it in the holder located on the right side of the plastic lid of the kit.

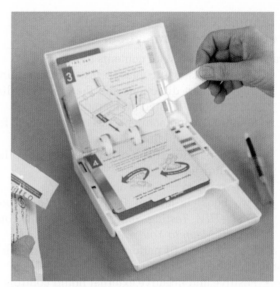

C, Step 3—Open foil wrap and remove the test stick; do not touch the pad with your fingers.

D, Step 4—Gently swipe the pad along your upper gums once and then your lower gums once.

E, Step 5—Put the test stick directly into the test tube located on the right of the plastic lid of the kit. And start the timer for 20 minutes.

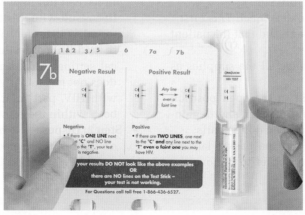

F, Steps 6 and 7—After 20 minutes, read the results by comparing the swab stick results (on the right) with the three keys (on the left) indicating negative and positive results. This test on the right shows a Negative Result.

(Continued)

PROCEDURE 7-5 HIV OraQuick Test—cont'd

Equipment, Supplies, and Patient Preparation—Preanalytical

OraQuick HIV self-test kit contents (see Figure A):

- Box and its white plastic test kit containing the flip chart directions and the following displayed items located in the pull-out drawer:
- Required manufacturer's insert and pencil for writing start and finish times
- Plastic bag for disposal of the test supplies when finished
- Foil-wrapped test stick and test tube
- Two booklets labeled *Please Read This Book First—HIV, Testing, and Me* and *What Your Results Mean to You!*

Additional items (if performing the HIV OraQuick test in the office):

- Positive and negative external liquid controls
- PPE to include gloves, face protection, gown, and OSHA-disposal equipment

Patient Preparation

1. Most people feel anxious when taking an HIV test. If the patient feels very anxious about taking the self-test, the patient may want to wait until he or she is calmer or get tested by the physician at a local clinic.
2. It is important not to eat, drink, or use oral care products (such as mouthwash, toothpaste, or whitening strips) 30 minutes before starting the test.
3. Remove dental products, such as dentures or any other products that cover the gums.
4. Find a quiet, well-lit place where you can be for at least 20 minutes.
5. You must follow the test directions carefully to obtain an accurate result.
6. Make sure you have a timer, watch, or any device that can time 20 to 40 minutes.

Procedure—Analytical

7. Sanitize the hands, and apply PPE.
8. Ensure that the pretest booklet, *"Read This First,"* has been given to the patient, and that the patient has read it.
9. Open kit drawer and arrange all the supplies as seen in Figure A.
10. With the white plastic lid in the open position proceed by following the directions and demonstrations on each of the numbered flip charts:

- **Step 1: Open test tube**—Find the packet labeled "Test Tube" and open the packet to remove the test tube.

- **Step 2: Setup**—Be careful! There is liquid at the bottom of the tube. Hold the tube upright. Then gently pop off the test tube's cap—do not twist (see Figure B). Then put the test tube in the holder labeled "Test Tube Holder" located on the right side of the plastic lid that is opened and upright.

- **Step 3: Open test stick**—Locate the packet labeled "Test Stick." Tear open the packet and remove the test stick, being careful not to touch the pad with your fingers (see Figure C).

- **Step 4: Swipe gums**—Make sure the timer is ready and set for 20 minutes but do not start it yet. Gently swipe the pad along the upper gums once and then the lower gums once (see Figure D). Make sure you swipe the pad between the gum and lips from one side all the way to the other on both the upper and lower gums.

- **Step 5: Drop in and start timing**—Put the test stick pad directly into the test tube located on the right side of the plastic lid and start the timer for 20 minutes as seen in Figure E. NOTE: The kit also provides a pencil and a place to enter the start time, the time after 20 minutes, and the time after 40 minutes.

- **Step 6: Wait 20 minutes**—The test kit provides a flap to cover the test area on the stick. The area will turn pink for a few minutes. This is normal. Do not read the results before 20 minutes (this may give a wrong result). Read the results between 20 and 40 minutes. After 40 minutes the test will no longer be accurate. While waiting for the results, the patient should read the second booklet, *What Your Results Mean to You!*

- **Step 7: Reading your results**—Move the flap that covered the test area to see the results. Compare the test stick to the pictures on the flip chart as in Figure F. If the results *do not* look like the examples on the flip chart *or* there are *no* lines on the test stick, the test is not working. For questions, call toll free: 1-866-436-6527. NOTE: A positive result with this test does not mean the person tested is definitely infected with HIV, but rather that additional testing should be done in a medical setting. Also, a negative result with this test does not mean that you are definitely not infected with HIV, particularly when exposure may have been within the previous 3 months.

- **Step 8: Dispose**—Remove the test stick, put the cap on the test tube, place all the contents in the disposal bag provided in the test kit, and dispose of the bag.

Advanced Concepts

Agglutination Reactions (Non–CLIA-Waived Tests)

Agglutination is the visible clumping of blood cells or other particulate matter, such as latex beads. Agglutination is caused by antibodies adhering to their antigens. This type of antibody is referred to as an *agglutinin*. An antibody/antigen reaction produces a visible, latticelike network of cells or beads that have agglutinated and fallen out of solution. The agglutination reaction can be seen on a slide or in a test tube and becomes visible to the naked eye as the slide or tube is tilted or centrifuged. Agglutination reactions require interpretation that is beyond the scope of CLIA-waived testing. They are therefore usually performed in hospital and reference laboratories.

Immunohematology

The most common antibody/antigen agglutination reactions are seen in immunohematology laboratories (also referred to as *blood banks*). Immunohematology uses agglutination testing to determine blood types for transfusions, paternity determinations, mother-baby blood compatibility, and forensic investigations.

ABO Blood Typing

The reasons for determining blood type are to provide safe blood transfusions, to prevent hemolytic disease in the newborn, to identify parentage, and for forensic (criminal) reasons. More than 300 types of inherited blood antigens are found on RBCs. The ABO and Rh blood types are most important because of their intense antigenic responses when transfused or transmitted into incompatible recipients.

Karl Landsteiner discovered the ABO blood groups in the early 1900s. He determined that two inherited antigens are present on the surface of RBCs: A and B. The presence or absence of each antigen produces the four blood types: A, B, AB, and O. Landsteiner also determined that individuals produce a natural antibody against any antigen absent on their RBC surface. Therefore a type A person has A antigens on his or her RBCs and produces anti-B antibodies in the plasma. A type B person has B antigens on his or her RBCs and anti-A antibodies in the plasma. A type AB person has both A and B antigens on his or her RBCs and no antibodies in the plasma. A type O person has neither A nor B antigens on his or her RBCs and has both anti-A and anti-B antibodies in the plasma. Table 7-2 provides a summary of these characteristics.

In the immunohematology department, agglutination testing is performed to determine blood types and the compatibility between the donor's blood and the recipient's blood. If a blood antigen comes in contact with its corresponding antibody, the result is agglutination (clumping) of the RBCs, which eventually leads to hemolysis (breakdown) of the RBCs. These dangerous reactions occur when the wrong type of blood is administered to a patient during a blood transfusion. For example, if a type A person is given type B blood, the recipient's blood, containing anti-B antibodies, would agglutinate the donor's RBCs containing the B antigen. The clumped RBCs would be unable to pass through the kidneys, which might lead to kidney failure. The universal ABO donor is type O because *no antigens* are present on the donor's RBCs, and the universal ABO recipient is AB because *no antibodies* are present in the recipient's plasma. (NOTE: The ideal transfusion is a perfect match. Universal donor and recipient transfusions are used only in "medical emergencies.")

Rh System

The Rh or D antigen is also found on the surface of RBCs. A person with the Rh antigen is referred to as *Rh positive (D+ or Rh+)*. All the previously discussed blood types (A, B, AB, and O) will be either Rh+ or Rh− independent of their ABO type. In the United States 85% of the population is Rh positive (Rh+). The remaining 15% of the population does not have the Rh antigen and are referred to as *Rh negative* (Rh− or D−). An *Rh negative* person has no naturally occurring anti-D *(Rh)* antibodies as in the ABO blood types. However, anti-D *(Rh)* antibody production may be induced *after* an *Rh negative* person is mistakenly transfused with *Rh positive* blood or after an *Rh negative* mother has carried an *Rh positive* baby.

Table 7-2	Summary of ABO Blood Types		
Blood Type	**Antigens on Cells**	**Antibodies in Plasma**	**Transfusion Compatibility**
A	A antigens	Anti-B antibodies	Can receive A or O
B	B antigens	Anti-A antibodies	Can receive B or O
AB	A and B antigens	No antibodies	Can receive A, B, AB, and O; Universal recipient
O	No antigens	Anti-A and anti-B	Can receive only O; Universal donor

In both cases the exposure to *Rh positive* cells has a strong antigenic effect in the *Rh negative* recipient. The *Rh negative* recipient starts producing anti-D (Rh) antibodies that hemolyze and destroy *Rh positive* cells.

Hemolytic Disease of the Newborn and RhoGAM

Hemolytic disease of the newborn (HDN), or **erythroblastosis fetalis**, is a hemolytic anemia in newborns resulting from maternal-fetal blood group incompatibility. Figure 7-8 illustrates the way an *Rh negative* mother becomes sensitized to her first baby's *Rh positive* blood cells after delivery. Subsequent pregnancies with *Rh positive* babies activate the anti-Rh antibody response. The anti-Rh antibodies cause the destruction of the baby's RBCs. The clinical manifestations in the *Rh positive* newborn include severe anemia, jaundice, and enlargement of the liver and spleen. These can lead to cardiac failure, respiratory distress, and death.

HDN can be prevented by the injection of anti-Rh gamma globulin (RhoGAM) during and after the pregnancy of an *Rh negative* mother. RhoGAM prevents the mother from becoming sensitized and slows her production of Rh antibodies to the Rh antigen.

Enzyme-Linked Immunosorbent Assay: Quantitative Analysis (ELISA)

The term **immunosorbent** pertains to the attachment of an antigen or antibody to a solid surface such as latex beads, wells in plastic dishes, or plastic cartridges (devices capable of absorbing the antigen or antibody). In the ELISA method, an antigen is fixed to a well in a plastic dish. A serum specimen is added to the well to test for a particular antibody. The well is then rinsed to remove anything that did not bind. Next, an enzyme/antibody complex is added that will further bind to the human antibody, if present, and the well is rinsed again to remove any enzyme/antibody that was not bound. The final step uses an enzyme color developer that reacts with the enzyme, if present, and produces a color change. If the serum contained the antibody specific to the antigen, a color change occurs. The more antibody present, the darker the color produced. This quantitative method of indirectly measuring antibodies is a non–CLIA-waived test and is performed in reference and hospital laboratories. NOTE: This is an "in vitro" lab testing method that is often used in allergy testing.

Fig. 7-8 Hemolytic disease of the newborn in the second pregnancy of an Rh negative mother carrying two Rh positive babies. **A,** Rh negative woman before first pregnancy, with Rh negative red blood cells (RBCs) and no anti-Rh antibodies. **B,** First baby with Rh positive RBCs begins to sensitize mother in utero, causing the production of anti-Rh antibodies *(blue squares).* **C,** After birth, more Rh positive cells enter the mother's bloodstream. **D,** Rh negative mother reacts, producing more anti-Rh antibodies *(blue squares).* **E,** Second baby's Rh positive RBCs are hemolyzed by the mother's antibodies *(blue squares). (From Stepp CA, Woods M: Laboratory procedures for medical office personnel, Philadelphia, 1998, Saunders.)*

Table 7-3   Common Immunology Tests

Tests	Clinical Significance
Bacterial Infections	
Group A *Streptococcus* (strep throat, fever)	The CLIA-waived rapid screening test detects the presence of group A *Streptococcus* antigens in a throat-swabbed specimen.
Helicobacter pylori (ulcers)	The CLIA-waived screening test detects the antibodies specific for *H. pylori* in the blood of an infected individual with ulcers.
Syphilis	Syphilis is a sexually transmitted disease. Three immunology tests for syphilis are rapid plasmin reagin, fluorescent treponemal antibody, and the Venereal Disease Research Laboratory (VDRL) test.
Chlamydia	*Chlamydia trachomatis* is the most common cause of sexually transmitted venereal infection in the world. Rapid lateral flow immunoassays are available for the qualitative detection of chlamydia directly from endocervical swab and cytology brush specimens.
Gardnerella vaginalis (vaginal infection)	This enzyme activity test is used to detect *G. vaginalis* in vaginal fluid specimens from patients suspected of having bacterial vaginosis, the most common vaginal infection.
Borrelia burgdorferi (Lyme disease)	Lyme disease is transmitted by ticks infected with *B. burgdorferi*. The immunology tests used are either the ELISA or the indirect fluorescent antibody test. If either of these tests is positive or uncertain, it is followed by the Western immunoblot.
Viral Infections	
Respiratory syncytial virus (RSV)	RSV is a highly contagious virus that causes acute respiratory illness. It is the most important cause of bronchiolitis and pneumonia in infants.
Epstein-Barr virus (EBV) (mononucleosis)	The CLIA-waived mononucleosis test detects the heterophile antibody associated with EBV infections.
Influenza A and B	The CLIA-waived rapid screening test detects the presence of influenza A and B in nasal-swabbed or nasal wash specimens.
HIV/AIDS	The CLIA-waived test detects antibodies in blood or oral cells that are specific for HIV-1.
Rubella (German measles)	The test is given to evaluate whether a woman is immune to rubella (as a result of childhood exposure or immunization) or presently infected with the disease. If a woman is not immune and becomes infected during pregnancy, the rubella virus could cause birth defects in the fetus.
Hepatitis C (bloodborne pathogen)	The "silent killer," hepatitis C is a growing public health concern. An at-home test provides a confidential hepatitis C result.
Varicella-zoster (chickenpox and shingles)	Immunofluorescence is a diagnostic technique used to identify antibodies to a specific virus. In the case of herpes zoster, ultraviolet rays are applied to a preparation composed of cells taken from the herpes blisters. The specific characteristics of the ultraviolet light as seen through a microscope identify the presence of the antibodies. This test is less expensive and more accurate than a culture, and the results are faster.
Other Antigenic Substances	
HCG hormone (pregnancy test)	HCG is produced by the placenta during pregnancy.
CA 125 (ovarian cancer)	This test detects the ovarian cancer antigen.
Prostate-specific antigen (PSA) (prostate cancer)	The PSA and percent-free PSA blood tests aid in the detection and treatment of prostate cancer.
Bladder tumor–associated antigen (BTA)	The BTA stat test was the first tumor marker test to be placed in the CLIA-waived category by the Centers for Disease Control and Prevention. The test detects BTA in the urine of persons being monitored for recurrent bladder cancer.
Rheumatoid factor (arthritis)	Rheumatoid arthritis is a chronic inflammatory disease that affects the connective tissue of the body and leads to crippling deformities. Most patients with this disease develop an antibody called *rheumatoid factor* that can be detected immunologically.
Fecal occult blood (screening for colon cancer)	The iFOB test is highly sensitive to blood on the feces. If positive, the patient will be evaluated as to what is causing the bleeding in the colon.

AIDS, Acquired immunodeficiency syndrome; *ELISA*, enzyme-linked immunosorbent assay; *HIV*, human immunodeficiency virus.

Antibody Titers

Reference and hospital laboratories perform both agglutination and ELISA tests with moderately complex equipment to determine the quantity of antibodies present in a specimen. Another quantitative method to determine the amount of a specific antibody in the blood is the **titer** (a quantitative test that measures the amount of antibody that reacts with a specific antigen). Quantitative antibody information can provide the physician with additional information regarding the extent of acquired immunity. For example, a physician might order a series of Rh titers to measure the number of anti-Rh antibodies in an Rh negative pregnant woman's serum. The Rh antibody titers could then be used to monitor the degree of sensitivity the mother might develop against her Rh positive baby's cells during the pregnancy. If the titer rises, she has an established immunity against the baby's Rh positive cells and appropriate measures to protect the baby must be taken.

Summary of Immunological Tests

The ability to detect specific antibodies and antigens associated with disease has made immunology a rapidly growing biomedical science. Table 7-3 describes CLIA-waived and non–CLIA-waived immunology tests commonly ordered for diagnosing bacterial, viral, and other immune-related disorders.

Review Questions

1. Which of the following is the causative agent of infectious mononucleosis?
   a. Variola major
   b. Epstein-Barr virus
   c. Cytomegalovirus
   d. Human immunodeficiency virus

2. Which of the following types of immunology tests involve the visible clumping of blood cells or latex beads caused by antibodies adhering to their antigens?
   a. Titer
   b. Lateral flow immunoassay
   c. Agglutination
   d. All the above

3. HCG is produced by the developing placenta during pregnancy with the levels peaking
   a. between the twentieth and eightieth days of pregnancy.
   b. between the thirtieth and seventieth days of pregnancy.
   c. between the tenth and sixtieth days of pregnancy.
   d. between the fiftieth and eightieth days of pregnancy.

4. Which of the following cells differentiate into plasma cells and memory cells, with the subsequent production of antibodies produced by the plasma cells?
   a. B cells
   b. T cells
   c. Natural killer cells
   d. All the above

5. Which of the following nonspecific immunity mechanisms involves the process of certain cells engulfing and destroying microorganisms and cellular debris?
   a. Normal flora
   b. Phagocytosis
   c. Intact skin and mucous membranes
   d. Inflammation

6. Which two of the five types of antibodies are elevated in acute allergic reactions and subsequent encounters?
   a. IgE
   b. IgM
   c. IgG
   d. IgA

7. Which antibody protects mucous membranes from bacterial and viral infections?
   a. IgG
   b. IgM
   c. IgE
   d. IgA

8. Type A blood consists of
   a. B antigens and anti-B antibodies.
   b. A antigens and anti-B antibodies.
   c. B antigens and anti-A antibodies.
   d. A antigens and anti-A antibodies.

9. Which of the following pregnancy scenarios could be a problem for the baby?
   a. Mother Rh positive and fetus Rh positive
   b. Mother Rh negative and fetus Rh negative
   c. Mother Rh positive and fetus Rh negative
   d. Mother Rh negative and fetus Rh positive

10. Name the antigens present in a B positive individual.

11. Name two specimens that are used in HIV CLIA-waived tests.

Websites

The National Primary Immunodeficiency Resource Center (NPI) is the central resource and clearinghouse on primary immunodeficiency, serving researchers, scientists, physicians, government, industry, patients, and their families. Click "related links" on the home page for access to additional sites related to the immune system and immunology:
www.info4pi.org/index.cfm?CFID=8903943&;CFTOKEN=22787603
Link to laboratory that performs IgA, IgG, and IgE testing for food and inhalant allergies:
www.usbiotek.com
Quidel-sponsored video on how to perform and read Quidel's CLIA-waived influenza test:
www.flutest.com/flu-facts/animation2b.htm
Links to all Quidel point-of-care test kits, including chlamydia, streptococcus A, *H. pylori* gII, influenza A and B, OneStep HCG urine, and infectious mononucleosis:
www.quidel.com/products/
Links to the Applied Biotech line of point-of-care products for testing for infectious diseases (mononucleosis, streptococcus, and *H. pylori*), pregnancy, and drug abuse:
www.invernessmedicalpd.com/point_of_care.aspx
Links to all Thermo BioStar kits for waived and moderately complex testing. The waived tests available are for HCG, streptococcus A, and mononucleosis:
www.pointofcare.net/vendors/thermobiostar.htm
Primary Care rapid diagnostic test products available from Beckman Coulter:
www.beckmancoulter.com/wsrportal/wsr/diagnostics/clinical-products/rapid-diagnostics/index.htm
Information on iFOB testing:
www.quidel.com/assets/swf/iFOBTrainingvideoHQ.htm

Microbiology

microorganism any tiny, usually microscopic, entity capable of carrying on living processes
morbidity the rate at which an illness occurs
mortality the rate of deaths
myalgia diffuse muscle pain
mycelium mass of hyphae that some fungi produce
peptidoglycan component made of polysaccharides and peptides that gives rigidity to the bacterial cell wall

Petri dish dish containing medium in which to grow microorganisms
prokaryotic pertaining to unicellular organisms that do not have a true nucleus with a nuclear membrane
purulent capable of forming pus
sensitivity test identification of the antibiotic of choice to treat an infection
sputum mucus expelled from the lungs

 ## Fundamental Concepts

Overview of Microbiology

Microbiology is the study of microorganisms, including bacteria, fungi, protozoa, and viruses. A **microorganism** is "any tiny, usually microscopic entity capable of carrying on living processes." Microorganisms were first discovered in 1676, when a Dutch linen merchant and self-made microbiologist named Anthony van Leeuwenhoek created a magnifying glass through which they could be observed.

Microorganisms are found everywhere—in the air, soil, and water. Some microorganisms are involved in the decomposition of waste and the natural recycling process of life and death. Microorganisms that are normally found in and on the human body are referred to as *normal flora* or *normal biota.* Normal flora assist in preventing the growth and spread of disease-causing microorganisms. An example of protective normal flora is the bacteria *Lactobacillus,* which creates an acidic environment in the female vagina. Certain antibiotics destroy *Lactobacillus,* thereby allowing opportunistic infections such as candidiasis (caused by the yeast *Candida albicans*) to take hold.

Research has determined that fewer than 1% of all microorganisms are pathogens. When pathogenic microorganisms invade the body and overcome its natural defense mechanisms, as discussed in Chapter 7, an **infection** occurs. Some infections are contagious, which means they can spread from person to person.

The role that pathogenic microorganisms play in causing disease should be understood, as well as the means to prevent the spread of these organisms. Table 8-1 shows a timeline of efforts to control infectious diseases throughout history.

When a patient contracts an infection, the first step is to identify the pathogenic organism that is causing the problem; then find the appropriate treatment to control the infection. The following is an overview of the ways in which microorganisms are classified.

Classification of Microorganisms

Although the more complex microorganism identification procedures are not performed in all laboratories, it is important to have a general knowledge of the classification, nomenclature, structure, and growth requirements of pathogenic microorganisms. Microorganisms are categorized as viruses, bacteria, fungi, or parasites.

Viruses

Viruses are the smallest microorganisms, consisting of either ribonucleic acid (RNA) or deoxyribonucleic acid (DNA) molecules. They are so small they can be seen only under a very high magnification using an electron microscope. They need to live in a host cell and use the host cell's metabolic machinery to multiply. Therefore, unlike bacteria and other microorganisms, viruses must be grown inside tissue cells rather than on typical culture **media** (liquid, semisolid, or solid substances containing nutrients needed to grow microorganisms).

Bacteria

Bacteria are classified as **prokaryotic,** which means they are unicellular organisms that do not have a true nucleus with a nuclear membrane. Bacteria do have a cell membrane and a cell wall. They reproduce by **binary fission,** asexual reproduction in which the cell splits in half. Bacteria can reproduce very rapidly on the culture media containing nutrients for their growth. They are able to form **colonies** (visible masses of bacteria formed on a culture medium by one bacterium growing and replicating itself). **Culture** is the reproduction of microorganisms in a laboratory culture medium. Bacteria are cultured (grown) to produce enough additional bacteria to allow testing for identification.

Fungi

Fungi (singular: fungus) are **eukaryotic,** which means they possess a true nucleus with a nuclear membrane. They lack chlorophyll, can be grown on media, and are generally classified as molds or yeasts. Yeasts are single cells that reproduce by budding, in which a new cell forms on the surface of the yeast, grows, pinches off, and becomes a separate cell. They form colonies with a smooth, creamy appearance on culture media. In contrast, molds are made up of **mycelium,** which consists of tubelike structures called **hyphae,** and have a fuzzy or woolly appearance.

Table 8-1	History of Infection Control
1300s	Quarantine practices began. Passengers on ships were not allowed to disembark for 40 days after anchoring to protect coastal cities from epidemics of plague. The Latin word *quaresma,* from which "quarantine" is derived, means 40.
1600s	Bubonic plague killed half the population of Europe. Latin as a spoken language disappeared as a result. During this period, infectious diseases were believed to be caused by poisonous vapors, sin, God, and foreigners.
1800s	The germ theory and Koch's postulates proved that microorganisms caused many diseases. Industrialization and immigration in the United States caused overcrowding in many cities. Inadequate waste disposal systems and unsafe drinking water led to outbreaks of diseases such as cholera, dysentery, tuberculosis, typhoid fever, yellow fever, and malaria.
	In 1878, after a yellow fever epidemic, the U.S. Congress passed the Federal Quarantine Legislation, which called for federal involvement in quarantine activities.
	In the late 1800s patients with infectious disease were isolated by disease in wards or floors. Although nursing books from this period discuss aseptic techniques, approximately 40% of maternal deaths were caused by pregnancy complications that occurred because aseptic procedures were not practiced.
1900s	In 1910 a cubicle system of isolation was introduced, consisting of multiple-bed wards, the practice of nurses changing gowns between patients, use of antiseptic hand-washing techniques, and disinfection of objects that patients had touched.
	In 1928 Alexander Fleming discovered penicillin. This antibiotic was first used in the 1940s by the U.S. military to treat sick and wounded soldiers. A 33-year-old woman was the first civilian to be treated with penicillin when her temperature rose to 107° F after she was hospitalized for more than a month with a streptococcal infection. She recovered from the infection, later met Sir Alexander Fleming, and died at the age of 90.
1950s	*Staphylococcus* infections acquired in the hospital were still causing the loss of limbs and death. Hospitals for infectious diseases began closing, except for tuberculosis sanatoriums.
1960s	Tuberculosis sanatoriums began to close.
1970s	In 1970 seven isolation categories for grouping patients with infectious diseases were developed by the Centers for Disease Control and Prevention (CDC). In 1975 hospitals across the nation developed infection-control manuals.
1980s	New nosocomial infections arose, such as those caused by multidrug-resistant organisms and new pathogens. In 1985 the human immunodeficiency virus (HIV) epidemic began, and Universal Precautions were introduced.
1990s	Multidrug resistance, increase in the number of tuberculosis cases, shorter hospital stays, overuse of antibiotics, and new diseases such as those caused by *Hantavirus* and Ebola virus were some of the medical issues of this decade.
	In 1991 the Occupational Safety and Health Administration (OSHA) Bloodborne Pathogens Standard was instituted.
	In 1997 the CDC revised isolation guidelines and introduced Standard Precautions (a combination of Universal Precautions and Body Substance Isolation) and Transmission-Based Precautions.
2000s	The CDC has stated that airplanes have replaced ships as the dominant vehicles for the international transmission of diseases.
	Emerging infectious diseases include bird flu (H5N1), swine flu (influenza A, H1N1), hepatitis C, MRSA (methicillin-resistant *Staphylococcus aureus*), *Clostridium difficile* (intestinal bacterial infection), and MERS-CoV (respiratory coronavirus similar to SARS).
	In 2013 HIV infection control using early detection and antiretroviral medication to prevent replication of virus reduces spread of HIV and progression to AIDS (but still no cure for HIV).
	Hospitals alerted to strongly enforce infection control (Standard Precautions) requiring vigilant hand sanitization and wearing of scrubs by physicians. High numbers of patients are contracting healthcare-acquired infections (HAIs) in health care facilities.
	HCV (hepatitis C virus) infection is highest in "Baby Boomers" who were born between 1945 and 1965, causing liver cancer to become the leading cause of cancer deaths.

Parasites

Parasites are organisms that live in or on a host and derive nourishment from the host. They can be one-celled protozoa (e.g., amoeba) or many-celled organisms such as helminths (roundworms, tapeworms, and flukes).

Nomenclature of Microorganisms

More than 250 years ago Carl von Linné, a Swedish botanist, created a nomenclature system for all living things. In this system each plant and animal has a name with two parts: genus (group) and species (kind). The standard rule is to capitalize the genus name and write the species name in lowercase. The genus and species names are always underlined or italicized, as in *Staphylococcus aureus*.

Structural Characteristics of Bacteria

Bacteria are classified and identified according to their shapes and growing patterns. Figure 8-1 illustrates three growing patterns of the circular cocci (diplococci, streptococci, and staphylococci), as well as rod-shaped bacilli and spiral-shaped spirilla.

Coccus

The coccus (plural: cocci) is a round bacterium that grows in a variety of formations, depending on the division pattern of the cocci and whether the cocci remain attached afterwards. Cocci are arranged in singles, in pairs (diplococci), in patterns of four (tetrads), in chains (e.g., *Streptococcus*), and in clusters (e.g., *Staphylococcus*, seen as grapelike clusters).

The most common species of *Staphylococcus* are *epidermidis* and *aureus*. *Staphylococcus epidermidis* is found normally on the surface of the skin and the mucous membrane of the mouth. *S. aureus,* on the other hand, is commonly associated with pathogenic conditions such as boils, carbuncles, pimples, impetigo, abscesses, wound infections, and even food poisoning.

Streptococci are cocci arranged in chains. Although some *Streptococci* are part of normal flora, some cause pathogenic conditions such as strep throat, scarlet fever, and rheumatic fever, which are discussed later in this chapter. In addition, *Streptococcus* can cause carbuncles, impetigo, pneumonia, puerperal sepsis (infection after childbirth), and erysipelas (infectious skin disease).

Bacillus

The bacillus (plural: bacilli) is rod shaped and can also be described as coccobacillus when it appears as a combination of cocci and bacilli (rod shaped but rounded on the ends) or diplobacillus (when it is arranged in pairs) (see Figure 8-1, *D*).

Bacilli cause diseases such as urinary tract infections, botulism, tetanus, gas gangrene, gastroenteritis, typhoid fever, pertussis (whooping cough), bacillary dysentery, diphtheria, tuberculosis, leprosy, and the plague.

Spirillum

Spirillum (plural: spirilla) is a spiral-shaped microorganism that can be a gently curved rod or look more like a corkscrew or a spring. Some spiral bacteria are *Treponema pallidum,* which causes syphilis, and *Vibrio cholerae,* which causes cholera.

Fig. 8-1 Classification of bacteria based on their shapes and groupings. **A,** Diplococci—pairs of circular cocci. **B,** Streptococci—chains of circular cocci. **C,** Staphylococci—clusters of circular cocci. **D,** Bacilli—rod-shaped bacteria. **E,** Spirilla—spiral-shaped bacteria.

Other Bacterial Structures

Some bacteria have the following additional structures:

- *Flagella* are projections that resemble whips and allow the organism to be motile. Flagella can be seen with the aid of certain stains.
- Some bacteria have *capsules* that surround the cell wall. Organisms with capsules are virulent because antibiotics have difficulty penetrating the capsule.
- Some bacteria produce *spores* when conditions become unfavorable for growth. Spores are resistant to heat, cold, chemicals, and certain conditions. They convert back to a reproductive stage when conditions improve. Some spores survive for many years. Examples of bacteria that can produce spores are *Clostridium tetani* (causes tetanus, or lockjaw), *Clostridium botulinum* (causes botulism), and *Bacillus anthracis* (causes anthrax).

Collecting, Transporting, and Processing Microbiology Specimens

Collection of microbiological specimens requires the use of infection-control techniques and precautions to prevent infecting yourself or others. The following precautions should be observed at all times:

- Wear the appropriate personal protection devices.
- Disinfect specimen containers after collection.
- Put the specimens in transport bags after collection.
- Wash the hands after specimen collection.

As with all specimen collections, the results are only as good as the specimen collected. The ideal time to collect a microbiological specimen is *before* antibiotics have been administered because the antibiotics will kill the microbes that are needed to be grown and identified.

Specific containers are used to transport a variety of specimens, such as blood cultures, body fluids, skin scrapings, exudates from deep wounds or abscesses, **sputum** from the lungs, and feces and urine specimens (Figure 8-2). The specific directions for collecting these specimens will be discussed later in the chapter.

Collecting a microbiological specimen from the following sites generally involves applying a swab to the infected area: eyes, rectum, urogenital areas, throat, nose, and wounds. The microbiology specimens must be processed as soon as possible. Transport systems provide the conditions microorganisms need to survive during the transport to the laboratory. These transport systems contain maintenance media that prevent the microorganisms from dying or multiplying. Two examples of transport systems are shown in Figure 8-3. The system at the top of the picture includes two blue-handled Dacron swabs on plastic sticks. When the specimen is obtained, the swabs are put into the holder and the bottom of the tube is squeezed, releasing the transport media onto the swab to maintain the organisms. The two swabs with the purple handle, at the bottom of the picture, each contain dried nutrient media. The transport system to be used will depend on the type of specimen collected or the specific organisms for which the culture was ordered.

Collecting a Throat Specimen

The swabbed throat specimen collection is one of the most common microbiology procedures performed in the physician's office laboratory (POL). The specimen may be tested for several different pathogens, but is most commonly used to test for streptococcal infections.

Fig. 8-2 Specimen containers from left to right: Ova and parasite containers (blue and red), sputum cup, skin scraping/biopsy container, and sterile urine cup and towelette.

Fig. 8-3 Two specimen transport systems for specimens collected on swabs.

The **Collecting a Throat Specimen** procedure check sheet is provided in the workbook and is demonstrated in Procedure 8-1, located at the end of this section.

Collecting a Nasal Specimen

Nasal specimens are most commonly collected when testing for influenza A and B. It is important to insert the foam swab at the base of the nostril as seen in Figure 8-4. The foam swab is then directly inserted along the base of the nostril at least 1 inch and is gently rotated while rocking it back and forth. More information is provided in Procedure 8-6: OSOM Influenza A and B Test Procedure.

Collecting a Blood Culture Specimen

Blood cultures are collected in containers such as BACTEC bottles (Becton Dickinson, Franklin Lakes, NJ) seen in Figure 8-5. Approximately 10 mL of blood is required for each bottle when collecting blood from an adult. NOTE: The aerobic bottle grows oxygen-dependent bacteria and must be collected first when using the butterfly method of draw. The anaerobic bottle grows bacteria that thrive best in the absence of oxygen. (It is drawn second when using a butterfly system.) Also displayed are the blood collection tubes with their light yellow caps. Pediatric patients generally need 1 to 3 mL collected into one aerobic bottle or culture tube. When a patient has a fever of unknown origin, the physician often orders a blood culture to determine whether microorganisms are

present in the blood. A specific aseptic preparation of the puncture site and the equipment is required when drawing blood cultures. The anaerobic bottle is filled first unless the butterfly method is used, in which case the aerobic bottle is filled first because of the air in the tubing.

Fig. 8-4 Nasal swab specimen. Note the proper angle to insert the foam swab when collecting a nasal specimen. The swab is inserted at least 1 inch along the base of the nostril on the side that has the most discharge. Once inside, the swab is rotated and rocked back and forth gently for 5 seconds to obtain a good specimen. *(Photo by Zack Bent.)*

Fig. 8-5 Blood culture equipment. *(a)* Aerobic bottle that grows oxygen-dependent bacteria is drawn first when using the butterfly method of draw. *(b)* Butterfly needle attached to a Vacutainer holder with yellow Vacutainer tube for blood culture testing. *(c)* Anaerobic bottle that grows bacteria in the absence of oxygen is collected second when using a butterfly needle system. *(d)* Blood culture Vacutainer tubes that have a light yellow stopper for pediatric patients. *(Photo by Zack Bent.)*

Collecting a Urine Culture Specimen

When a urinary tract infection is present, the physician will typically order a urine culture and **sensitivity test** to determine the type of pathogen causing the infection and the antibiotic that will most effectively treat the infection. The patient is instructed to collect a clean-catch midstream urine into a sterile specimen container, as described in Chapter 3. If the urine specimen must be transported to the microbiology lab, the urine can be transferred into a sterile Vacutainer tube with the appropriate preservatives, as seen in Figure 8-6, *A* and *B*.

Collecting a Chlamydia Specimen

Another type of transport media is used for *Chlamydia* organisms. Chlamydia is a sexually transmitted disease caused by *Chlamydia trachomatis,* a tiny **gram-negative** (having the pink/red color of the counterstain used in Gram's method of staining microorganisms) intracellular bacterium that requires a host cell for growth. Women with this disease may have no symptoms or may have any of the following: dysuria, itching, irritation of the genital area, and an odorless, yellowish vaginal discharge. Left untreated, chlamydia can cause pelvic inflammatory disease and

Fig. 8-6 Preparing a clean-catch midstream urine specimen for transport. **A,** The white sterile "straw" and Vacutainer holder with a needle inside are inserted into the urine. The Vacutainer tube is pushed into the needle, causing the urine to fill the tube. **B,** The filled Vacutainer tube is then labeled and sent to the lab. *(Photo by Zack Bent.)*

infertility. The symptoms in men are mild dysuria and a thin, watery discharge from the penis. If not treated in men, the disease can cause epididymitis, which could result in infertility. Using a sterile swab, the physician collects a specimen from the female endocervical canal or the male urethra. The swab is placed in a tube containing a transport medium to preserve the specimen during transport and is sent to a reference laboratory for testing. Testing for *Chlamydia* is most frequently done using a DNA-probe test (test based on DNA detection).

Collecting a Gonorrhea Specimen

The JEMBEC transport system (Becton Dickinson) (Figure 8-7) consists of a JEMBEC plate, a small white pill, and a plastic bag. It is used for transporting and growing *Neisseria gonorrhoeae,* the gram-negative diplococcus that causes gonorrhea. When activated, the pill creates a 10% carbon dioxide atmosphere that this organism needs for growth. Gonorrhea is a sexually transmitted disease of the genitourinary tract. Women either show no symptoms or have dysuria and a yellow discharge. If untreated, the infection can result in pelvic inflammatory disease, which could lead to infertility. Men infected with gonorrhea have dysuria and may have a whitish discharge from the penis that may become thick and creamy. Epididymitis may occur in untreated men, which can lead to infertility. Like *Chlamydia, N. gonorrhoeae* can be diagnosed with a DNA probe, which tests for the presence of the gonorrhea gene. The collection procedure is the same as that for *Chlamydia.*

Collecting a Fecal Specimen for Ova and Parasites

Collection kits for transporting ova and parasite specimens are available and consist of two containers—one with formalin and one with polyvinyl alcohol (Figure 8-8). The containers must be filled to the designated line with a fecal specimen. The kit is used for the preservation of fecal parasites.

Transporting Specimens by Mail

When specimens are transported by mail, they must be packed in the correct container (Figure 8-9). The specimen is placed in a container, which is then placed inside a mailing container. A biohazard emblem must be affixed to every container, including the outside one.

Fig. 8-7 JEMBEC transport system for growing *Neisseria gonorrhoeae* that causes gonorrhea (a sexually transmitted disease). *(From Mahon CR, Manuselis G:* Textbook of diagnostic microbiology, *ed 4, St Louis, 2011, Saunders.)*

Fig. 8-8 Ova and parasite collection kit for fecal specimens. *(From Proctor D, Adams A:* Kinn's the medical assistant: an applied learning approach, *ed 12, St Louis, 2014, Saunders. Courtesy Meridan Bioscience, Inc.)*

Fig. 8-9 Specimen mailing containers. *(From Proctor D, Adams A:* Kinn's the medical assistant: an applied learning approach, *ed 12, St Louis, 2014, Saunders.)*

Microbiology Smears, Stains, and Wet Mounts

After the microbiology specimen is collected, the next step is to identify the infectious microorganism microscopically. A portion of the specimen is generally smeared directly onto a slide or mixed into a solution on a slide. The smeared specimen is then dried and fixed to the slide followed by staining it to demonstrate its characteristics.

Gram Stain

More than 100 years have passed since the **Gram stain** was developed by Dr. Hans Christian Gram. The Gram stain is a "method of staining microorganisms as a primary means of identifying and classifying bacteria." The Gram stain reaction is still used today to distinguish between **gram-positive** organisms that retain a purple color and gram-negative organisms that retain a pink/red color. Table 8-2 lists the four reagents used in Gram staining and the positive (dark purple) and negative (pink/red) results that can occur.

Medical assistants should be able to perform a Gram stain on a specimen that has been smeared and fixed on a slide. Although medical assistants will not interpret Gram stains, it is important that they understand why the identification of bacterial shapes and growth patterns is important, as well as understand the significance of whether an organism is gram-positive (purple) or gram-negative (pink/red). (See Tables 8-4 and 8-5 at the end of this chapter for the lists of pathogenic bacilli and cocci, with their Gram reactions in column 3 of the tables.)

Smear Preparation

The bacterial specimen must be smeared onto a glass slide, fixed, and then stained to identify it as gram-positive or gram-negative. The specimen is obtained from the following three possible sources:

1. A direct smear is made by rolling a specimen swab onto a glass slide. All areas of the swab must touch the slide.
2. A colony of bacteria growing on a culture plate is transferred to a glass slide. This is done by taking a colony and rubbing it into a drop of normal saline on the glass slide.
3. A smear may be made from a liquid media culture. Either a sterile swab or a sterilized inoculating needle is dipped in the culture broth, and then rolled or placed on the glass slide.

The smear is allowed to dry and is then heat fixed either by running it through a natural gas Bunsen burner or by placing the slide on an electric incinerator for a few seconds (do not overheat because this could cause distortion of the bacterial cells). Heat fixing kills the microorganisms and causes the swabbed material to stick to the slide before the staining procedure. The methanol fixative, used in blood smears, may also be used to affix the smear to the slide.

The Gram stain procedure consists of the four basic steps seen in Table 8-2. First, crystal violet is applied to the slide, and then it is rinsed off. Second, Gram's iodine is applied, and then rinsed off. Third, a decolorizer is used, and then rinsed off. Fourth, a counterstain, safranin, is applied, and then rinsed off.

The most critical step in the Gram stain procedure is the decolorizing step. If the decolorizing is not done for a sufficient length of time, all the bacteria will be purple, and, conversely, if decolorizing is done for too long a duration, all the bacteria will be pink/red.

Table 8-2   Gram Stain Reactions

Stain Step	Staining Reagent	Color of Gram-Positive Organism	Example Gram-Positive Cocci (GPC)	Color of Gram-Negative Organism	Example Gram-Negative Bacilli (GNB)
1. Primary stain	Crystal violet	Purple	● ● ●	Purple	
2. Mordant	Gram's iodine	Purple	● ● ●	Purple	
3. Decolorizer	Acetone or ethyl alcohol	Purple	● ● ●	Colorless	
4. Counterstain	Safranin	Purple	● ● ●	Pink/red	

Gram-positive organisms stain purple because they have a large **peptidoglycan** layer present in their cell walls that holds the crystal violet stain. Peptidoglycan is a component that gives rigidity to the bacteria's cell walls. Gram-negative organisms, on the other hand, have a small layer of peptidoglycan. In addition, they have an outer layer that is soluble in the decolorizing solution. When the decolorizer is applied, it punches holes in the lipid portion of the gram-negative outer layer, allowing the crystal violet to leak. A counterstain of red safranin stains all the material that is not stained by the crystal violet. At the end of the staining procedure, the gram-positive organisms are purple and the gram-negative organisms are pink/red.

The Gram reaction and shape of the pathogen give the microbiologist the necessary information to help identify the bacteria that are causing the infection in question. For example, gram-positive cocci (GPC) are seen as purple, circular bacteria (Figure 8-10), and gram-negative bacilli (GNB) are seen as pink/red, rod-shaped bacteria (Figure 8-11). *N. gonorrhoeae* (Figure 8-12) are gram-negative cocci (GNC) that appear as pairs of pink/red diplococci shaped like kidney beans and facing each other.

The Gram stain procedure check sheet is provided in the workbook and is demonstrated in Procedure 8-2, located at the end of this section.

Acid-Fast Stains

The acid-fast stain is used to microscopically search for microorganisms in the *Mycobacterium* genus referred to as acid-fast bacilli (AFB), which resist decolorization with acid alcohol. *Mycobacterium tuberculosis* causes tuberculosis (TB), a lung infection in which tubercles (nodules) are formed. Symptoms include night sweats, pulmonary hemorrhage, and **expectoration** (coughing up of sputum and mucus from the trachea and lungs) containing **purulent** (pus filled) sputum. Another pathogen, *Mycobacterium avium* complex, disseminates throughout the body in patients with acquired immunodeficiency syndrome (AIDS). Both mycobacterial diseases have been on the increase with the spread of AIDS.

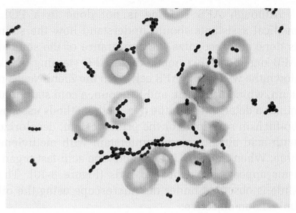

Fig. 8-10 Purple stained gram-positive cocci (GPC) in chains (streptococci) seen with red blood cells. *(From Proctor D, Adams A:* Kinn's the medical assistant: an applied learning approach, *ed 12, St Louis, 2014, Saunders.)*

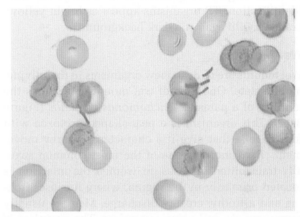

Fig. 8-11 Pink/red stained gram-negative bacilli (GNB) seen with red blood cells. *(From Proctor D, Adams A:* Kinn's the medical assistant: an applied learning approach, *ed 12, St Louis, 2014, Saunders.)*

Fig. 8-12 Pink/red gram-negative cocci (GNC) in pairs (diplococci) seen with epithelial cells. *(From Mahon CR, Manuselis G:* Textbook of diagnostic microbiology, *ed 4, St Louis, 2011, Saunders.)*

Although AFB staining is not done in a POL, medical assistants should understand how the stain is done and recognize the appearance of the stained AFB organism. Two methods of AFB staining break down the wax in the AFB cell wall: the Ziehl-Neelsen stain, which uses heat; and Kinyoun, a cold stain that mixes a detergent with the dye. Both methods use carbolfuchsin solutions for the primary stain, decolorize with acid alcohol, and counterstain with methylene blue. When the stain is complete, the acid-fast organisms appear as red beaded rods (Figure 8-13). The slide is observed under the microscope using the oil immersion objective.

Fluorescent staining is another method used to identify pathogens. Auramine or auramine-rhodamine fluorochrome stain is used. It is viewed under a fluorescence microscope equipped with the appropriate filter system for this type of stained smear. The stain may be screened at a lower magnification, which allows more fields to be examined in a shorter period of time. Higher magnification is needed for final identification. TB organisms appear as bright yellow-orange bacilli against a dark background.

Wet Mounts

Wet mounts are done to view organisms in their living, mobile state. One type of wet mount determines the motility of a parasite, *Trichomonas vaginalis* (Figure 8-14). This organism is a pear-shaped protozoa with four flagella that give it a characteristic jerky movement. *T. vaginalis* is one of the most common sexually transmitted diseases. In women the infection is located primarily in the vagina, where it causes itching and a frothy, creamy discharge. Men are usually asymptomatic and serve as carriers. The organism is found in urine or vaginal specimens in women and in urine or prostatic sections in men.

Wet mounts are also done to detect the presence of "clue cells," vaginal epithelial cells covered with *Gardnerella vaginalis*, a gram-negative coccobacillus. This organism is found in almost 100% of women who have bacterial vaginosis. Infected women produce a watery exudate that lacks white blood cells and usually has a fishy odor, and the clue cells are covered by the *Gardnerella* organism.

The **Wet Mount** procedure check sheet is provided in the workbook and is demonstrated in Procedure 8-3, located at the end of this section.

KOH Preparation

Another type of microbiology slide identification is the KOH (potassium hydroxide) preparation. KOH is an alkaline solution that breaks down protein material, facilitating the identification of any fungus that may be present in skin scrapings, vaginal specimens, or mucus. A KOH preparation shows fungal hyphae from skin dermatophyte infections, as well as yeast such as *Candida albicans*. Although the KOH preparation may be done by a medical assistant, it is interpreted by a trained laboratorian or physician.

The **KOH Preparation** procedure check sheet is provided in the workbook and is demonstrated in Procedure 8-4, located at the end of this section.

Fig. 8-13 Red rod-shaped *Mycobacterium tuberculosis* in acid-fast stain. *(From Proctor D, Adams A:* Kinn's the medical assistant: an applied learning approach, *ed 12, St Louis, 2014, Saunders.)*

Trichomonas vaginalis

Fig. 8-14 *Trichomonas vaginalis*—a single celled protozoan with flagella. *(From Stepp CA, Woods M:* Laboratory procedures for medical office personnel, *Philadelphia, 1998, Saunders.)*

Fig. 8-15 Cellulose tape procedure for collecting pinworm eggs. *(From Proctor D, Adams A: Kinn's the medical assistant: an applied learning approach, ed 12, St Louis, 2014, Saunders.)*

Pinworm Specimen Collection and Microscopic Results

Enterobius vermicularis is a tiny roundworm commonly known as *pinworm*. The female pinworm normally lays her eggs during the nighttime hours in the anal area of the human host. This causes itching, and the host scratches this area, infecting the hands and fingernails. Pinworm infections are common among young children in preschools (or day care centers) as a result of sharing toys contaminated with pinworm eggs. The identification test is performed by using either swabs coated with petroleum jelly or cellulose tape.

The *cellulose tape test* consists of placing cellulose tape (sticky side) over the patient's anal area and then placing the tape sticky-side-down on a glass slide (Figure 8-15). A physician or trained laboratorian examines the tape microscopically for *E. vermicularis* eggs (Figure 8-16).

Fig. 8-16 *Enterobius vermicularis* (pinworm) egg as seen under the microscope. *(From Proctor D, Adams A: Kinn's the medical assistant: an applied learning approach, ed 12, St Louis, 2014, Saunders.)*

✳ **PROCEDURE 8-1** Procedure for Collecting a Throat Specimen

A, Have the patient sit with head back. Use a sterile tongue depressor to hold down the tip of the tongue and have the patient say "ahh" while inserting the two sterile swabs to the back of the throat. *(Photo by Zack Bent.)*

Equipment and Supplies

- Gloves
- Sterile Dacron swabs (not cotton because it inhibits *Streptococcus* growth)
- Swab container
- Tongue depressor

Procedure

1. Sanitize the hands, and apply gloves.
2. Aseptically (following techniques that prevent contamination) remove the sterile swab from the package, holding it by the tip.
3. Have the patient sit with the head back. Use a sterile tongue depressor to hold down the tip of the tongue, and have the patient say "ahh" (Figure A).
4. Rotate the swab on the back of the throat (Figure B) in a circular motion or figure-eight pattern, and

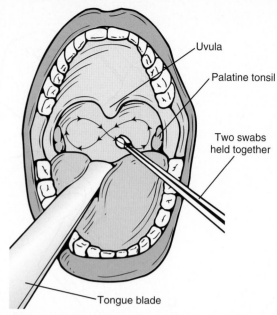

B, Figure-eight technique for obtaining a throat specimen. *(From Stepp CA, Woods M:* Laboratory procedures for medical office personnel, *Philadelphia, 1998, Saunders.)*

place it in the appropriate container. Do not touch the teeth or the back of the tongue because these areas have normal flora. Two swabs may be used at the same time, as seen in Figure A.

5. Depending on the microbiology requisition, one swab may be used for a Rapid Strep test and the other will be placed in a sterile culture transportation tube as seen in Figure 8-3.
6. Remove gloves (unless the rapid test is done immediately after specimen collection), sanitize the hands, and document the collection procedure.

✳ PROCEDURE 8-2 Gram Stain Procedure

A, Gram stain equipment. *a,* Crystal violet; *b,* Gram's iodine; *c,* decolorizer; *d,* safranin; *e,* rinse water; *f,* staining rack; *g,* bibulous paper.

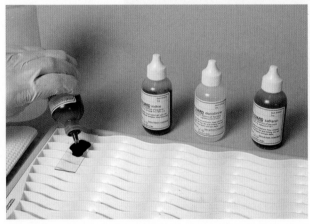

B, Apply crystal violet onto the smeared fixed slide, and time for 1 minute.

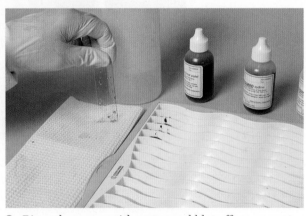

C, Rinse the smear with water, and blot off excess water.

D, Apply Gram's iodine and time for 1 minute, then rinse and blot.

E, Apply decolorizer approximately 3 to 5 seconds until the unbound purple dye is removed (seen at the bottom of the slide when the purple run-off becomes clear).

(Continued)

8-2

PROCEDURE 8-2 Gram Stain Procedure—cont'd

F, Immediately rinse with water to stop the decolorizing reaction.

G, Apply the safranin counterstain for 1 minute; then rinse and blot dry.

Equipment and Supplies (Figure A)

Gram stain reagents:
- Crystal violet
- Gram's iodine
- Decolorizer
- Safranin
- Rinse water
- Staining rack
- Bibulous (highly absorbent) paper
- Gloves (not pictured)

Procedure

1. Sanitize the hands, and apply gloves.
2. Pour crystal violet over the smeared and fixed slide, and leave it on for 1 minute (Figure B). Using the rinse water bottle, flood the slide with water. Then, use gloves or forceps to tip the slide and blot the end of the slide onto the absorbent paper to remove water (Figure C). At this stage, both gram-positive and gram-negative organisms are purple.
3. Pour Gram's iodine over the slide (Figure D), and leave it on for 1 minute. Rinse the slide with water. Again, at this stage both gram-positive and gram-negative organisms are purple. Iodine acts as a mordant to hold the crystal violet dye in gram-positive organisms.
4. Holding the slide vertically, pour decolorizer, which consists of alcohol or acetone, over the slide, and allow it to run off the slide (Figure E). Watch carefully to note when the purple dye stops flowing (3 to 5 seconds). Rinse the slide immediately with

PROCEDURE 8-2 Gram Stain Procedure—cont'd

the water to stop the reaction (Figure F). The crystal violet is removed from gram-negative organisms during this step.

5. Apply the red dye, safranin (Figure G). This dye acts as a counterstain and should be left on for 1 minute. Rinse the slide with water. The safranin stains everything red that was no longer stained purple.

6. Blot the slide dry with bibulous paper. Gram-negative organisms are pink/red, and gram-positive organisms are purple at this end stage of Gram staining.
7. Position the slide under the microscope for the physician to view.
8. Remove gloves, sanitize the hands, and document the procedure.

 ## PROCEDURE 8-3 Wet Mount Procedure

Equipment and Supplies

- Glass slide or slide with a well carved into it
- Coverslip
- Gloves
- Drop of saline
- Specimen

Procedure

1. Sanitize the hands, and apply gloves.
2. Place a small amount of the specimen on the slide or in the slide well.
3. Place a drop of saline (normal, 0.9%) on the specimen and a coverslip over the specimen.
4. Position the slide under the microscope for the physician to view.
5. Remove gloves, sanitize the hands, and document the procedure.

 ## PROCEDURE 8-4 KOH Preparation Procedure

Equipment and Supplies

- Glass slide
- Coverslip
- KOH
- Scalpel
- Swabs
- Specimen
- Gloves

Procedure

1. Sanitize the hands, and apply gloves.
2. Clean the specimen area with 70% alcohol.

3. The sample of hair, skin, or nail is scraped with a scalpel by the physician. A vaginal swab specimen may also be obtained by the physician for yeast determination.
4. Place a drop of 10% KOH on the glass slide.
5. Position the specimen in the KOH on the slide.
6. Place a coverslip on the specimen, and let it sit for 30 minutes. The 10% KOH will dissolve all protein material, leaving any fungus to be seen microscopically.
7. Position the slide under the microscope for the physician to view.
8. Remove gloves, sanitize the hands, and document the procedure.

CLIA-Waived Microbiology Tests

Streptococcus Group A Testing

Streptococcus species are gram-positive cocci in chains. Some streptococci are capable of producing hemolytic toxins, which hemolyze red blood cells (RBCs) when grown on blood agar. Part of the identification of *Streptococcus* depends on which of the following types of hemolytic reactions (breaking down red blood cells) occur on blood agar:

- Alpha hemolysis, incomplete hemolysis of RBCs, is seen as a green color around the colonies.
- Beta hemolysis, complete hemolysis of RBCs, is seen as a clear area around the colonies. *Streptococcus pyogenes,* the bacteria that cause strep throat, demonstrates beta hemolysis (Figure 8-17).
- Gamma hemolysis occurs when no toxin is present and therefore no hemolysis is seen around the colonies.

Streptococcus species can also be divided into groups A through O according to the antigenic properties (the ability to induce the formation of specific antibodies) in their cell walls. This system of classification is named after Dr. Rebecca Lancefield, who identified the various groups. *S. pyogenes* is beta hemolytic and serologically types in group A. This organism, which is often called group A *strep,* causes strep throat, a contagious disease passed from one person to another through droplets of saliva or nasal secretions. The symptoms of strep throat are a very sore throat, a bright red pharynx, white patches on the tonsils, swollen glands in the neck, a tired feeling, and muscular aches.

Some complications of strep throat are scarlet fever, rheumatic fever, and glomerulonephritis. Scarlet fever is a contagious disease characterized by symptoms such as sore throat, fever, enlarged lymph nodes in the neck, flushing of the face, strawberry tongue, and a bright red rash. Rheumatic fever is a systemic inflammatory disease that may affect the brain, heart, joints, skin, or subcutaneous tissues. This disease, which usually occurs in children, may be caused by a delayed reaction to an inadequately treated *S. pyogenes* group A infection. Glomerulonephritis is an inflammation of the glomerulus of the kidney characterized by decreased urine production, edema, and protein and blood in the urine.

Rapid Strep Testing (CLIA-Waived)

There are many CLIA-waived group A strep kits that test directly for the extracted *Streptococcus* A antigen using a throat swab specimen. An example is the Acceava kit (Thermo Electron Corp.).

The **Acceava Strep A Test** procedure check sheet is provided in the workbook and is demonstrated in Procedure 8-5, located at the end of this section.

Bacitracin Method

If the Rapid Strep test is negative, a culture (with a bacitracin disk) may be done at a reference lab. The specimen might not have contained enough organisms to be detected by the Rapid Strep test. Preparing the culture consists of swabbing a blood agar culture plate with the throat specimen. The agar is streaked for isolation. A disk impregnated with a specified amount of the antibiotic bacitracin ("A" disk) is then placed on the swabbed area. The plate is incubated overnight at 37° C. After 24 hours the plate is observed for **S. pyogenes group A**, which will cause beta hemolysis (clearing of the RBCs) on the blood agar plate. It will also show a zone of no growth or beta hemolysis around the bacitracin disk, because strep A is sensitive to the antibiotic. In Figure 8-18, the positive results of beta hemolysis and inhibited growth around the bacitracin disk are seen on the left, and the negative result of no hemolysis and

Fig. 8-18 Bacitracin group A test. Notice how the beta hemolysis is on the left side but not present around the bacitracin disk: this is a positive test for Strep A. The bacterial growth on the right shows no beta hemolysis and is not inhibited by the bacitracin disk: this is a negative result for Strep A. *(From Mahon CR, Manuselis G: Textbook of diagnostic microbiology, ed 4, St Louis, 2011, Saunders.)*

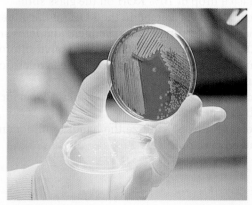

Fig. 8-17 Beta hemolysis showing complete clearing of the blood plate where *Streptococcus* group A is growing. *(From Proctor D, Adams A:* Kinn's the medical assistant: an applied learning approach, *ed 12, St Louis, 2014, Saunders.)*

no inhibited growth around the disk is on the right. If the positive culture is smeared and stained, the bacteria should appear as gram-positive cocci in chains.

Influenza

Influenza is commonly known as the flu. It is caused by a virus that affects the respiratory tract. Symptoms, which last 1 to 2 weeks, are fever (100° to 103° F, higher in children), cough, sore throat, runny or stuffy nose, headache, muscle aches, and fatigue. Gastrointestinal symptoms are rare.

Some individuals with the flu develop complications such as pneumonia. The elderly and people with chronic problems are at greater risk for complications. Three types of influenza exist: A, B, and C. Types A and B cause the winter epidemics that occur almost every year. Type C influenza is milder.

Influenza viruses have the capacity to mutate. One type of mutation is called *antigenic drift*, which refers to a gradual change in the virus strain. Antigenic drift occurs in viruses from one season to another. Another type of mutation, *antigenic shift*, involves an abrupt change in the antigenic properties of the virus. When an antigenic shift occurs, it causes a pandemic, in which large numbers of people contract the disease. The following are examples of past influenza pandemics:

- From 1918 to 1919 the "swine flu," also known as *Spanish flu* H1N1 because Spain was 1 of the countries most seriously affected, killed 675,000 people in the United States and 50 million worldwide. This was probably the most devastating epidemic ever to affect the human race.
- In 1957 the "Asian flu" H2N2 caused 70,000 deaths in the United States.
- In 2005 the "avian flu" became widespread in humans and affected 50 countries in Asia, Europe, and Africa.
- In 2009 the "swine flu," which was referred to as *H1N1,* was considered pandemic.
- In 2013 the World Health Organization (WHO) identified a serious threat of H7N9 bird flu based on 126 cases diagnosed in China with a 20% fatality rate.

Influenza Testing (CLIA-Waved)

The OSOM influenza A and B test (Genzyme Corp.) is a qualitative lateral flow immunoassay. The kit detects the presence of influenza types A and B (direct immunoassay test).

A nasal swab specimen is collected by inserting a soft foam swab approximately 1 inch into the nose (or until resistance is felt). The swab can then be placed in a dry, closed container for up to 8 hours.

The **OSOM Influenza A and B Test** procedure check sheet is provided in the workbook and is demonstrated in Procedure 8-6.

✳ PROCEDURE 8-5 Acceava Strep A Test Procedure

A, Acceava group A strep kit. *a,* Acceava test kit box; *b,* reagents 1 and 2; *c,* positive and negative liquid external controls; *d,* testing tubes; *e,* test sticks and their air-tight container; *f,* sterile swab.

(Continued)

PROCEDURE 8-5 Acceava Strep A Test Procedure—cont'd

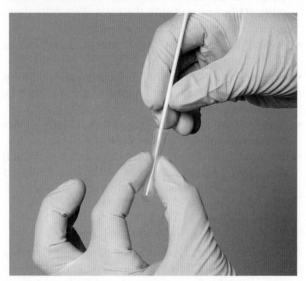

B, Place throat specimen in tube with extraction fluid.

C, Reading results. *1*, Strip before testing; *2*, positive result; *3*, negative result.

Equipment and Supplies (Figure A)

- Acceava group A *Streptococcus* test kit box
- Reagents 1 and 2
- Liquid external controls, positive and negative
- Soft plastic testing tubes
- Test sticks and their container
- Sterile rayon swab taken from wrapper (NOTE: Cotton swabs may inhibit *Streptococcus* growth)
- Personal protective equipment—gloves and face mask

Procedure

1. Sanitize the hands, and apply gloves.
2. Just before testing, add 4 drops of reagent 1 and 4 drops of reagent 2 into a test tube. (The solution should turn light yellow. If it does not, do not proceed with the test.) Immediately put the rayon swab (from the test kit) containing the patient's specimen in the extract solution.
3. Vigorously mix the solution by rotating the swab forcefully against the side of the tube at least 10 times. The best results are obtained when the specimen is vigorously extracted in the solution.
4. Allow the tube containing the swab to stand for 1 minute, and then squeeze the swab against the sides of the tube while withdrawing the swab (Figure B). Discard the swab in a biohazard container.
5. Remove a test stick from the container, and recap immediately. Place the absorbent end of the test stick into the extracted sample in the tube.
6. After 5 minutes read and record the results (Figure C). A positive test result shows as a blue line indicating the presence of *Streptococcus pyogenes*

antigen. A pink line indicates that the specimen flowed up the entire strip and activated the internal control. A negative test result will show no blue line in the test area. The pink line indicates that the internal control worked.
7. Discard all the test materials in the appropriate biohazard containers.
8. Remove and discard gloves in a biohazard container, sanitize the hands, and document the procedure.

Quality Control Procedures

Internal controls are built into each test strip. The appearance of the pink line indicates that the extracted solution passed through the test area and reacted with the pink antigenic control. If the pink line does not appear, the test is considered invalid.

External positive and negative liquid controls must be performed when a new kit is used. In addition, each operator of the test kit should perform a positive and negative control once with each test kit method to confirm that the testing technique is correct. The controls should be documented.

The liquid control procedure is performed in the same way as the patient procedure, except for the step in which the patient swab is added to the extract solution. Instead of the patient swab, add 1 drop of well-mixed positive control to the plastic tube along with a sterile swab. Follow the directions in the patient procedure, starting with step 3. Observe and record the results in 5 minutes. Repeat the procedure with a drop of well-mixed negative control.

PROCEDURE 8-6 OSOM Influenza A and B Test Procedure

A, OSOM influenza A and B test kit supplies. *a,* OSOM kit; *b,* gloves and face mask; *c,* foam swab; *d,* plastic test tube; *e,* extract solution; *f,* test strip; *g,* control swabs; *h,* air-tight strip container with key to results.

B, Collect the nasal specimen by inserting the foam swab 1 inch into the nostril displaying the most discharge, and gently rotate while rocking it back and forth for five seconds.

C, After mixing the nasal swab in the buffer extract solution, extract all the solution from the swab by squeezing the swab with the plastic tube while removing it from the tube.

(Continued)

8-6

PROCEDURE 8-6 OSOM Influenza A and B Test Procedure—cont'd

D, Place the testing strip into the extracted fluid in the patient's tube, and wait 10 minutes. NOTE: The tubes to the right of the patient's test are the negative and positive controls.

Keys to interpretation

Positive control for Influenza A

Positive control for Influenza B

Negative control for Influenza

Patient tested positive for Influenza A

E, Using the interpretation key on the container and the control results, determine the patient's reaction.

Equipment and Supplies (Figure A)

OSOM influenza A and B test kit supplies:

(A) OSOM kit containing all supplies

(B) Personal protective equipment (face mask and gloves)

(C) Sterile foam swab provided in kit to collect nasal specimen

(D) Plastic testing tube provided in kit

(E) Extract solution provided in kit

(F) Testing strip provided in kit

(G) Control swabs for influenza A and B

(H) Air-tight container of testing strips with diagram showing how to interpret results

Procedure

1. Sanitize the hands, and apply gloves and face mask.

2. Before running the first patient test from a new test kit, run a negative control test and both of the positive A and the positive B controls to see whether they react correctly. If they are correct, then proceed with the patient testing.

3. Insert the foam swab provided in the test kit into the patient's nostril displaying the most secretion. Using a gentle rotation, push the swab until resistance is met at the level of the turbinates (at least 1 inch into the nostril; see Figure B). Rotate the swab a few times against the nasal wall, and gently rock it back and forth, and hold swab in place for 5 seconds to ensure maximum absorbency.

(Continued)

PROCEDURE 8-6 OSOM Influenza A and B Test Procedure—cont'd

4. Place the nasal swab into the plastic tube containing the designated amount of extraction buffer solution, and vigorously twist the swab against the sides and bottom of the tube at least 10 times. This disrupts the virus particles and releases the internal viral nucleoproteins into the solution.

5. Extract all the solution from the swab by squeezing the plastic tube against the swab while removing it from the tube, as seen in Figure C. Dispose of swab properly.

6. Dip the influenza test strip into the tube with the extraction buffer solution with the arrows on the strip pointing down, as seen in Figure D. It takes 10 minutes for the sample to be absorbed by the strip. During this time the liquid sample migrates across the test areas and control area of the strip, and the colored reactions develop. The nucleoproteins from the virus will react with the reagents on the test strip.

7. Read the test results for influenza A and B (Figure E). A positive test result is shown by a pink or purple line in the "A" or "B" test area and a pink line in the internal control area. A negative test result shows no color change in the test area and a pink line in the internal control area.

8. Discard all the test materials in the appropriate biohazard containers.

9. Remove and discard gloves and mask in the biohazard container, sanitize the hands, and chart the results.

Quality Control Procedure

Internal quality controls are built into each strip. The appearance of a pink line in the control area of the strip is the positive control demonstrating that sufficient flow has occurred and the functional integrity of the test strip has been maintained. If the pink line does not appear, the test is considered invalid. A clearing of the background color is the negative internal control and verifies that the test was correctly performed. If background color appears, it will interfere with test interpretation and render the test results invalid.

External quality controls include one influenza A positive control swab and one influenza B positive control swab. The control swabs supplied in the kit are tested following the swab procedure described previously. See Figure E for the three external control results.

- The presence of a light pink to purple line in the "A" test line position and at the "Control" line position when the influenza A positive control swab is tested indicates that the influenza antigen binding property of the test stick is functional.
- The presence of a light pink to purple line in the "B" test line position and at the "Control" line position when the influenza B positive control swab is tested indicates that the influenza antigen binding property of the test stick is functional.
- The influenza A control swab acts as a negative control for the influenza B antigen, and, conversely, the influenza B control swab acts as a negative control for the influenza B antigen.

External positive and negative liquid controls must be performed when a new kit is used. In addition, each operator of the test kit should perform a positive and negative control once with each test kit method to confirm that the testing technique is correct. The control results should be documented.

Photos A through E by Zack Bent.

Advanced Concepts

When a microbiology specimen is sent to a reference laboratory, various steps are followed in the growth, identification, and sensitivity testing of the microorganisms.

Growth Requirements of Bacteria

Identification of bacteria is made on the basis of their growth requirements, particularly their need for oxygen, carbon dioxide, and specific nutrients.

Oxygen Requirements

Of the three gases that are needed for growth—oxygen, carbon dioxide, and nitrogen—oxygen has the greatest impact on an organism's ability to adapt. Organisms can be classified into the following two types:

- **Aerobic** organisms require oxygen for growth. *Salmonella* (some species cause enteric dysentery) is an example of an aerobe.
- **Anaerobic** organisms can grow and function in the absence of oxygen. *Clostridium tetani* is an anaerobe

found in soil. If this organism penetrates a wound deep in the tissue, it will grow and produce a deadly neurotoxin that causes tetanus or lockjaw. Therefore all patients with a puncture wound should receive a tetanus injection.

Nutrient Requirements

The nutrients that most pathogenic bacteria require outside the body are meat extracts, peptone (a nitrogen compound), mineral salts such as sulfates, chlorides, and calcium and sodium phosphates. Some organisms are **fastidious**, which means they require specific nutrients and conditions for growth. An example of a fastidious pathogen is *N. gonorrhoeae,* which requires blood serum, some amino acids, vitamins, and 10% carbon dioxide.

Media Used for Growing Bacteria

Bacteria are grown and isolated on culture media for identification purposes. Media contain essential nutritious substances that allow microorganisms to grow and multiply. Media can be solid, semisolid, or liquid. Solid media contain **agar**, a gelatinous substance obtained from seaweed that is liquid when heated and becomes solid when cooled in a **Petri dish** (Figure 8-19). When a bacterium is placed on a solid medium, it will grow and replicate until it forms a visible mass of bacteria, or a colony. Liquid media such as thioglycolate broth are used to grow most bacteria, including anaerobes.

Microbiology Equipment

Several types of equipment used in a microbiology laboratory are very large and are not usually found in a POL.

Fig. 8-19 Three types of culture media for growing specific bacteria based on their nutrient requirements.

Larger equipment commonly used in a microbiology laboratory includes the following:
- Incubator (37° C)—used for growing cultures at body temperature
- Safety hood—built-in area with a fan to pull the airflow away from the operator
- Autoclave—destroys microorganisms by applying steam under pressure
- Refrigerator—for storage of culture plates and supplies
- Microscopes—used to identify microorganisms

Equipment Used to Inoculate Culture Plates

The most common equipment used to transfer microorganisms from specimens to various culture media are **inoculation** loops and needles. The inoculating loop has a bubble wand at the end that varies in size. One type of inoculating loop is a reusable wire type that is sterilized before and after each use. Another type is a sterile disposable loop (Figure 8-20). Loops can be calibrated to collect a precise amount of specimen. An example is the urine culture loop, made of platinum, which is calibrated to collect either 0.01 or 0.001 mL of urine for culturing. The inoculating needle is straight at the end and is used to collect colonies of bacteria.

Fig. 8-20 Disposable inoculating loops for transferring liquids to culture plates. *(From Proctor D, Adams A:* Kinn's the medical assistant: an applied learning approach, *ed 12, St Louis, 2014, Saunders. Courtesy Simport Plastics, Beloeil, Quebec.)*

Equipment Used for Incineration

The incineration equipment used to sterilize loops and needles are Bunsen burners and electric incinerators (Figure 8-21). Bunsen burners produce a flame by igniting natural gas that is connected to the burner. This method is dangerous because of the fire hazard and because the organisms could splatter as they are heated. The electric incinerator is much safer because it prevents splattering.

Culturing Methods

Inoculation of Media

If a patient's clinical signs and symptoms indicate that a bacterial infection is present, the physician orders a "culture and sensitivity" to determine what bacteria

Fig. 8-21 Reusable metal loops (for transferring liquids and inoculating culture plates) being "sterilized" using the electronically heated incinerator. *(From Stepp CA, Woods M:* Laboratory procedures for medical office personnel, *Philadelphia, 1998, Saunders.)*

are present (culture) and what antibiotics will kill them (sensitivity).

After microbiology specimens are collected, they are placed on the correct media according to the source of the specimen. If the specimen is sent to the laboratory on a swab or a sterile swab is dipped into the specimen (e.g., sputum), the swab is rolled in the upper quadrant of a solid-medium Petri dish so that all sides of the swab touch the medium. If the specimen is liquid, an inoculating loop is used. The loop must be sterilized first by placing it in a Bunsen burner or incinerator until it is red and then allowing it to cool. The sterilized loop is placed in the liquid specimen and applied to the upper quadrant of the solid culture medium.

The following two techniques are used for spreading a specimen:

- The isolation technique, or *quadrant technique,* consists of using the sterilized loop to spread the specimen over four areas of the plate to establish isolated colonies of bacteria that can be used for identification (Figure 8-22). Better isolation is achieved if the streak lines are kept close together and the loop is sterilized between quadrants.
- The *colony count,* or *lawn technique,* involves streaking the entire plate (Figure 8-23). The lawn method is used for antibiotic sensitivity testing and consists of using a swab that has been dipped in a broth containing only one kind of organism (pure culture) and swabbing the entire plate (see following section titled Sensitivity Testing). In the urine colony count method, the whole plate is streaked with a calibrated loop so that the colonies that grow on the plate can be counted.

Fig. 8-22 Quadrant streaking method used for inoculating a swab specimen on a culture plate to establish isolated colonies for further identification and testing of the pathogenic organism.

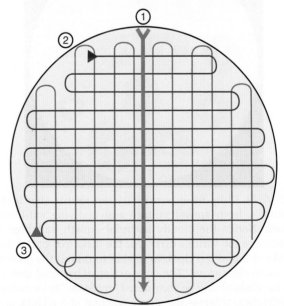

Fig. 8-23 Lawn spread or colony count streaking used when testing a pure bacterial culture for antibiotic sensitivity testing, or for counting colonies that form when applying a urine specimen using a calibrated loop.

After the specimens are streaked onto the appropriate media plates, the plates are placed in an incubator with the correct amount of atmospheric gases to grow the organisms. The temperature of the incubator is usually 37° C, which is body temperature.

Sensitivity Testing

Physicians often order sensitivity tests to determine the type of antibiotics that would be most effective at treating patients' bacterial infections. One of the methods used for sensitivity testing is the Kirby-Bauer method. A liquid nutrient broth is inoculated with a pure culture of the bacteria grown to a specific turbidity, or cloudiness. The bacteria are then spread over the whole plate (lawn method) of the appropriate media. The Kirby-Bauer apparatus fits over the media plate and drops disks, with each disk containing a specific amount of antibiotic on the bacteria. After the plates are incubated overnight, each disk on the plate is checked for zones of inhibition. The zones are measured in millimeters, compared with the manufacturer's values, and recorded as *S* (sensitive), *I* (intermediate), or *R* (resistant) (Figures 8-24 and 8-25).

For the physician the best antibiotic is the one that is most sensitive, showing no growth of bacteria (clear) around the white disk. It should also be the least toxic to the patient and the patient's normal flora, and it should be the most cost-effective.

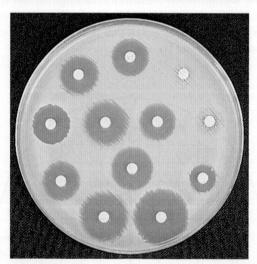

Fig. 8-24 Kirby-Bauer sensitivity test results after incubating a lawn spread culture and applying antibiotic disks. Notice the cloudy bacterial growth and how it reacted to the various disks. All the disks except the two disks at 2 and 3 o'clock were able to inhibit the growth (seen as clear areas). The nonreaction of bacterial growth to the disks would be considered "resistant" to those two antibiotics, whereas the strong reaction at 5 o'clock and the "no growth" rings around the others would be considered "sensitive" to those antibiotics. *(From Mahon CR, Manuselis G: Textbook of diagnostic microbiology, ed 4, St Louis, 2011, Saunders.)*

Urine Culture

A urine culture is commonly ordered to evaluate urinary tract infections. It involves sending the urine to the laboratory to perform a colony count as described previously. The urine must be collected by the midstream clean-catch method and should be the first morning specimen.

There are also rapid urine culture tests that may be performed in the medical office. See Procedure 8-7 at the end of this advanced concepts section and in the workbook for the Uricult rapid screening for urine culture.

Pathogenic Organisms Seen Frequently in Physician Office Laboratories

Medical assistants should understand some of the common causes of diseases frequently seen in patients in physicians' offices. See Atlas of Common Pathogenic Organisms (Figures 8-26 to 8-31).

Pathogenic Bacteria

The following are bacterial infections most commonly seen in the POL:
- Strep throat—*Streptococcus pyogenes group A*, gram-positive cocci in chains (see Figure 8-10)
- Urinary tract infections—*Escherichia coli, Proteus* spp., *Klebsiella* spp., *Pseudomonas aeruginosa;* all gram-negative bacilli (see Figure 8-11)
- Pneumonia—*Streptococcus pneumoniae*, gram-positive diplococci (look like cat eyes) (see Atlas Figure 8-26)
- Wound infections—*Staphylococcus aureus*, gram-positive cocci in clusters (see Atlas Figure 8-27).

Fig. 8-25 Reading a Kirby-Bauer sensitivity test using calipers to measure whether the bacteria is *S* (sensitive), *I* (intermediate), or *R* (resistant) to the antibiotic. *(From Mahon CR, Manuselis G: Textbook of diagnostic microbiology, ed 4, St Louis, 2011, Saunders.)*

Common Pathogenic Organisms

Fig. 8-26 *Streptococcus pneumoniae* Gram stain. *(From Mahon CR, Manuselis G:* Textbook of diagnostic microbiology, *ed 4, St Louis, 2011, Saunders.)*

Fig. 8-27 *Staphylococcus aureus* Gram stain. *(From Mahon CR, Manuselis G:* Textbook of diagnostic microbiology, *ed 4, St Louis, 2011, Saunders.)*

Fig. 8-28 *Neisseria gonorrhoeae* Gram stain. *(From Mahon CR, Manuselis G:* Textbook of diagnostic microbiology, *ed 4, St Louis, 2011, Saunders.)*

Fig. 8-29 *Giardia lamblia* smear. *(From Mahon CR, Manuselis G:* Textbook of diagnostic microbiology, *ed 4, St Louis, 2011, Saunders.)*

Fig. 8-30 Body louse. *(From Stepp CA, Woods M:* Laboratory procedures for medical office personnel, *Philadelphia, 1998, Saunders.)*

Fig. 8-31 Pubic louse, also called crab louse. *(From Mahon CR, Manuselis G:* Textbook of diagnostic microbiology, *ed 4, St Louis, 2011, Saunders.)*

NOTE: Because of the danger of methicillin-resistant *Staphylococcus aureus* (MRSA), strict aseptic technique is necessary to prevent nosocomial infections.

- Gonorrhea—*N. gonorrhoeae*, gram-negative diplococci (kidney-bean shape, facing each other) (see Atlas Figure 8-28)
- Chlamydia—*C. trachomatis*, gram-negative group of bacteria that can reproduce only in a cell

Pathogenic Fungi

The following are fungal infections commonly seen in POLs:

- Yeast infections—*C. albicans*, oval-shaped organisms that absorb crystal violet and can be seen budding
- Dermatophyte infections (athlete's foot, jock itch, ringworm)—*Trichophyton* spp., *Microsporum* spp., and others (see hyphae in KOH preparation)

Parasites and Protozoa

The following are pathogenic parasites frequently seen in the POL:

- Pinworm—*E. vermicularis*
- Giardiasis—*Giardia lamblia*, protozoan flagellate that causes gastrointestinal symptoms (see Atlas Figure 8-29)
- Trichomonas—*T. vaginalis* (see Figure 8-14)
- Lice—*Pediculus humanus* (body louse) (see Atlas Figure 8-30), *Phthirus pubis* (crab louse, or crab) (see Atlas Figure 8-31)

Emerging Infectious Diseases

The relation between microorganisms and diseases is not fixed. New infectious diseases may emerge suddenly, whereas others seem to disappear and then reemerge. According to most experts, the rate at which infectious diseases emerge and reemerge has risen in recent years. Some of the most important reasons for this trend are the growth of human populations, the increase in international travel, and the effect of environmental changes. Table 8-3 lists some emerging diseases and the microorganisms that cause them (causative agents).

Bioterrorism

As a result of the bioterrorism threats that occurred in the aftermath of 9/11, all laboratories (including POLs) should perform a risk assessment. Laboratories must identify procedures and methods that have the potential to produce **aerosols** (fine particles suspended in the air). The use of biosafety cabinets or hoods when performing tasks is one way to avoid exposure to aerosols. The Centers for Disease Control and Prevention recommends referring any suspicious organisms or substances to the proper authorities and practicing the proper biosafety techniques at all times.

Most of the bacteria, viruses, and toxins used as bioterrorism agents can be spread by an aerosol route, which is very stable. They also produce high **morbidity** (rate of illness) and **mortality** (rate of deaths). Other bioterrorism agents are transmitted person to person, and some are difficult to treat.

Agents Used in Viral Bioterrorism

Smallpox

Some historians believe that smallpox has killed more people than any other disease (300 million deaths in the twentieth century). *Variola major* is the most virulent strain and causes severe blistering and high fever that kills approximately half of those affected. *Variola minor* is a milder form, with a death rate of less than 1%. As of 1980, smallpox was declared eradicated, thanks to vaccination programs around the world. This victory over smallpox could be in jeopardy if it were to be used as a weapon of bioterrorism.

Viral Hemorrhagic Fever

Viral hemorrhagic fever is thought by some to be the most lethal disease known to man. The Ebola virus is one of the causes of the fever and is spread by direct contact with infected blood or body parts. The disease is characterized by high fever, extensive bleeding, and destruction of internal organs.

Biological Toxin Used in Bioterrorism

Botulism

Clostridium botulinum produces a neurotoxin, botulinum, which is the most poisonous natural substance known. It causes dry mouth, dilated pupils, and a progressive muscle weakness that leads to respiratory failure and death. There are seven types of botulism toxin, but types A, B, and E are most commonly associated with human disease. Toxin A is the most potent.

Agents Used in Bacterial Bioterrorism

Plague

In the Middle Ages between a quarter and a third of the population of Europe was killed by the plague. In 1891 approximately 6 million people died as a result of the plague in India. Currently, only a dozen cases are reported in the United States each year. The plague is known as the "black death" because in its later stages, in untreated patients, the blood vessels are destroyed and subcutaneous bleeding leads to black spots on the skin.

Yersinia pestis is the causative agent of the plague. The disease primarily affects rodents, but it is transferred to human beings by flea bites. Two forms of the plague are the following:

- Bubonic plague results from flea bites.
- Pneumonic plague is spread person to person by respiratory droplets. If the disease is not treated, the death rate is 100%.

Table 8-3   Some Emerging Infectious Diseases

Disease	Causative Agent	Description
Influenza—Swine	Influenza A (H1N1)	On June 11, 2009, the World Health Organization (WHO) signaled that a pandemic of 2009 H1N1 flu was under way. The virus had mutated genes from former flu viruses that normally circulated in pigs in Europe and Asia and in bird (avian) genes and human genes. Scientists called this a "quadruple reassortant" virus.
Influenza—Avian	Influenza A (H5N1)	In 1997 a novel strain of flu virus was discovered in poultry in South Asia and China. In 2005 it became widespread in humans, including those in 50 countries in Asia, Europe, and Africa.
C. diff colitis	*Clostridium difficile*	Major cause of colitis and antibiotic-induced diarrhea. It produces two toxins, which cause inflammation of the intestinal wall (colitis) along with diarrhea, abdominal pain, and fever. It is one of the most common hospital (nosocomial) infections around the world. As of 2009, it was becoming resistant to most antibiotics. Treatment is by discontinuing antibiotics and starting specific anticlostridial antibiotics, such as metronidazole.
MRSA	Methicillin-resistant *Staphylococcus aureus*	In 2005 the Centers for Disease Control and Prevention reported more deaths attributed to MRSA than to acquired immunodeficiency syndrome (AIDS). This superbug caused nosocomial wound infections such as toxic shock syndrome, scalded skin syndrome, scarlet fever, erysipelas, impetigo, and pneumonia. The antibiotic-resistant staph also emerged in the community, causing skin infections, such as pimples and boils, to occur in otherwise healthy people.
Severe acute respiratory syndrome (SARS)	Coronavirus	During November 2002 through July 2003, a total of 8098 people worldwide became sick with SARS, which was accompanied by either pneumonia or respiratory distress syndrome (probable cases), according to the World Health Organization.
MERS-CoV	New corona respiratory virus	This deadly respiratory virus (similar to SARS) was discovered in India in 2013.
Ebola	Ebola virus	Ebola was first discovered in 1977 after two simultaneous outbreaks in Africa (Sudan and Congo). It causes fever, extensive bleeding, and destruction of internal organs.
Hantavirus pulmonary syndrome	Sin nombre virus	Hantavirus was first isolated in 1993 in the southwestern United States from patients with highly fatal respiratory tract infections.
Hepatitis C	Hepatitis C virus	Hepatitis C virus infects up to 3% of the world's population. It was identified in 1989. In 2013 80% of cases were the "baby boomers" born between 1945 and 1965.
Hemolytic uremic syndrome	*Escherichia coli* 0157:H7	First detected in 1982, hemolytic uremic syndrome is a life-threatening condition characterized by severe anemia and kidney failure.
HIV/AIDS (acquired immunodeficiency syndrome)	Human immunodeficiency virus	HIV, first discovered in 1981, is the cause of AIDS.

Tularemia

Tularemia is caused by *Francisella tularensis,* a gram-negative bacillus. Human beings are usually infected after being bitten by infected rabbits or ticks. The disease is characterized by fever and flulike symptoms. The patient may develop ulcerated skin lesions with localized lymph node enlargement as the result of direct contact.

Pneumonic tularemia may result from exposure to aerosols. The incubation period is 3 to 5 days, with the abrupt onset of chills, fever, headache, **myalgia**, and nonproductive cough. The death rate is 30% if the disease is untreated and less than 10% if treated.

Anthrax

Anthrax, caused by *Bacillus anthracis,* is a very old disease—the fifth plague of the Bible (Figure 8-32). It is a disease of livestock, which become infected after feeding on plants contaminated with the organism. Human beings contract the disease mostly through contact with infected animals or animal products. The organism is a gram-positive bacillus. *Endospores,* as seen in the spore stain, can live for 40 years (Figure 8-33). The spores must be ground into a very fine powder before they can penetrate deep into the lungs and cause infection.

Three forms of anthrax can be contracted in human beings: cutaneous, inhalation (or pulmonary), and gastrointestinal.

- *Cutaneous anthrax*—Blisters form and develop into blackened craters, called *eschars* (Figure 8-34). These may heal spontaneously or be treated with penicillin. If the anthrax organism enters the blood and produces substantial quantities of toxin, however, antibiotics are no longer effective.
- *Inhalation or pulmonary anthrax*—Naturally occurring pulmonary anthrax is rare. In September and October 2001, pulmonary anthrax was spread through letters in the mail. The cutaneous form developed in a number of people, and at least 10 people contracted the inhalation form. Six of those 10 survived, probably because they were treated early with combinations of antibiotics—ciprofloxacin or doxycycline along with one or more other antibiotics effective against anthrax.
- *Gastrointestinal anthrax*—Intestinal eschars, similar to those produced by cutaneous anthrax, are characteristic of this disease. It can progress to generalized toxemia. The death rate is 50% to 100% despite treatment.

Reference Tables for Common Infectious Diseases Categorized

The following tables are an excellent resource for locating information on the most common infectious diseases, with descriptions of the organisms that cause each disease, ways the disease is transmitted, symptoms of the disease, test specimens required for diagnosis of the disease, and actions that will help prevent infection (see Tables 8-4 to 8-9).

Fig. 8-32 *Bacillus anthracis* Gram stain. *(From Mahon CR, Manuselis G:* Textbook of diagnostic microbiology, *ed 4, St Louis, 2011, Saunders.)*

Fig. 8-33 *Bacillus anthracis* acid-fast stain showing endospores within the bacilli. *(From Mahon CR, Manuselis G:* Textbook of diagnostic microbiology, *ed 4, St Louis, 2011, Saunders.)*

Fig. 8-34 Cutaneous anthrax eschar. *(Courtesy Centers for Disease Control and Prevention.)*

Table 8-4 Common Diseases Caused by Bacilli

Disease	Organism	Description	Transmission	Symptoms	Tests/Specimens	Prevention and Immunization
Tuberculosis	*Mycobacterium tuberculosis*	Acid-fast branching bacilli, anaerobic	Inhalation	Pulmonary: cough, hemoptysis, sweats, weight loss; May affect other systems	Sputum for culture, radiographs, skin tests	BCG vaccine (not routinely given in United States)
Urinary tract infections	*Escherichia coli,* *Proteus* spp., *Klebsiella* spp., *Pseudomonas aeruginosa*	Gram-negative bacilli, many flagellated	Ascends urethra; catheterization	Cystitis: frequency, burning, blood in urine; Pyelonephritis: flank pain, fever	Clean-catch urine for culture and analysis	Good personal hygiene (always wipe from front to back)
C. diff infection	*Clostridium difficile*	Spore-forming, gram-positive, anaerobic bacilli	Nosocomial: direct contact with contaminated equipment and hands; patients receiving antibiotic therapy are susceptible	Diarrhea, fever, nausea, belly pain, colitis	Stool culture and toxin confirmation followed by endoscopy	Antibiotics taken only as prescribed; proper washing of hands and equipment after bowel movement
Legionnaires' disease	*Legionella pneumophila*	Gram-negative bacillus (stains poorly with usual methods)	Grows freely in water (air-conditioning systems)	Pneumonia-like symptoms	Sputum, blood	Isolation
Tetanus (lockjaw)	*Clostridium tetani*	Gram-positive spore-forming bacilli; anaerobic	Open wounds, fractures, punctures	Toxin affects motor nerves; muscle spasms, convulsions, rigidity	Blood	DPT vaccine in childhood; T or Td every 10 years
Gas gangrene	*Clostridium perfringens*	Gram-positive spore-forming bacilli; anaerobic	Wounds	Gas and watery exudate in infected wound	Swab, aspirate of wound for culture	Proper wound care
Botulism	*Clostridium botulinum*	Gram-positive spore-forming bacilli; anaerobic	Improperly cooked canned foods	Neurotoxin affects speech, swallowing, vision; paralysis of respiratory muscles; death	Contaminated food, blood	*Botulinum* antitoxin; canned goods boiled for 20 minutes before tasting or eating
Diphtheria respiratory secretions	*Corynebacterium diphtheriae*	Gram-positive bacilli; club shaped		Sore throat, fever, headache, gray membrane in throat	Swabs; Gram stain, culture; Schick test for immunity	DPT in childhood
Whooping cough	*Bordetella pertussis*	Gram-negative bacilli	Respiratory tract secretions	Upper respiratory tract symptoms; high-pitched crowing "whoop"	Swabs for culture	DPT in childhood
Plague	*Yersinia pestis*	Gram-negative bacilli	Flea bite from infected rodents	Fever and chills, delirium; enlarged, painful lymph nodes	Sputum for culture, blood	Vaccine, rodent control

Modified from Proctor D, Adams A: *Kinn's the medical assistant: an applied learning approach,* ed 12, St Louis, 2014, Saunders.
BCG, Bacille Calmette-Guérin vaccine; *DPT,* diphtheria-pertussis-tetanus vaccine; *T,* tetanus (toxoid); *Td,* tetanus and diphtheria (toxoids).

Table 8-5 Common Diseases Caused by Cocci

Disease	Organism	Description	Transmission	Symptoms	Specimens	Tests	Prevention
Pneumonia	Streptococcus pneumoniae	Gram-positive encapsulated cocci in pairs	Direct contact, droplets	Productive cough, fever, chest pain	Sputum, bronchoscopy secretions	Culture, Gram stain	Vaccine
Strep throat	Streptococcus pyogenes (group A strep)	Gram-positive cocci in chains	Direct contact, droplets, fomites	Severe sore throat, fever, **malaise**	Direct swab	Rapid Strep test, throat culture	None
Wound infection, abscesses, boils	Staphylococcus aureus and methicillin-resistant Staphylococcus aureus (MRSA)	Gram-positive cocci in clusters	Direct contact, fomites, carriers; poor hand washing	Area red, warm, swollen; pus; pain; ulceration or sinus formation	Deep swab, aspirate of drainage	Culture and sensitivity (aerobic and anaerobic)	None
Staphylococcal food poisoning	Staphylococcus aureus	Gram-positive cocci in clusters	Poor hygiene and improper refrigeration of foods	Vomiting, abdominal cramps, diarrhea	Suspected food, stool	Culture of food (organism will not be found in stool)	Properly refrigerated food to prevent toxin production
Toxic shock	Staphylococcus aureus	Gram-positive cocci in clusters	Use of absorbent pack materials (e.g., tampons, nasal packs)	Fever, headache, nausea, vomiting, delirium, low blood pressure	Swab, blood	Culture and serology	Frequent changing of tampons, packing material
Gonorrhea	Neisseria gonorrhoeae	Gram-negative cocci in pairs; intracellular in white blood cells	Sexually transmitted	Women: pelvic pain, discharge; may be asymptomatic Men: urethral drip, pain on urination	Swab of cervix, urethra; rectal and pharyngeal swabs in homosexuals	Gram stain, culture	Avoidance of unprotected sex
Meningococcal meningitis	Neisseria meningitidis	Gram-negative diplococci	Respiratory tract secretions	High fever, headache, projectile vomiting, delirium, neck and back rigidity, convulsions, petechial rash	Nasopharyngeal swabs, cerebrospinal fluid, blood	Gram stain, culture, cell counts and chemistries	Vaccine, prophylactic antibiotics

Modified from Proctor D, Adams A: *Kinn's the medical assistant: an applied learning approach*, ed 12, St Louis, 2014, Saunders.

Table 8-6	Common Diseases Caused by Spirilla

Disease	Organism	Description	Transmission	Symptoms	Tests/ Specimens	Prevention and Immunization
Syphilis	*Treponema pallidum*	Spirochete	Sexually, congenitally	Primary: painless sore (chancre) Secondary: generalized rash involving palms and soles of feet Congenital: birth defects	Blood for serological tests: VDRL, RPR, FTA-ABS	Avoidance of unprotected sex
Lyme disease	*Borrelia burgdorferi*	Spirochete	Tick bite	Fever, joint pain, red bull's-eye rash	Swab for culture	Avoidance of tick-infested areas
Pyloric ulcers	*Helicobacter pylori*	Gram-negative, spiral-shaped	Unknown, possibly food and water	Burning pain in stomach, especially between meals	Stomach biopsy for staining and culture; stool for EIA testing	Unknown
Food poisoning (most common cause in United States)	*Campylobacter jejuni*	Paired gram-negative curved rods forming a seagull shape	Contaminated food, water, and milk	Bloody or watery diarrhea	Stool for dark field microscopy	Sanitary food preparation and control of water and milk supplies

From Proctor D, Adams A: *Kinn's the medical assistant: an applied learning approach,* ed 12, St Louis, 2014, Saunders.
EIA, Enzyme immunoassay(s); *FTA-ABS,* fluorescent treponemal antibody absorption (test); *RPR,* rapid plasma reagin (test); *VDRL,* Venereal Disease Research Laboratory.

Table 8-7	Diseases Caused by *Rickettsia, Chlamydia,* and *Mycoplasma*

Disease	Organism	Transmission	Symptoms	Tests/Specimens
Rocky Mountain spotted fever	*Rickettsia rickettsiae*	Tick bite	Headache, chills, fever, characteristic rash on extremities and trunk	Blood for serological tests, skin biopsy for direct fluorescent microscopy
Typhus	*Rickettsia prowazekii*	Tick bite	Fever, rash, confusion	Blood for serological tests
Atypical (walking) pneumonia	*Mycoplasma pneumoniae*	Respiratory tract secretions	Fever, cough, chest pain	Blood, sputum
Nongonococcal urethritis and vaginitis	*Chlamydia trachomatis*	Sexual	May be asymptomatic	Swabs for culture and serological testing
Inclusion conjunctivitis, pneumonia		Congenital	Severe conjunctivitis in newborns; afebrile pneumonia in newborns	

From Proctor D, Adams A: *Kinn's the medical assistant: an applied learning approach,* ed 12, St Louis, 2014, Saunders.

Table 8-8   Common Diseases Caused by Fungi

Disease	Organism	Predisposing Conditions and Transmission	Symptoms	Tests/Specimens
Thrush (oral yeast), vulvovaginal candidiasis, or *Monilia* (vaginal yeast)	*Candida* spp. (yeast)	Oral: during birth; other: after antibiotic therapy, oral birth control, severe diabetes	White, cheesy growth	Swab for KOH prep, culture
Athlete's foot, jock itch, ringworm (tinea)	*Trichophyton* spp., *Microsporum* spp., and others (skin fungi)	Opportunistic; direct contact; clothing; prolonged exposure to moist environment	Hair loss, thickening of skin, nails; itching; red, scaly patches	Skin scraping for KOH prep; skin, hair for culture
Histoplasmosis	*Histoplasma capsulatum*	Inhalation of dust contaminated with bird or bat droppings	Mild, flulike to systemic	Serological, culture of biopsy material
Cryptococcosis	*Cryptococcus neoformans*	Contact with poultry droppings	Cough, fever, malaise; can become systemic	Sputum culture
Sporotrichosis	*Sporothrix schenckii*	Farmers, florists, people exposed to soil	Skin lesions that spread along lymphatics; can become systemic	Cerebrospinal fluid culture, India ink direct examination, scrapings, serological KOH (potassium hydroxide)
Pneumocystis pneumonia	*Pneumocystis jirovecii*	Widely prevalent in animals; occurs in debilitated persons, immunosuppressed; common in patients with acquired immunodeficiency syndrome (AIDS)	Pneumonia-like	Biopsy

From Proctor D, Adams A: *Kinn's the medical assistant: an applied learning approach,* ed 12, St Louis, 2014, Saunders.

Table 8-9	Common Protozoan and Parasitic Diseases			
Disease	**Organism**	**Transmission**	**Symptoms**	**Tests/Specimens**
Malaria	*Plasmodium* spp. (protozoa)	Bite of *Anopheles* mosquito	Chills, fever (cyclic)	Blood: examination of stained blood for parasites
Toxoplasmosis	*Toxoplasma gondii* (protozoa)	Fecal contamination (cat litter), congenital	Febrile illness, rash; congenital: jaundice, enlarged liver and spleen, brain abnormalities	Skin test
Amoebic dysentery	*Entamoeba histolytica* (protozoa)	Fecal contamination of food and water	Bloody diarrhea, cramping, fever	Stool for O&P
Giardiasis	*Giardia lamblia* (protozoa)	Common in intestinal tract, opportunistic; contaminated surface water	Asymptomatic to severe diarrhea and abdominal discomfort	Stool for O&P, intestinal biopsy, string test
Trichinosis	*Trichinella spiralis* (roundworm)	Ingestion of undercooked pork or bear meat	Nausea, fever, diarrhea, muscle pain and swelling, edema of face	Biopsy, blood tests
Tapeworm	*Taenia* spp., *Diphyllobothrium latum*	Undercooked meats (beef and pork) Undercooked fish; common among Norwegians, Japanese	Abdominal discomfort, diarrhea, weight loss; as above, may become anemia	Stool for O&P Stool for O&P
Pinworm	*Enterobius vermicularis* (roundworm)	Fecal-oral	Severe rectal itching, restlessness, insomnia	Adhesive tape applied to perianal region for ova
Scabies	Itch mite: *Sarcoptes scabiei*	Direct contact, clothing, bedding	Nocturnal itching, skin burrows	Skin scrapings for parasites
Lice	*Pediculus humanus, Pthirus pubis* (crabs)	Direct contact, clothing, bedding, furniture (can transmit other diseases by bite)	Intense itching, skin lesions	Finding adult lice or eggs (nits) on body or hair

O&P, Ova and parasites.

✳ PROCEDURE 8-7 Rapid Urine Culture Test

A, Uricult testing supplies. *a,* Uricult box kit containing the following: *b,* vial with agar-coated slide attached to plastic screw top; *c,* reference chart to compare growth results after 18 to 24 hours; *d,* midstream clean-catch urine specimen (preferably first morning specimen); *e,* gloves. *(From Bonewit-West K: Clinical procedures for medical assistants, ed 9, St Louis, 2015, Saunders.)*

B, After unscrewing the agar-coated slide from the vial, dip the slide into the urine specimen, making sure all the surfaces have made contact with the urine, and then replace the slide into the vial and screw cap loosely. *(From Bonewit-West K: Clinical procedures for medical assistants, ed 9, St Louis, 2015, Saunders.)*

C, Incubate specimen vial for 18 to 24 hours at a temperature of 93° to 100° F (35° to 38° C). *(From Bonewit-West K: Clinical procedures for medical assistants, ed 9, St Louis, 2015, Saunders.)*

D, Read and record the color results on the slide using the reference chart from the kit. *(From Bonewit-West K: Clinical procedures for medical assistants, ed 9, St Louis, 2015, Saunders.)*

PROCEDURE 8-7 Rapid Urine Culture Test—cont'd

Purpose

Testing for bacterial growth in a urine specimen

Equipment and Supplies

Clinical incubator,
Uricult kit containing vial with agar-coated slide and reference chart (Figure A)
Gloves

Procedure

1. Sanitize and glove your hands, and assemble the equipment. Check the expiration date on the reagent kit.
2. Into the appropriate sterile container, have the patient produce a freshly voided clean-catch midstream urine specimen that has been in the bladder for a minimum of 4 to 6 hours. Be sure to mix the urine sample thoroughly before testing.
3. After you unscrew the agar-coated slide from the vial, do not touch the agar.
4. Make sure the agar on both sides of the slide is completely immersed into the urine, but do not immerse more than several seconds (Figure B). (NOTE: If the urine volume in the cup is too small to dip, the urine may be poured over the agar surfaces.)

5. Place the urine-dipped specimen back into the vial and screw the cap on loosely. Label the vial with the patient's name, date, time, and your initials. Then place in the incubator (Figure C).
6. Read the results using the reference chart supplied with the kit after 18 to 24 hours of incubation (do not exceed 24 hours) (Figure D). Results are interpreted as follows:
   - *Normal:* Color that reads as less than 10,000 bacteria/mL of urine indicates the absence of infection.
   - *Borderline:* Color that reads 10,000 to 100,000 bacteria/mL of urine may indicate a chronic or relapsing infection, and it is recommended that the test be repeated.
   - *Positive:* More than 100,000 bacteria/mL of urine indicates complete coverage of the agar surface with bacterial colonies.
7. Replace the agar slide in the vial and discard in a biohazard bag.
8. Remove the gloves, and sanitize your hands.
9. Document the procedure, indicating the results, the brand name of the test used, the date, the time, and the name of the person testing and charting (or record results on the preprinted requisition/report).

8-7

Review Questions

1. Which of the following statements is incorrect (false)?
   a. The most important step in the Gram stain procedure is the decolorizer step.
   b. If too much decolorizer has been applied, at the end of the Gram stain procedure all the organisms will be pink/red.
   c. At the end of the decolorizer step, the gram-positive organisms are purple and the gram-negative organisms are colorless.
   d. If too little decolorizer has been applied, at the end of the Gram stain procedure all the organisms will be pink/red.

2. Which of the following organisms is gram-positive? (HINT: Check "Pathogenic Bacteria" and/or Tables 8-4 and 8-5.)
   a. *Escherichia coli*
   b. *Proteus*
   c. *Staphylococcus*
   d. *Pseudomonas*

3. Which of the following statements about *Neisseria gonorrhoeae* is incorrect (false)?
   a. *Neisseria gonorrhoeae* is a sexually transmitted disease.
   b. *Neisseria gonorrhoeae* requires 10% carbon dioxide for growth.
   c. *Neisseria gonorrhoeae* organisms are gram-positive cocci in pairs.
   d. The JEMBEC transportation system is used to transport and grow *Neisseria gonorrhoeae*.

4. Which of the following statements about normal flora is incorrect (false)?
   a. Normal flora inhabit parts of the body.
   b. Normal flora are never pathogenic.
   c. Normal flora assist in preventing the colonization of pathogens.
   d. If normal flora are destroyed in a part of the body, opportunistic pathogens can invade the area.

Review Questions—cont'd

5. When collecting a throat specimen for a Rapid Strep test, which of the following steps is incorrect (false)?
   a. Use a cotton swab.
   b. Have the patient sit with head back.
   c. Use a sterile tongue depressor to hold down the tongue, and have patient say "ahh."
   d. Rotate the swab on the back of throat in a circular motion or figure-of-eight pattern.

6. In the aftermath of the 9/11 bioterrorism threats, all laboratories (including POLs) should do which of the following?
   a. Identify procedures and methods that have the potential to produce aerosols.
   b. Refer any suspicious organisms or substances to the proper authorities.
   c. Use proper biosafety techniques at all times.
   d. All of the above are true.

7. Which of the following statements about pinworm testing is incorrect (false)?
   a. The female pinworm normally lays her eggs during the night in the anal area of the human host.
   b. The cellulose tape test consists of pressing cellulose tape (sticky side) over the patient's anal area.
   c. The tape is placed with the tape sticky-side-down on a glass slide.
   d. A physician or trained laboratorian microscopically examines the tape for *Giardia lamblia* eggs.

8. Which of the following statements concerning bioterrorism organisms is incorrect (false)?
   a. Anthrax has three forms: cutaneous, pulmonary, and gastrointestinal.
   b. The causative agent of plague is *Yersinia pestis*.
   c. Bioterrorism smallpox is caused by the bacteria *Variola minor*.
   d. Tularemia is caused by *Francisella tularensis*, a gram-negative bacillus.

9. Name the three sources from which smears on slides are made.

10. Which of the following associations is incorrect (false)?
    a. Eukaryotic/contains a nucleus
    b. Aerobe/oxygen
    c. Aerosols/particles suspended in air
    d. Morbidity/rate of deaths

Websites

The Public Health Image Library is a great site for microbiology pictures. Click "continue" to enter the PHIL directory and search for microbiology pictures:
http://phil.cdc.gov/Phil/home.asp

American Society for Microbiology:
www.asm.org/

Information on group A streptococcal infections from the National Institute of Allergy and Infectious Diseases:
www.niaid.nih.gov/factsheets/strep.htm

Information on MRSA:
www.cdc.gov/mrsa/mrsa_initiative/skin_infection/index.html

Great slideshow on MRSA:
www.medicinenet.com/mrsa_picture_slideshow/article.htm

Information on Swine Flu (H1N1):
www.cdc.gov/h1n1flu/qa.htm

World Health Organization:
www.who.int/en/

Information on bioterrorism from Centers for Disease Control and Prevention:
www.bt.cdc.gov/bioterrorism/

Toxicology

Fundamental Concepts

Overview of Toxicology

The toxicology department in the medical laboratory tests the levels of both therapeutic drugs and drugs of abuse to determine their presence and/or their harmful or "toxic" effect on the body. These departments may also test for other poisons, such as lead. In the toxicology laboratory, tests are generally performed using blood or urine specimens and sometimes saliva, sweat, or stomach contents. A toxicology test may be used to denote the presence of 1 specific drug or more than 20 drugs.

Drugs may be accidentally or deliberately injected, inhaled, swallowed, or absorbed through the skin or mucous membranes. Toxicity is the level at which a drug becomes poisonous in the body.

The medical assistant may be responsible for collecting the urine or blood specimen, which is then sent to the toxicology lab, also for testing the specimen for screening or monitoring purposes. The following are common reasons for performing drug screening tests:

- To determine the cause of bizarre behavior, unconsciousness, or life-threatening symptoms in an emergency situation in which drug overdose may be a possibility

- To test for drug use in the workplace or in schools, particularly among bus and truck drivers, child-care workers, and public safety workers. These professions generally require a urine or blood drug test as part of the application process and may also require employees to undergo periodic drug testing (especially after an accident that occurred during work activities).
- To test athletes for drugs that enhance their athletic ability

The Fundamental Concepts section of this chapter includes an overview of the common drugs of abuse that can become toxic and/or addictive when taken incorrectly. It then describes proper collection of urine and blood specimens used for drug testing. When testing for drugs of abuse, the medical assistant must ensure that collection of the specimen adheres to the legal "chain of custody" guidelines certifying that the collection of the specimen was witnessed and there was no opportunity for the specimen to be tampered with in any way.

The CLIA-Waived Drug Screening Tests part of this chapter presents in-office drug screening tests and the procedure for monitoring patients on **buprenorphine** (a Food and Drug Administration [FDA]–approved drug for treating drug addiction).

The Advanced Concepts section presents the principles of therapeutic drug monitoring and collecting a blood specimen for lead poisoning.

Drugs of Abuse

There are thousands of drugs available worldwide. Over-the-counter (OTC) drugs fill the shelves of pharmacies and are useful for many minor medical conditions. Unfortunately, these drugs may have toxic effects on the body if taken incorrectly. Three causes of drug toxicity with OTCs are overdosage, interactions with other drugs, or **idiosyncrasy** (an abnormal susceptibility to a drug or other agent that is peculiar to the individual). The medical assistant should be mindful of these possibilities and faithfully record any OTC drugs that are being taken.

Any drug can be abused, but "drugs of abuse" are considered to be those that are illegally obtained for recreational purposes or to satisfy an addiction. Some therapeutic drugs may be misused or become addictive over time.

Each of the drugs produces a specific **metabolite**, the substance produced by the **metabolism** (breaking down) of the drug in the body. The metabolite is then excreted in the urine. A **qualitative drug screening** (test of the drug) is performed to see if the metabolite is present in the same way that the urine dipstick tested for various analytes (e.g., glucose, protein). Urine is generally the specimen of choice for screening drugs of abuse because it is easily obtained and it is relatively simple to perform

multiple drug tests at the same time. Table 9-1 lists the time intervals for detecting various drugs in urine (also see Procedure 9-1 located at the end of this section).

If a **quantitative drug screening** (test of the drug) is necessary to determine the amount of the drug that is in the patient, a blood specimen would also be used (along with the saved urine specimen) because its dilution stays constant. The dilution of the drug in the urine volume varies depending on water intake and

Table 9-1	Typical Time Intervals for Detecting Drugs in Urine
Drug	**Time Found in Urine**
Alcohol	6 hours to 1 day
Amphetamines	4 hours
Barbiturates	24 hours to 4 days
Benzodiazepines	Short-term therapeutic use: 3 days; long-term chronic use: 4 to 6 weeks
Cannabinoids	1 hour to 3 days
Cocaine	2 to 3 days
Codeine	4 hours
LSD	1 to 4 days
Marijuana (THC)	Casual use: up to 7 days; chronic use: up to 30 days or longer
MDMA (Ecstasy)	1 to 4 days
Methadone	1 to 7 days
Methamphetamine	1 to 4 days
Opiates	1 to 4 days
PCP	Casual use: up to 7 days; chronic use: up to 30 days
Tricyclic antidepressants	1 to 9 days

Modified from Stepp CA, Woods M: *Laboratory procedures for medical office personnel,* Philadelphia, 1998, Saunders.

Table 9-2	Approximate Ethanol Content in Alcoholic Beverages
Beverage	**Ethanol Content (%)**
Beer	3-6
Ciders	4-5
Wines	8-15
Sherry, Madeira, Port	18-20
Whiskey, gin	40-45
Vodka	40-50
Brandy	45-50
Rum	50-70

From Calbreath DF: *Clinical chemistry,* 1992, Philadelphia, Saunders.

output. The blood specimen is commonly ordered by law enforcement officials who need to know the actual amount of a specific illicit drug after it has tested positive in the urine.

The most common legal drug of abuse in America is ethanol, also known as grain alcohol. It is found in beer, wine, and distilled liquors. Table 9-2 lists the approximate ethanol content in alcoholic beverages. Ethanol depresses the central nervous system and may lead to coma, progressing to death at the following "panic" (possibly lethal) levels:

>2000 µg/mL in the blood, or >1600 µg/mL in the urine

Alcohol is one of the few drugs that has a direct correlation between blood levels and impaired driving ability. Drug alcohol testing for prosecution of an accused drunk driver is strictly regulated by law (see Procedure 9-2).

✳ PROCEDURE 9-1 Assisting with Urine Collection for Drug Screening

A, a, Urine drug screening collection kit specimen cup; b, temperature indicator on collection cup; c, urine specimen containers to be sent to the lab; d, plastic sealable pouch for the two urine specimen containers and the chain of custody documents.

Equipment and Supplies for Collecting and Processing Urine Specimen (Figure A)

- Urine drug screening collection kit specimen cup
- Temperature indicator on collection cup
- Urine specimen containers to be sent to the laboratory
- Plastic sealable pouch for the two urine specimen containers and the chain of custody documents

Procedure

1. Prepare the bathroom before the patient collects urine by turning off the water and adding blue dye to the toilet bowl.
2. Call in the patient and explain the purpose of the test and the procedure to be followed for a midstream clean-catch specimen collection (see Chapter 3). Also, explain that no personal belongings may be taken into the bathroom and that patient may lock belongings in a provided locker.

3. Sanitize hands, and apply gloves.
4. Obtain a signed consent form from the patient.
5. A trained professional must witness the actual voiding of at least 50 mL of urine into the specimen cup provided in the urine collection drug kit.
6. Originate the chain of custody document at the time of the sample collection. The person who witnessed the voiding must sign the document, as must every other person who handles the sample.
7. After the collection, verify the temperature of the urine as seen on the indicator at the bottom of the cup, and document it. NOTE: If the temperature of the urine specimen is out of range (too cold), a second specimen must be collected. If the donor refuses to provide the second specimen under direct observation, the collection would be considered "refusal to test."
8. Transfer the specimen to the two containers that must be labeled with the following information:
   - Full name of the patient
   - Date and time of collection
   - Your initials
   - Initials of the witnessing officer
9. Place the two sample containers into the sealed plastic pouch, mark it with a notary-style seal or with tamper-proof tape to protect the integrity of the sample, and send the specimen to the toxicology laboratory.
10. If you are trained and qualified to do the testing, proceed with the testing according to laboratory and state regulations.
11. After both the initial and the confirmatory testing are complete, mark the urine sample, reseal it, and securely store it for a minimum of 30 days or for the length of time specified by laboratory protocols.
12. Clean or discard all equipment and supplies according to safety guidelines.
13. Remove gloves, and wash hands.

9-1

✳ PROCEDURE 9-2 Assisting with Blood Collection for Alcohol Testing

Equipment and Supplies

- Gray-topped Vacutainer tubes
- Venipuncture needle and holder (or syringe and transfer device)
- Nonvolatile disinfectant (e.g., benzalkonium [Zephiran] or aqueous thimerosal [Merthiolate])
- Gauze
- Tourniquet
- Gloves
- Legally authorized transportation envelope, container, or plastic pouch

Patient Preparation

1. An officer of the law will be present to act as a witness to the procedure.
2. The patient will probably still be under the influence of alcohol, so explain what you will be doing in as brief and concise a manner as possible. NOTE: Do not allow yourself to become irritated by the speech or mannerisms of the patient. Treat the patient with the respect and dignity with which you treat all your patients.

Blood Collection Procedure

NOTE: The Department of Justice for each state has established uniform standards for the collection, handling, and preservation of blood samples used for alcohol testing. If you are authorized to obtain specimens for forensic analysis, check your laboratory's procedure manual so that you perform the collection *exactly* as required by the uniform standards established for your state.

3. Sanitize hands, and apply gloves.
4. Prepare the draw site using Zephiran, aqueous Merthiolate, or another aqueous disinfectant.

Do not use alcohol or other volatile organic disinfectants to clean the skin site.

5. Complete the blood draw, filling both tubes with sufficient blood to permit duplicate blood alcohol determinations (see Chapter 5).
6. Label the two gray-stoppered tubes with the following information:
   - Full name of the patient
   - Date and time of collection
   - Your initials
   - Initials of the witnessing officer
7. Give the labeled blood samples to the witnessing officer, who will immediately complete the required information on the transportation envelope, container, or plastic pouch. The officer will then seal it securely. Information on the envelope or container should include the following:
   - The full name of the patient
   - Whether the patient is alive or dead
   - The submitting agency
   - The geographical location where the blood was drawn (e.g., hospital, clinic, jail)
   - The name of the person drawing the blood sample
   - The date and time the blood sample was drawn
   - The signature of the witnessing officer
8. Once the envelope or container is sealed, it must not be opened, except for analysis. Each person who is subsequently in possession of the sealed sample must sign his or her name in the space provided on the envelope or container (chain of custody). The integrity of the sample *must* be safeguarded.
9. Remove gloves, and wash hands.

CLIA-Waived Drug Screening Tests

Some offices may perform drug screening tests for companies as part of preemployment physicals or as a requirement for insurance or government mandates (e.g., the federally mandated testing of transportation workers, and after a workplace accident).

Although plasma samples provide the best diagnostic and quantitative results, CLIA-waived urine test kits are available to provide an initial screening for the presence of a variety of drugs, including amphetamines, marijuana (**cannabinoid**), cocaine, and **opiates** (e.g., methadone and morphine). The urine drug testing kits generally contain a rapid drug screening device and a wide-mouth collection container. Be sure to read the step-by-step instructions on the package inserts. Generally, the instructions require that the operator dip the testing device into the urine and observe the qualitative reactions in a specified time. The results are reported as positive, negative, or inconclusive (which requires an additional confirmation test utilizing the same urine sample). Be sure to follow the shipping instructions if the screening device indicates the presence of drugs in the sample or if the results are inconclusive.

CLIA-waived saliva alcohol tests are also available for facilities that screen clients or patients for alcohol.

These qualitative tests generally consist of a test strip that turns shades of green or blue if alcohol is present in the subject's saliva.

A growing number of drug screening products are also FDA approved for home use. (For a list of the drugs that may be detected in urine, saliva, hair, and breath, see the website at the end of the chapter.) Schools, employers, and the Department of Transportation (DOT) may also use these products to randomly monitor their students and employees. NOTE: If performing drug testing for the DOT in the office, the physician must be a certified Medical Review Officer (MRO). As an MRO, the licensed physician is responsible for receiving laboratory results and interpreting and evaluating an individual's positive test result.

Most rapid urine drug tests are immunoassay tests based on the principle of competitive binding. Drugs that may be present in the urine specimen compete against their respective drug conjugate for binding sites with their specific antibody. During testing the urine specimen migrates upward on the test strip by capillary action. If the drug in question has a sufficiently high concentration, it will saturate all the binding sites of the antibody so that it will not react in the drug-protein conjugate test area of the strip. Therefore, if the drug is present in the urine, the test area will show no reaction. (NOTE: The immunoassay results discussed in Chapter 7 had an opposite positive reaction.) Conversely, if the drug is not present, it will not saturate the antibody sites and the antibody will then react in the test area, causing a colored line to appear. The control area *(C)* of the strip indicates that the proper volume of urine migrated through the test area and that the color change was caused by antibody conjugation. (NOTE: The colored line in the internal control area does not represent a positive reaction, as in other immunoassays, because a positive reaction in this method inhibits the formation of a colored band.) See Figure D in Procedure 9-3, which demonstrates drug screening test results.

Physicians who treat opioid addiction using buprenorphine must monitor their patients using CLIA-waived urine drug screening test kits. These physicians are authorized by the FDA and the Substance Abuse and Mental Health Services Association (SAMHSA) to treat and monitor up to 30 patients. (For more information on buprenorphine treatment, see the websites at the end of this chapter.) The urine test cassettes detect the presence of nine addictive drugs in addition to buprenorphine and assist the physician in monitoring the patient's drug use and treatment progress. NOTE: The presence of buprenorphine ensures that the patient is taking the therapeutic drug and not selling it. Table 9-1 lists each drug with its three- or four-digit testing code along with the drug's street name, source, method of administration, medical use, side effects, and overdose information. Table 9-2 shows the time intervals for detecting various drugs in urine.

✳ PROCEDURE 9-3 Urine Drug Panel Testing Procedure

A, *a,* Gloves; *b,* test card with multiple test strips (five tests are on each side of the card); *c,* fresh urine specimen, or specimen that has been stored at 2° to 8° C (refrigerated) for up to 48 hours and then brought to room temperature; *d,* metal pouch that stored the card at 2° to 30° C (refrigerator or room temperature).

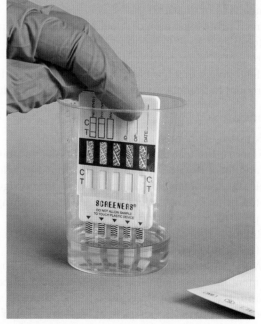

B, Immerse the strips to at least the level of the wavy lines on the strips but not above the arrows on the test card for 10 to 15 seconds.

(Continued)

PROCEDURE 9-3 Urine Drug Panel Testing Procedure—cont'd

C, Results after 5 minutes from both sides of the card showing six negative results (testing area shows two colored bands) and four positive results (the testing areas have only one colored band in the control area).

Equipment and Supplies (Figure A)
- Gloves
- Test card with multiple test strips (five tests are on each side of the card)
- Fresh urine specimen or specimen that has been stored at 2° to 8° C for up to 48 hours and then brought to room temperature
- Metal pouch that has been stored at 2° to 30° C also brought to room temperature (check expiration date)

Procedure

1. Sanitize the hands, and apply gloves.
2. Remove the test device from its protective pouch, and label it with the patient's identification. NOTE: If the specimen has been stored in the refrigerator, bring it to room temperature before opening to prevent condensation.
3. Remove the cap from the end of the test card (Figure A).
4. With the arrows pointing toward the urine specimen, immerse the strips of the test card vertically into the urine specimen for at least 10 to 15 seconds. **Immerse the strips to at least the level of the wavy lines on the strips but not above the arrows on the test card** (Figure B).

D, Close-up on first three drug results: *COC* = cocaine is negative; *AMP* = amphetamine is negative; *mAMP* = methamphetamine is positive.

5. Place the test card on a nonabsorbent surface, and wait for the colored lines to appear.
6. At 5 minutes, read and record the results (Figure C).
   - Positive test result: One distinct pink band appears in the control region *(C)* and no line in the test region *(T)*
   - Negative test result: Two pink bands appear, one pink band in the control region *(C)* and one pink band in the patient test region *(T)*
   - Invalid: Pink bands are absent from the control region; repeat the test with a new device; if the problem persists, call for technical assistance.
7. See Figure D for close-up results on the following three drugs:
   - COC = Cocaine is negative
   - AMP = Amphetamine is negative
   - mAMP = Methamphetamine is positive
8. See Table 9-3: Common Drugs of Abuse on pp. 291-292.

Quality Control Procedure

In addition to the internal control region built into the test device, external positive and negative liquid controls should be performed when a new kit is used. Also, each operator of the test should perform a positive and negative control once with each testing method to confirm that his or her testing technique is correct. The results of the control tests should be logged in the drug screening control log.

The positive liquid control procedure is performed in the same way as the patient procedure, with a new testing card. Observe and record the results within 5 minutes. Repeat the procedure with a drop of well-mixed negative control.

9-3

Table 9-3 **Common Drugs of Abuse Detected on Multiple Drug Urine Screening Tests***

Drug (Test Code)	Street Name	Source/Route	Medical Use/Brand Names	Side Effects, Risks/Overdose
1. Cocaine (COC)	Rock, crack, coke, blow, nose nachos, hooter, yeyo	Coca bush leaves refined/Nasal administration, smoked	Topical anesthetic, natural stimulant, anesthetic, vasoconstrictor, pain killer, appetite suppressant, altitude sickness/Less addictive derivatives for anesthesia: benzocaine, lidocaine, Cepacol, Dermoplast, Lanacane	Perforation of nasal septum, renal failure, hyperthermia, cardiac arrest, seizures, dermatitis, tetany, septicemia, respiratory arrest, dehydration, sleep disorders, depression, impulsiveness, hostility, impaired memory/**Overdose:** fever, unresponsiveness, difficulty breathing, unconsciousness, stroke, death
2. Amphetamine (AMP)	Black beauties, Christmas trees, dexies, speed, double trouble, gaggler, beanies	Made in illegal laboratories/Smoked, injected, snorted	Appetite suppressant, central nervous system stimulant/Adderall, Citramine, DexAlone, Tamphetamin, Zamitam	Dependence, increased blood pressure, increased respiration, dilated pupils, sweating, tremors/**Overdose:** seizures, cardiac arrest
3. Methamphetamine (mAMP) Ecstasy XTC (MDMA)	Cat, crank, glass, speed, ice, love, Disco biscuits, Molly	Made in illegal laboratories/Oral, powder inhalant, crystals smoked	Nasal decongestant/Desoxyn No medical use	Dependence, psychosis, decreased appetite, restlessness, anxiety, heart failure, extreme fatigue, hunger, mental depression, dysrhythmias, lethargy, skin pallor, fits of rage/**Overdose:** seizures, cardiac arrest
4. Marijuana (THC) Hashish	Pot, weed, joint, reefer, roach, dope Hashish, hash oil, ganja	*Cannabis sativa,* hemp plant flowers and leaves/Smoked, eaten, injected	Pain relief (colitis), treatment of glaucoma, appetite stimulant, reduction of nausea from chemotherapy, euphoria, detachment, relaxation/Marinol, Dronabinol	Talkativeness, slowed time perception, inappropriate hilarity, paranoia, confusion, anxiety, short-term memory loss/**Overuse:** impaired lung structure, chromosomal mutation, micronucleic white blood cells, cancer, lack of motivation
5. Methadone (MTD)	Fizzies, chocolate chip cookies, juice, wafer	Laboratory manufactured/Oral, injection, powder	Treatment for narcotic addiction, pain/Methadose, Dolophine	Also addictive/**Danger** of respiratory and cardiac arrest and death if stopped suddenly
6. Opiates (OPI 2000) (also see MOP 300)	Smack, horse, chiva, junk, black tar, gunpowder, courage pills, bomb	Poppy refined/Nasal, oral, intravenous injection, dermal patch	Potent pain killer, heroin, morphine, codeine, fentanyl/Demerol, Darvon, Vicodin, Dilaudid	Addiction in hospitals, constipation, dermatitis, malnutrition, hypoglycemia, dental caries, amenorrhea/**Danger** of acquired immunodeficiency syndrome (from sharing needles)
7. Oxycodone (OXY)	Oxy, OC, blues, killers, kickers hillbilly percs	Semisynthetic similar to codeine/Oral, injection	Moderate to heavy pain relief/OxyContin, Percodan, Percocet	Addiction in patients on long-term pain therapy

(Continued)

Table 9-3   **Common Drugs of Abuse Detected on Multiple Drug Urine Screening Tests*—cont'd**

Drug (Test Code)	Street Name	Source/Route	Medical Use/Brand Names	Side Effects, Risks/Overdose
8. Barbiturates (BAR)	Barbs, pinks, blockbusters, Christmas trees, goofballs, red devils, reds and blues, yellowjackets	Laboratory manufactured/Oral, intravenous injection	Depressant, sedative, hypnotic, anticonvulsant/Seconal, Amytal, Nembutal	Dullness, apathy, dependence/**Overdose:** respiratory arrest, coma, death
9. Benzodiazepines (BZO)	Roofies, downers, tranks, benzos	Laboratory manufactured/Oral, injection	Treatment for anxiety, seizures, sleeplessness, muscle relaxant/Valium, Xanax, Restoril, Versed	Carefree, detached, sleepy, disoriented, unconsciousness, amnesia, diminished reflexes/**Overdose:** coma, can be lethal when combined with alcohol
10. Buprenorphine (BUP)	Bupe, Subs	Laboratory manufactured	Analgesic, treatment for opioid addiction/Buprenex, Suboxone, Subutix	Euphoria, respiratory depression, sedation/**Overdose:** causes severe respiratory depression when combined with benzodiazepines
11. Tricyclic antidepressants (TCA)	Yellow	Laboratory manufactured/Oral, injection	Treatment for depression, attention-deficit/hyperactivity disorder, migraines/Adapin, Norpramin, Anafranil, Pamelor, Tofranil, Elavil	Blurred vision, constipation and dry mouth, anxiety, restlessness, difficulty urinating, weight gain, drowsiness, muscle twitches, weakness, sweating, nausea, dizziness, cognitive and memory difficulties, increased heart rate, irregular heart rhythms/**Overdose:** panic attacks, hostile/angry feelings, impulsive actions, severe restlessness, very rapid speech
12. Lysergic acid diethylamide (LSD)	Acid, the Beast, California sunshine	Illicit laboratories, peyote (mescaline), psilocybin mexicana (mushroom), fungus on grains/Ingested orally	No medical use	Hallucinations, anxiety, depression, confusion, paranoia, panic attacks, impaired memory, inability to reason, flashbacks, increased blood pressure, high temperature, dilated pupils, increased heart rate/**Overdose:** psychosis, flashbacks
13. Phencyclidine (PCP)	Angel dust, peace pill, rocket fuel, wack, ozone, fry	Illegal laboratories/Oral, intravenous, sniffed, smoked	No medical use	Hallucinations, acute anxiety, dulled thinking, poor memory, depression, severe brain damage, hepatitis, respiratory arrest, panic reaction, confusion, blurred vision, high blood pressure/**Overdose:** violence, psychoses, self-injurious behavior, suicide

*Numbers 1 through 9 are the screened drugs for patients taking number 10, buprenorphine therapy (see Procedure 9-3).

Advanced Concepts

Therapeutic Drug Monitoring

Therapeutic drug monitoring (TDM) is the process of measuring either the effects of a drug on a patient or the actual levels of a drug being administered to a patient. For example, we have already discussed monitoring the *effect* of insulin therapy by performing blood glucose levels, and we monitored the *effect* of Coumadin therapy by testing the patient's protime and international normalized ratio (INR). In this chapter we will learn the importance of monitoring therapeutic drug levels in the patient's blood and/or urine.

Most prescribed drugs have a therapeutic range that must be maintained for successful therapy. If a patient's drug level falls outside of the range, it may become ineffective if too low or toxic if too high. Table 9-4 lists therapeutic ranges and toxic levels for various drugs. Therapeutic ranges and the subsequent monitoring of the drug levels in the body give the physician guidelines for prescribing the medication and fine-tuning the exact effective amount of medication to keep the patient within the range.

It is very important to collect the blood sample for TDM at a certain time—either before or after administering the drug. Otherwise, the test results will be useless and unreliable, or even worse, they may prompt the physician to initiate inappropriate treatment.

Table 9-4	Drug Categories Showing Therapeutic Ranges and Toxic Levels	
Drug	**Therapeutic Range**	**Toxic Level**
Antibiotics		
Ampicillin	20-25 mcg/mL	35 mcg/mL
Gentamicin	4-8 mcg/mL	12 mcg/mL
Kanamycin	20-25 mcg/mL	35 mcg/mL
Tobramycin	2-8 mcg/mL	12 mcg/mL
Anticonvulsants		
Carbamazepine (Tegretol)	2-10 mcg/mL	12 mcg/mL
Ethosuximide (Zarontin)	40-80 mcg/mL	100 mcg/mL
Phenobarbital (Luminal)	10 mcg/mL	>55 mcg/mL
Phenytoin (Dilantin)	10-20 mcg/mL	>20 mcg/mL
Primidone	1 mcg/mL	>10 mcg/mL
Antidepressants and Antipsychotics		
Amitriptyline (Elavil)	100-250 ng/mL	>300 ng/mL
Diazepam (Valium)	5-70 ng/mL	>70 ng/mL
Imipramine (Tofranil)	100-250 ng/mL	>300 ng/mL
Lithium (Lithonate)	0.8-1.4 mEq/L	1.5 mEq/L
Antirheumatics		
Salicylate (aspirin)	2-30 mg/dL	>40 mg/dL
Acetaminophen (Tylenol)	0-25 mg/mL	>150 mcg/mL
Barbiturates		
Amobarbital (Amytal)	7 mcg/mL	30 mcg/mL
Pentobarbital (Nembutal)	10 mcg/mL	55 mcg/mL
Secobarbital (Seconal)	3 mcg/mL	10 mcg/mL
Cardiotonics		
Digoxin	0.5-2 mcg/mL	>2.5 mcg/mL
Disopyramide	2-4.5 mcg/mL	>9 mcg/mL
Lidocaine	2-6 mcg/mL	>9 mcg/mL
Procainamide (Pronestyl)	4-8 mcg/mL	>12 mcg/mL
Quinidine	2.3-5 mcg/mL	>5 mcg/mL

Modified from Stepp CA, Woods M: *Laboratory procedures for medical office personnel,* Philadelphia, 1998, Saunders.

Common Therapeutic Drugs That Are Tested for Toxicity

Amikacin	Paracetamol
Caffeine	Phenobarbitone
Carbamazepine	Phenytoin
Cyclosporine	Primidone
Digoxin	Salicylic acid
Ethosuximide	Theophylline
Gentamicin	Tobramycin
Lithium	Valproic acid
Methotrexate	

Pharmacokinetics

For a better understanding of how drugs are utilized by the body, here is a brief look at the five stages of **pharmacokinetics** (the movement of drugs through the body from the time of introduction to elimination).

Liberation

Liberation is the release of a drug from its dosage form. For a drug to be liberated, it must first enter the body by way of a solution. For example, eye drops go into solution in the tears of the eye. Swallowed medication goes into solution in the gastric fluid. Liquid injections are inserted into the skin, muscle, or vein.

Absorption and Distribution

Absorption is the movement of a drug from a body surface (e.g., the skin or mucous membrane) through the tissues and into the blood (also called *uptake*). The blood then carries the drug through the body **(distribution)** until it finds its target (e.g., antibiotics find the pathogen, anticonvulsants and antidepressants find the brain, cardiotonics find the heart and vessels).

Metabolism and Elimination

Next, the drug needs to be broken down (metabolism), which generally occurs in the liver. Once it is broken down, the drug metabolite is *eliminated* by way of bile from the liver or urine from the kidneys. Drug metabolites may also be excreted through the skin by way of sweat, the lungs by way of expired air, or the salivary or mammary glands.

Drug Half-Life and Specimen Collection

The amount of time necessary to eliminate 50% of a drug is referred to as its *half-life*. The half-life cycle varies for each individual depending on sex, age, body weight, and health status. For example, children and the elderly are more prone to experiencing toxic levels of therapeutic drugs because of their body size and/or altered metabolic rates. All these factors have an effect on whether a drug is prescribed, when to test for the drug, and what type of specimen is tested (e.g., urine, blood).

Drugs of abuse are generally tested using urine specimens for the qualitative result and blood for the quantitative result. Therapeutic drug monitoring generally uses blood specimens taken in a gold gel tube (serum separator tube) or a light green heparin tube with gel (plasma separator tube). NOTE: Do *not* use a lithium heparin tube when monitoring blood lithium levels. Be sure to refer to the laboratory manual when collecting toxicology specimens that are sent to the toxicology department of reference labs and hospitals. See the website listed at the end of the chapter for additional information on TDM testing and specimen collection.

Other Toxicology Tests

Other conditions in which a medical assistant may be asked to collect specimens for toxicology or perform drug screening tests are as follows:

- Chronic lead poisoning from the lead-based paint found in old homes. Figure 9-1 shows the royal blue–topped tube needed for a lead test specimen. NOTE: The royal blue–topped tube has a red strip on the label indicating that it has no additive (similar to the red-topped tubes) and should therefore be drawn in the same order as red-topped tubes. Also, refer to the laboratory manual for any other directions regarding collection and processing of the specimen.
- Acute iron poisoning in children who have taken adult iron tablets is a stat test.
- Chronic exposure to mercury and arsenic poisoning tests
- Forensic drug tests for court purposes
- Urine screening testing on pregnant mothers for drugs of abuse
- Urine and blood drug testing for on-the-job injuries to rule out an impaired employee

Fig. 9-1 Royal blue Vacutainer tube for lead toxicology test. Note the red band on the label, which indicates it has no additives and is therefore drawn in the order of a red Vacutainer tube. *(Photo by Zack Bent.)*

Summary

We are constantly exposed to harmful and poisonous substances. Even prescription medications may be harmful if not used as directed. The physician needs to know whether a drug is at its therapeutic level or whether the drug level is becoming toxic. Toxicology is the study and monitoring of these drugs as well as the identification of drugs of abuse. The medical assistant must be aware of the proper timing and specifics of collecting toxicology specimens, as well as the legal processing of specimens that may contain illicit drugs (i.e., chain of custody protocol).

Review Questions

True or False

Indicate if the following statements are true or false:

1. Therapeutic drug monitoring (TDM) is a way for the physician to measure the effects and levels of a drug being administered to a patient.

2. Pharmacokinetics is the study of drugs.

Fill in the Blanks

Complete the following statements:

3. _____ is the term meaning the release of the drug from its dosage.

4. The movement of a drug from solution to the blood is called _____.

5. The transport of a drug throughout the body by way of the blood is called _____.

6. The term for the breakdown of a drug within the body is _____.

7. The two main organs that eliminate drugs are the _____ and the _____.

8. The time it takes to eliminate 50% of any drug is called its _____.

9. Poisonous metals may include _____, _____, _____, and _____.

10. The most widely used and abused legal drug in society is _____.

11. Methamphetamine is also known as _____ or _____.

12. Two examples of opiate-derived drugs are _____ and _____.

Multiple Choice

Circle the letter that represents the single best answer:

13. Drugs may be excreted through all of the following *except:*
    a. skin
    b. sweat
    c. stool
    d. tears
    e. lungs

14. Forensic laboratories often prefer _____ for quantitative drug testing.
    a. urine
    b. serum
    c. plasma
    d. whole blood
    e. breath

Websites

DEA—Drug Enforcement Administration—Drug Fact Sheets: An excellent website for finding fact sheets on drugs of abuse, it provides an updated alphabetical index of the drugs and chemicals of concern:
www.justice.gov/dea/druginfo/factsheets.shtml

Drug abuse signs and symptoms (updated as of June 2013):
www.helpguide.org/mental/drug_substance_abuse_addiction_signs_effects_treatment.htm

Drugs that may be detected in urine, saliva, hair, and breath:
www.drugalcoholtestkits.com/fs_search.asp?testtypes=urine&;portalid=GOO

Substance Abuse and Mental Health Services Administration (SAMHSA) for alcohol and drug abuse information:
http://ncadi.samhsa.gov/

Information on drug addiction treatment using buprenorphine (still active):
http://buprenorphine.samhsa.gov/bwns_locator/dr_facilitylocatordoc.htm

Website for Screeners Dip Drug Test Kit (still active):
www.lifelinemedical.net/ddd_dip_drug_test.html

Website with links to therapeutic drug monitoring (TDM) testing and specimen collection information:
www.questdiagnostics.com/testcenter/testguide.action?dc=WP_DrugHalfLife

10 Electrocardiography and Spirometry

electrodes the 10 "sensors" placed on the limbs and chest that pick up the electrical activity of the heart

Holter monitoring ambulatory ECG monitoring

intercostal between the ribs

peak flow rate a test that measures how fast a person can exhale

precordial leads chest leads

pulmonary circulation blood flowing to the lungs and back to the heart

Purkinje fibers network that transmits electrical impulses to the ventricles, causing them to contract.

septum a muscular wall that divides the right and left sides of the heart

sinoatrial (SA) node node that transmits an electrical impulse that starts the heartbeat

sinus rhythm heart rhythm that is within normal limits

spirometer instrument that measures the volume and flow of air that is breathed

spirometry measurement of the volume and flow of air that is breathed

standard limb leads Einthoven's first leads known as bipolar leads – I, II, III

sternum breastbone

systemic circulation blood flowing to the body and back to the heart

systole the contraction phase of the heart when the cardiac muscle is being stimulated by electrical impulses

tachycardia fast heart rate

ventricles pump the blood out of the heart to the lungs and the body

ABBREVIATIONS

COPD	chronic obstructive pulmonary disease
ECG	electrocardiogram
FET	forced expiratory time—the horizontal length of the line showing how long the patient exhaled in seconds (ideally the line should continue to 6 seconds)
FEV₁	forced expiratory volume in the first second; expressed in liters

FVC	forced vital capacity—the total volume of air exhaled in 6 seconds
PAC	premature atrial contraction(s)
PEF	peak expiratory flow
PFM	peak flow meter (a portable, hand-held device used in ambulatory monitoring)
PVC	premature ventricular contraction(s)

Fundamental Concepts

This chapter is unique from the other laboratory testing chapters in that it does not use a specimen from the body to test. Instead it utilizes various instruments applied to the body itself to evaluate cardiac and pulmonary function. Consequently, these cardiopulmonary tests are referred to as "diagnostic tests" rather than "laboratory tests." In this section, the heart and lung will each be reviewed anatomically followed by discussions of the ways the electrocardiogram and the spirometer are able to display various graphs and interpretations of the patient's heart and lung health status.

Anatomy of the Heart

In Chapter 4, we studied the blood vessels in the cardiovascular system. This chapter focuses on the heart and how it is able to rhythmically and continuously pump the blood to the **pulmonary circulation** (lungs) and to the **systemic circulation** (upper and lower body), and return the blood to the heart after each circulation (Figure 10-1).

Chambers and Vessels of the Heart

Anatomically, the heart is divided into right and left sides by a muscular wall referred to as the **septum**. Both sides contain upper chambers, **atria**, that receive blood from the body (right atrium) and from

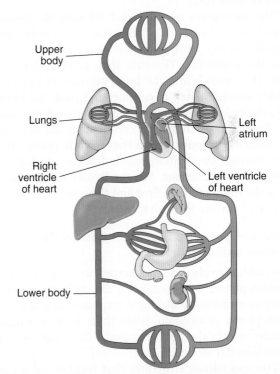

Fig. 10-1 Note how the right side of the patient's heart receives blood from the upper and lower body. The right ventricle then pumps the deoxygenated *(blue)* blood to the **pulmonary circulation** (lungs) and then back to the left side of the patient's heart. The oxygenated *(red)* blood in the heart's left ventricle is pumped to the **systemic circulation** (upper and lower body). *(From Frazier M: Human diseases and conditions, ed 5, St Louis, 2013, Saunders.)*

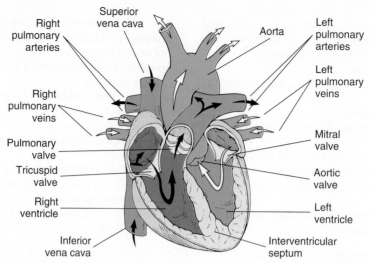

Fig. 10-2 Close-up view of blood circulation through the heart. *(From Frazier M:* Human diseases and conditions, *ed 5, St Louis, 2013, Saunders.)*

the lungs (left atrium). The lower chambers on each side are **ventricles** that then pump the blood out of the heart. The right ventricle sends the blood to the lungs, and the left ventricle pumps the blood to the body (Figure 10-2).

The movement of the blood through the heart's chambers is the result of the muscles in both atria simultaneously contracting and pushing the blood into the ventricles. The atria then relax and fill up with the blood while the large muscles of the ventricles are stimulated to contract and push the blood into the pulmonary artery on the right, and the aorta on the left. These muscular contractions are initiated by electrical impulses from the nervous system that flow through the cardiac muscle from top to bottom, creating each heartbeat. See the Evolve animation to view the route of blood flow and the movement of the electrical current through the heart.

Cardiac Cycle and Electrical Conduction System in the Heart

The **cardiac cycle** is a sequence of two phases: a contraction phase, or **systole**, when the cardiac muscle is being stimulated by electrical impulses; and a relaxation phase, or **diastole**, when there is no electrical activity within the cardiac muscle. On average, each cycle lasts 0.8 second.

The specialized structures that regulate each cardiac cycle include the sinoatrial (SA) node, the atrioventricular (AV) node, the bundle of His, the right and left bundle branches, and the Purkinje fibers (Figure 10-3).

During each cardiac cycle, the electrical impulses and muscular contractions flow as follows:

1. The **sinoatrial (SA) node** transmits an electrical impulse that starts the heartbeat and sets its rhythm, or pattern. The SA node is also known as the "pacemaker."
2. The electrical impulse from the SA node moves through the atria, causing them to contract first.
3. From the atria, the impulse travels to the **atrioventricular (AV) node.** Here, the impulse is slightly delayed to give the atria time to fully contract and fill the ventricles with blood.
4. Then the AV node transmits the electrical impulse to the **bundle of His.**
5. Next, the impulse splits and travels down the **right and left bundle branches.**
6. The impulse continues along the branches to the **Purkinje fibers.** This network of fibers transmits the impulse to the ventricles, causing them to contract.

Brief History of the Electrocardiogram (ECG)

Willem Einthoven invented the first practical electrocardiogram (ECG or EKG) in 1903 and received the Nobel Prize in Medicine in 1924 for it. His research included placing his two arms into salt solutions and his right foot into a bucket to provide an electrical ground. He then measured the electrical activity that took place between his arms using a crude galvanometer that moved a stylus up and down on a moving background. The first picture of the heartbeats between the arms was labeled *"Lead I."*

He also measured the electrical activity between his right arm and left leg and saw that the picture of the electrical impulse that flowed through the heart from top to bottom created a more defined picture, and it was labeled *"Lead II."* A typical lead II recording is seen on the right side of Figure 10-4. Note the positive upward and negative downward deflections

Fig. 10-3 The electrical conduction system in the heart flows as follows: *(1) The SA node* initiates the cycle, sending impulses that excite the atria. *(2) The atria* contract while *(3) the AV node* becomes stimulated and sends impulse to *(4) the bundle of His*, which sends the impulse down *(5) the right and left bundle branches*, which continue to branch into *(6) the Purkinje network* of fibers that excite *(7) the ventricles*, causing them to contract.

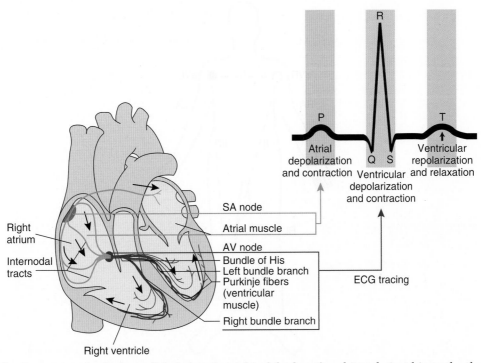

Fig. 10-4 Conduction system in the heart (labeled to the right of the heart) and its relationship to the three color-coded phases seen on the electrocardiogram. *(From Gould B:* Pathophysiology for the health professions, *ed 4, Philadelphia, 2011, Saunders.)*

called "waves" that were produced with each heartbeat cycle during lead II. The waves were labeled P through T. The three color-coded areas (P, QRS, and T) relate to the following electrical activities in the heart:

- The *P wave* on the graph shows **atrial depolarization.** This wave occurs when the nervous impulse starts in the SA node, causing the atria to contract.
- The *QRS complex* of three waves shows **ventricular depolarization.** These waves occur as the impulse moves through the heart's AV node, bundle of His, and Purkinje fibers, causing the ventricles to contract.
- The *T wave* shows **repolarization.** This state occurs during a period of electrical recovery. Then the ventricles relax briefly before the cycle resumes.
- NOTE: A small *U wave* may appear after the *T wave* for some patients. The cause is often unknown.

Einthoven also measured the left arm and left leg and created another picture of heartbeats that became known as *"Lead III."* Collectively, these three leads were referred to as the **bipolar limb leads** because they were measuring the electrical impulses that occurred between two limbs that were dipped into the two salt solutions. These first three "limb" leads are still referred to as "Einthoven's Triangle" (Figure 10-5).

Modern ECG Monitors and Tracings

Einthoven's initial invention to detect the electrical activity in the heart has evolved into modern electrocardiograph instruments and computers that are now able to record and analyze 12 leads in less than 15 seconds by recording 3 leads at the same time. See the ECG report in Figure 10-6. Each of the 12 leads, seen in the top 3 rows, shows a view of the heart from 12 different angles with the bottom graph showing a continuous lead II for rhythm analysis known as the **"Rhythm strip."** Together the leads give an overall picture of the electrical activity in the entire heart. By analyzing different leads, the physician is able to pinpoint the source of certain problems.

Electrodes

Einthoven's 3 salt solutions in buckets have been replaced by 10 disposable **"electrodes,"** or *sensors,* that are placed on the patient's limbs and chest. The disposable electrodes have an electrolyte gel and adhesive backing that are applied to the four limbs and six locations on the chest. They simultaneously detect the electrical impulses produced when the heart contracts (Figure 10-7).

From the electrodes, the impulses from the heart are then transmitted through their 10 designated "lead" wires that are connected to a patient cable that attaches to the electrocardiograph instrument as seen in Figure 10-8. The signal is amplified and sent to the galvanometer, which changes the electrical impulse into mechanical motion. The motion is then recorded on moving graph paper or to a computerized graph.

Fig. 10-5 Einthoven's Triangle: Note the four limb electrodes: RA *(white),* LA *(black),* RL *(green),* and LL *(red).* The right leg functions as a "ground" and the other three limbs form Einthoven's triangle, which is able to take six limb lead pictures of the heart: three bipolar leads (I, II, and III) and three augmented unipolar leads (aVR, aVL, and aVF).

Name : Jane Doe
ID : 34
Date : 04/06/73   Time : 11:37
Age : 20   Sex : Female
Hgt : 64 IN   Wgt : 130 LBS

Vent rate : 81   SINUS RHYTHM
                    WITHIN NORMAL LIMITS
- - Durations - -
P : 84   SUMMARY: NORMAL
QRS : 92

I   aVR   V1   V4
II   aVL   V2   V5
III   aVF   V3   V6
II

Speed: 25 mm/s   Freq: 60~ .05-30Hz   E350i Rev.1.26 GRI 10.1
Gain : Limb 10   Chest 10 mm/mv

Fig. 10-6 A three-channel ECG report showing the six limb lead recordings on the left and the chest lead recordings on the right. Also notice the "rhythm strip" at the bottom showing lead II uninterrupted, and the interpretation of the recording on the upper right. *(From Bonewit-West K:* Clinical procedures for medical assistants, *ed 9, St Louis, 2015, Saunders.)*

Fig. 10-7 Electrode card with 10 stick-on electrodes (4 will be placed on the limbs and 6 will be placed on the chest). Also, notice the blue-tipped alligator clips seen under the card that are attached to brown "lead" wires. The alligator clips will clamp on to the electrodes after they have been placed on the patient.

Fig. 10-8 Electrodes, lead wires, and ECG recorder. *1,* Right arm limb electrode; *2,* chest electrodes; *3,* lower limb lead wires; *4,* patient cable *5,* amplifier; *6,* galvanometer; *7,* recording stylus; *(8)* moving ECG paper *9,* power cord.

Limb Lead Wires

The lead wires that connect to the electrodes are labeled and color coded as follows:

- **RA** designates right arm—white
- **LA** designates left arm—black
- **RL** designates right leg—green
- **LL** designates left leg—red

Standard Limb Leads

The first three leads recorded on a routine ECG are called **standard limb leads**. They are Einthoven's first leads known as *bipolar leads* because they each monitor two limb electrodes. They show the following electrical activity between the electrodes:

- Lead I shows the voltage changes between the right arm and left arm.
- Lead II shows the voltage changes between the right arm and left leg.
- Lead III shows the voltage changes between the left arm and left leg.

Augmented Limb Leads

The next three limb leads are called **augmented limb leads**. They are known as *unipolar leads* because they each directly monitor only one limb electrode. Each lead shows the electrical activity between one limb electrode and a point midway between the other two limb electrodes in the triangle.

The electrical impulses recorded by these leads are small. As a result, the ECG machine must augment, or *increase,* their size in order for the tracing to be readable. These leads are labeled aV, denoting "augmented voltage."

- **Lead aVR** shows the voltage difference between the *right arm* and the midpoint of the left arm and left leg.
- **Lead aVL** shows the voltage difference between the *left arm* and the midpoint of the right arm and left leg.
- **Lead aVF** shows the voltage difference between the *left leg* and the midpoint of the right arm and left arm.

Refer back to Figure 10-5, Einthoven's triangle, showing all six limb leads: I, II, III, aVR, aVL, and aVF.

Note the placement of the electrodes (sensors) on the lower limbs with the color-coded lead wires attached in Figure 10-9. The electrode placed on the right leg (green) is not used as part of the recording. Instead, it functions as an electrical ground and reference point.

Fig. 10-9 Note the disposable electrodes with color-coded wires for the grounded right leg (green-tipped wire) and the lead wire for the left leg (red-tipped wire). *(Photo by Zack Bent.)*

Precordial Chest Lead Wires

In addition to the limb leads, there are six **precordial leads**, or *chest leads*. They are also unipolar leads that monitor the heart from one chest electrode at a time. Each precordial lead shows the electrical activity between a central point within the heart and a specific site on the front of the chest based on skeletal structures.

Six electrodes are placed across the chest in a specific pattern based on the patient's skeletal structures. The precordial lead wires are each labeled with the letter V or C and a lead number 1 through 6. They monitor electrodes at the following sites:

- **V1:** fourth **intercostal** space on the right side of the **sternum**
- **V2:** fourth intercostal space on the left side of the sternum
- **V3:** midway between the V2 and V4 positions
- **V4:** fifth intercostal space on the left mid-clavicular line
- **V5:** horizontal to V4 at the left anterior axillary line
- **V6:** horizontal to V4 at the left midaxillary line

See Figure 10-10, *A-D*, which shows the four steps taken to locate the six chest leads using skeletal landmarks.

Fig. 10-10 **A,** *Step 1:* Locate V1 by palpating the top three intercostal spaces and then placing the electrode on the next fourth intercostal space on the right side of the patient's sternum.

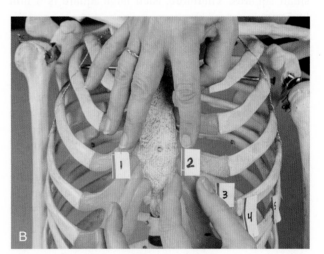

Fig. 10-10 **B,** *Step 2:* Place V2 directly across from V1 over the fourth intercostal space on the left side of the patient's sternum.

Fig. 10-10 **C,** *Step 3:* Locate V4 by drawing an imaginary line from the mid-**clavicle** to the fifth intercostal space; then place V3 midway on an imaginary straight line between V2 and V4.

Fig. 10-10 **D,** *Step 4:* Place V5 in line with V4 at the anterior/lateral "corner" of the chest. And then place V6 in line with V5 at the midaxillary line on the left side of the chest.

Standardization and Interpretation of the Electrocardiograph

Standardization

All electrocardiographs (instruments) must be standardized in order to produce a consistent electrocardiogram (picture) that records the electrical deflections produced by each person's heartbeats over time. All ECG tracing paper is divided into squares that form graph lines. The size and pattern of the squares are standard. As a result, physicians throughout the world are able to read and compare a patient's tracings in the same way (Figure 10-11).

Two sizes of squares are in the graph, small and large. Each small square is 1 millimeter (mm) by 1 millimeter (mm). A large square is made up of 25 small squares. Therefore, each large square is 5 mm by 5 mm.

- The vertical lines on the graph measure voltage, or the strength of the electrical impulse. One small square represents 0.1 millivolt (mV), and two large squares (10 mm) represent 1 mV.
- The horizontal lines on the graph measure time. One small square represents 0.04 second, and five large squares (25 mm) represent 1 second.

The upward and downward deflections produced on the moving graph paper are standardized to a sensitivity showing 1 mV of electricity producing a 10-mm deflection on the graph paper as seen in Figure 10-11. NOTE: The standardized pulses were also seen at the beginning and end of each of the leads in Figure 10-6. The sensitivity may also be set at ½ when a large heartbeat needs to be diminished on the graph, or at 2 times to magnify the recording of a small heartbeat.

The time it takes to produce each cardiac cycle is also standardized by setting the speed of the graph paper to move horizontally at a speed of 25 mm per second.

Interpretation of ECG

Physicians are now able to analyze the electrical patterns (vertical waves) and the specific timing (horizontal measurements) of each wave (P, Q, R, S, T, and the occasional U) (see Figure 10-11).

Cardiologists (and interpretive ECGs) also measure the following (as seen in Figure 10-11):

- The timing of the **QRS complex** related to ventricular stimulation and contraction
- The timing (or duration) of two *segments:* the **P-R segment,** showing the time when the impulse is delayed at the AV node before traveling down the bundle of His; and the **ST segment,** showing the time between ventricular depolarization and repolarization
- The timing (or duration) of two *intervals* related to atrial activity **(P-R interval)** and ventricular activity **(Q-T interval)**

Fig. 10-11 Enlarged ECG graph paper showing the large boxes that have been divided into 5 × 5 1-mm small boxes. Notice the normal standardization pulse on the left: 1 millivolt charge should cause the stylus to jump up 10 mm (2 large squares) while the paper is moving, creating a 2-mm horizontal line that returns to the baseline. Notice how the waves (P, Q, R, S, and T) are identified and measured by the up and down movement of the stylus showing voltage. The "segments" and "intervals" of each ECG cycle are also analyzed and measured based on the horizontal movement of the paper over time.

The **baseline** on the ECG is when the heart is at rest between beats, and no electrical activity is taking place. Cardiologists and computerized interpretive ECGs are able to calculate the rate and rhythm of the heartbeat per minute by observing the distance between the peaks of the R waves of each **ECG cycle**. See Figure 10-12, which displays an interpretation of **"Sinus Bradycardia"** (slow heart rate) with a ventricular rate of 58 beats/minute, and compare the distance of the ECG cycles seen at the bottom of the ECG in Figure 10-6, which displays an interpretation of **"Sinus Rhythm"** (within normal limits) with a ventricular rate of 81 beats/minute. If the cardiac cycles were very close together on the bottom "rhythm strip," the result would be **"Sinus Tachycardia."**

Name : Jane Doe		
ID : 27		
Date : 08/28/03	Time : 04:17	
Age : 48	Sex : Female	
Hgt : 67 IN	Wgt : 150 LBS	
Med1 :		
Med2 :		
Ccl1 :		
Ccl2 :		
Cmnt :		

Vent rate : 58

- - Durations - -
P   : 82
QRS : 92
- - Intervals - -
PR   : 110
QT   : 426
QTc : 423
- - Axes - -
P   : -15
QRS : 34
T   : 33

SINUS BRADYCARDIA
SUPRAVENTRICULAR EXTRASYSTOLES
    ST junctional depression
NON SPECIFIC ST CHANGES

SUMMARY: BORDERLINE NORMAL

Speed: 25 mm/s   Freq: 60~ .05-30Hz
Gain : Limb 10   Chest 10 mm/mv

E350i Rev.1.15 GRI 10.1

Fig. 10-12 ECG recording with interpretation at the top showing "sinus bradycardia." Notice how much farther apart the R spikes are compared to those in Figure 10-6. *(From Bonewit-West K:* Clinical procedures for medical assistants, *ed 9, St Louis, 2015, Saunders.)*

Anatomy of the Lungs

Lung function tests are able to measure how much and how fast air is inhaled and exhaled from the lungs. They are generally used in primary care to identify breathing obstructions and restrictions in the respiratory system airways. A review of the structures in the respiratory tract and common obstructive diseases related to each are listed below and are seen in Figure 10-13.

Note the upper respiratory tract at the top and the lower respiratory tract with its bronchial tubes (primary, secondary, and tertiary, and terminal) branching out like a tree until it terminates in alveoli (seen enlarged at the bottom), where gas exchange occurs.

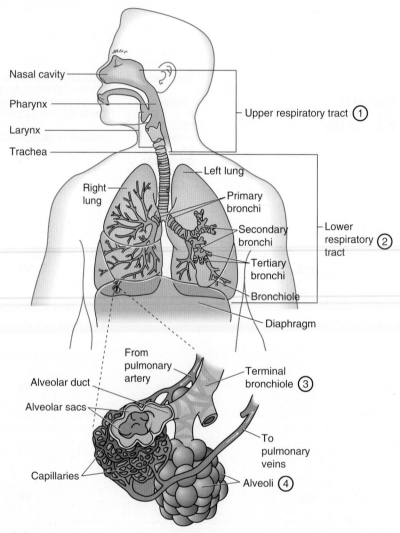

Fig. 10-13 Structures of the respiratory tract. *(From Warekois R, Robinson R: Phlebotomy: worktext and procedures manual, ed 3, St Louis, 2012, Saunders.)*

Respiratory Structures	Common Obstructive Diseases
1. **Upper respiratory tract** (nasal cavity, pharynx, larynx, trachea)	**URI**—upper respiratory tract infections such as colds, flu, allergies
2. **Lower respiratory tract** (primary bronchi, secondary bronchi, tertiary bronchi)	**Bronchitis**—acute infection may follow URI; chronic form typically caused by smoking, toxic fumes, or other irritants
3. **Terminal bronchioles** (muscles capable of dilation or constriction)	**Asthma**—bronchioles are inflamed (swollen) and thick mucus forms, causing difficulty during inspiration and expiration
4. **Alveoli** (air sacs where oxygen and carbon dioxide exchange takes place)	**Emphysema**—walls of alveoli break down; most commonly caused by smoking

Spirometry Testing

The spirometer test in the ambulatory setting is usually a screening test that is given when a patient's pulmonary dysfunction is known or suspected (e.g., chronic obstructive pulmonary disease [COPD] patients), or if a patient's respiratory system is at risk from inhaling toxins such as toxic gases or smoke.

The **spirometer** is an instrument that measures the volume and flow of air that is breathed. In ambulatory settings, the most common screening test is the **FVC** (forced vital capacity). In this diagnostic test, the patient is asked to fully inflate the lungs followed by exhaling the air from the lungs into the spirometer's disposable mouthpiece as fast and as forcibly as possible.

The FVC test requires the patient to complete the following three-step "forced expiratory maneuver":

Step 1—While holding the disposable mouthpiece that is attached to the spirometer, the patient uses full inspiration to fill the lungs and then holds his or her breath while sealing the lips around the disposable mouthpiece.

Step 2—The patient then exhales fast and hard to exhale most of the air within the first second of exhalation.

Step 3—The patient continues to exhale any remaining air for as close to 6 seconds as possible.

When the maneuver is performed correctly, the spirometer produces two graphs along with an analysis and interpretation of the results as seen in Figure 10-14.

Volume/Time Chart

The graph in the lower right of the report (Figure 10-14) provides the physician with the following information:

1. **FET**, or forced expiratory time, is the horizontal length of the curved line, which shows how long the patient exhaled in seconds (ideally the line should continue to 6 seconds).
2. **FVC**, or forced vital capacity, is the vertical height of the line, which shows how much air was exhaled in liters. (Note: The total volume will vary with patient based on size, age, gender, and race.)
3. FEV_1 is the forced expiratory volume in the first second and is expressed in liters.
4. FEV_1/**FVC ratio**—A healthy person is predicted to exhale 80% to 90% of their total volume (FVC) within the first second (FEV_1). This percentage is calculated by dividing the FEV_1 volume by the total FVC volume.

A good maneuver will show a volume/time chart with a quick rise within the first second and then a steady upward rise plateauing for up to 6 seconds. Note: A patient with an obstructive disorder will not be able to exhale rapidly in the first second and will consequently have a predicted percentage less than 80%.

Flow/Volume Chart—"Peak Flow Chart"

The graph in the lower left of the report (Figure 10-14) provides the physician with the following information:

- **PEF,** or peak expiratory flow, is the highest point on the graph representing maximum flow during the maneuver.
- $FEF_{25-75\%}$ is the breakdown of flow at 25%, 50%, and 75% of the maneuver.

A good maneuver should show a fast rise in the beginning of the graph with a gradual curve downward that ends on the baseline.

Predicted Values and Percentiles

A computerized, interpretive spirometer will also provide **predicted values** to compare the patient's results with a control group of others who share the same age, height, weight, gender, and race. This allows the physician to readily see when a patient lags behind predicted values (i.e., below 80% of predicted values), which may then necessitate more extensive pulmonary function tests.

Quality Control–Spirometer Calibration

The spirometer needs to be calibrated on each testing day using a large 3-L syringe as seen in Figure 10-15. A mouthpiece is applied to the syringe and the air is pushed into the spirometer in a rapid steady motion. The spirometer then provides feedback if the calibration is successful (results will show a total exhaled volume within 3% of 3 L). If not, refer to the instruction manual for recommended ways to adjust the instrument. A typical adjustment is to enter the temperature and elevation settings (barometric pressure) for the testing area. Both of these variables affect the accuracy of the test. See the spirometer video on the Evolve website for a demonstration on calibrating the spirometer with the 3-L syringe.

Spirometry Report

Name:		Age:	37 years	Race:	Caucasian
ID:		Height:	73 inches	Weight:	Unspecified
Sex:	Male	Indication:			
Smoker:	No	Medications:			
COPD risk	Low	Lung age:	< 37 years		

Requested by:		Performed by:	MG
Test date:	03/15/13 14:35:28	Sensor S/N:	543679
Test date post:		Sensor calibrated:	01/30/12 14:10:58
Press/Temp:	760 mmHg/79 degrees F	Spiro control ver:	8.5.0
Bronchodilator:		Normals/interp:	Crapo/ATS (1991)

Measurement	Units	Predicted	Pre-Bronchodilator Trial					
			1		2		3	
			Actual	% pred.	Actual	% pred.	Actual	% pred.
FVC	L	5.68	5.95	105 %	5.83	103 %	5.80	102 %
FEV1	L	4.58	4.32	94 %	4.49*	98 %	4.44	97 %
FEV1/FVC	%	81 %	73 %	90 %	77 %	95 %	77 %	95 %
FEF25%	L/S	9.40	7.90	84 %	8.40	89 %	8.52	91 %
FEF50%	L/S	5.79	3.70	64 %	4.29	74 %	4.20	73 %
FEF75%	L/S	2.41	1.55	64 %	1.81	75 %	1.82	75 %
FEF25-75%	L/S	4.51	3.24	72 %	3.80	84 %	3.70	82 %
PEF	L/S	10.14	8.87	87 %	9.93	98 %	10.02	99 %
Exp. time	SEC.		5.93		3.60		3.38	
V ext.	L		0.14		0.09		0.09	

Test #1
Test #2 (Best)
Test #3

= Best FVC test
★ = Best Pre FEV1

Pre-BD FVC: 3 attempted, 3 accepted, 2 matches.

Interpretation: Normal spirometry

Observations:

Unconfirmed report

Midmark Diagnostics Group   Software Version: 8.5.0   Printed: 03/15/13   14:35:34   Page 1 of 1

Fig. 10-14 Spirometry report showing "normal spirometry." The volume/time graph (on the right) has a quick rise within the first second and then a steady upward rise plateauing for the next 6 seconds.

Fig. 10-15 Spirometer calibration syringe showing the right hand pushing 3 L of air through the mouthpiece held by the left hand. The spirometer result must register 3 L within ±3% to be in control.

 ## Diagnostic Procedures: ECG and Spirometry

In this chapter, the ECG and the spirometer are recording the results produced by the patient's heart and breathing rather than lab specimens. It is therefore necessary to prepare patients properly and to coach them with helpful instructions throughout the procedures in order to produce accurate reports. It is also important to identify and correct any **artifacts** (tracings other than from the heart or lungs that will interfere with the interpretation of the ECG or spirometer recordings) before submitting a final report to the physician.

ECG Patient Preparations, Instructions, and Identification of Artifacts

Patient Preparation

Call the patient into the room and sanitize your hands while confirming the patient's name with the same methods that were covered in Chapter 4: Ask each patient to spell his or her last name, provide his or her date of birth, and give one more identifier, such as phone number or address, or show a driver's license.

Be aware of patients' anxiety level and assure them that the ECG test is "routine" and that when they are being connected to the lead wires, the procedure is not forcing any electricity into them. The wires are simply attaching to the sticky "sensors" (electrodes) that are placed on various places on their body in order to "take pictures" of the electrical activity generated by the heart and any other muscle in the body. Explain that it is important that they are very comfortable and relaxed so that the only muscular activity during the test should be from their hearts. Show them the gowns and have them disrobe from the waist up; then tell them you will return to their room when they are ready.

When you return, help them recline on their back with their head placed comfortably on the pillow

Fig. 10-16 Computer monitoring of all 12 leads. Notice the "artifacts" (erratic tracings attributable to patient movement) on three of the limb tracings. These artifacts would need to be corrected before printing the final report.

and their arms rested on their sides in a comfortable position. NOTE: If a large person's body does not allow enough room for their arms on the table, have the person tuck their thumbs under their legs. This will reduce the muscular interference caused by using their arm muscles to keep their arms on the table. Also, make sure the patients' legs are relaxed by allowing their feet to turn outward.

When running the test let the patient know when the ECG is recording and encourage them to be very still and relaxed with no talking or moving for the 15 seconds of recording.

Identifying and Correcting ECG Artifacts

When the patient's electrocardiogram tracing is printed on the 3-channel ECG paper, or "captured" on the computer screen, it is the medical assistant's responsibility to analyze the tracings on each of the 12 leads and identify any artifacts. See Figure 10-16, which shows a computer readout of all 12 leads. Notice the hand pointing at the erratic tracings on 3 of the 12 lead tracings. You may also notice that the erratic tracings appeared and then stabilized to the right of the artifacts, which means that the patient moved an arm during that part of the tracing. Obviously, you would not want to have that part of the tracing in the final report.

Figure 10-17, *A* through *D* illustrates four examples of the most common artifacts found on ECG tracings (somatic tremors, wandering baseline, AC interference, and interrupted baseline). The four artifacts shown in the accompanying table explain the possible causes of each artifact.

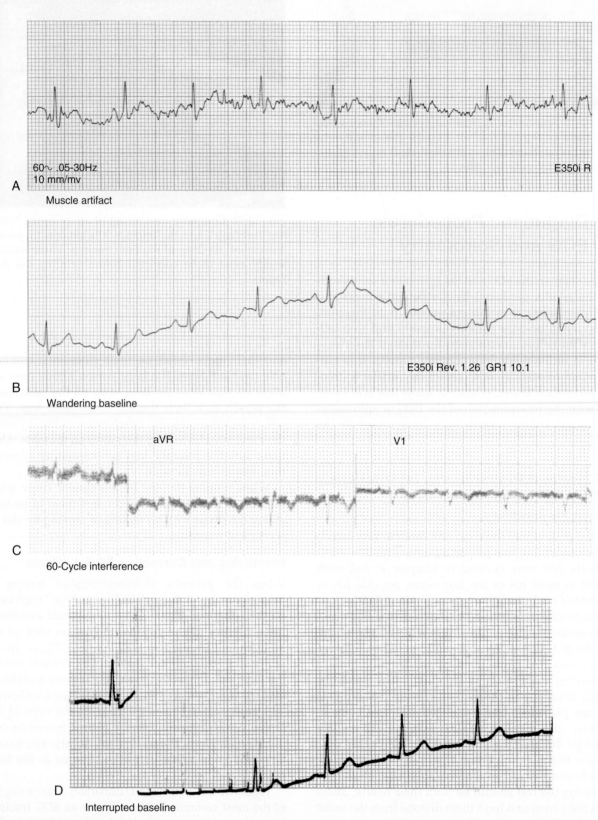

Fig. 10-17 ECG artifacts (tracings caused by sources other than the patient's heart) that need to be corrected. Refer to the table on p. 311 showing the possible causes and ways to correct and/or eliminate each of these artifacts *(From Bonewit-West K: Clinical procedures for medical assistants, ed 9, St Louis, 2015, Saunders, with reference to Long BW: Radiography essentials for limited practice, ed 3, 2010, Saunders.)*

ECG ARTIFACTS	WAYS TO CORRECT
A. Muscle Artifact "Somatic Tremor"	1. Check to ensure patient is comfortable and relaxed. 2. Provide a blanket if patient is cold. 3. Provide patient with a pillow. 4. Elevate the back of the exam table until patient is comfortable. 5. Check if the patient's arms are slipping off the exam table. (Have patient tuck their thumbs under their legs for better passive support.) 6. Explain that patient should not talk, chew, or move during the 15-second procedure. 7. If the patient has Parkinson's disease with involuntary muscle tremors in their limbs, place the electrodes on their trunk by the shoulders instead of the arms, and the hips instead of the legs. Note the new locations on the recording and in the patient's medical record.
B. Wandering Baseline	1. Check to see if the patient cable and/or the lead wires are dangling and unsupported. The lead wires should follow the contour of the body and not cross one another. 2. Have the patient hold his or her breath for 15 seconds if patient's rising and falling chest is causing the drifting baseline.
C. 60-Cycle Interference "AC Interference"	1. Check if the power cord is running under the exam table. If it is, find another plug or move the table. 2. Check if high-voltage wiring is running parallel in the walls or overhead (e.g., x-ray equipment uses high voltage). If this is true, turn the exam table at a 90-degree angle to the wiring.
D. Interrupted Baseline	1. This is seen frequently when an electrode becomes dislodged (especially on the chest leads). Correct the problem by applying hypoallergenic tape to reinforce the electrodes. 2. The electrode is not making contact because of hair on the legs or chest. Shave the site and reapply a new electrode. 3. The cable showing the interrupted pattern may be damaged and in need of replacement.

If the medical assistant spots artifacts on any of the limb leads (I, II, III, aVR, aVL, or aVF), the problem needs to be located and corrected. Knowledge of Einthoven's triangle is helpful in locating the limb producing the artifact. For example, if there are muscle tremors or poor electrode contact on lead I and III but not on lead II, it can be deduced that the problem stems from the left arm because leads I and III both involve the left arm, and lead II does not.

If the problem is seen on one of the chest leads (V1, V2, V3, V4, V5, or V6) then go directly to the lead wire and its electrode location on the chest to correct it.

When all the artifacts have been corrected and a new acceptable final tracing is printed, the physician will then check the tracing and give his or her approval before having the lead wires and electrodes removed from the patient. It should be noted that most patients are anxious about the results, knowing that their heart is a very vital organ. So, be aware how you relate to patients during and after the procedure. Also, remember that you are not authorized to tell the patient the results of the ECG and that the physician will be sharing the findings with the patient along with the whole picture of the patient's health status.

You are now ready to perform the ECG. You will want to view the ECG video on the Evolve website before lab, and read Procedure 10-1 at the end of this section.

Spirometer Patient Preparations, Instructions, and Identification of Artifacts

Similar to ECG testing, patients may be anxious to know the results of their spirometer test in hopes of "passing" the test. The success of their test requires an understanding of exactly what they need to do during the maneuver, and good coaching from the assistant or technician running the test.

Patient Preparation

When making the appointment for the **spirometry** test, the patient should be instructed to make the following preparations:

- Wear loose clothing.
- Avoid smoking and eating anything heavy 8 hours before the procedure.
- Do not use the bronchodilator 4 hours before the test based on the physician's recommendations.

On the day of the test, explain the procedure in a simple, clear manner, emphasizing that you will be performing a lung measurement test that does not hurt, but will require effort and cooperation in order to produce two reproducible records for the physician to interpret. Explain and demonstrate the three steps of the maneuver using a mouthpiece that is not connected to the spirometer:

1. **Fully inflate** your lungs and then hold your breath while sealing your lips around the mouthpiece.
2. **Fully exhale** into the mouthpiece as fast and as hard as possible.
3. Give **full effort** to exhale the remaining air in your lungs for another 5 seconds without inhaling until the time has expired.

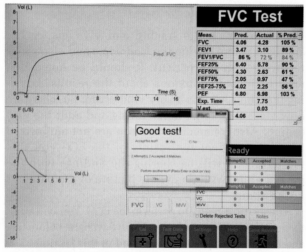

Fig. 10-18 Spirometer results on a computer showing a "Good test" maneuver. Note the upper time/volume curve shows a sharp rise within the first second and then a slight steady rise for the next 2 to 6 seconds. The lower volume/flow curve shows a fast rise in the beginning of the graph with a gradual curve downward that ends on the baseline.

Show and explain the importance of standing upright during the maneuver and that the patient will have 1 minute to sit and rest between a minimum of three attempts.

Coaching the Maneuver

Watch the patient as he or she performs the maneuver, making sure you see all three steps: inspiration, rapid exhalation, and extended exhalation. Praise the patient for maneuvers performed well and communicate positive ways to improve the next maneuver. Do not give negative feedback. The following chart provides examples of positive versus negative comments.

Positive Corrective Feedback	Negative Corrective Feedback
"I need you to blow out really hard."	"You didn't blow hard enough."
"I need you to seal your lips firmly around the mouthpiece so all your breath is captured."	"You're not putting the mouthpiece far enough into your mouth."
"I need you to blow until I say stop."	"You didn't blow long enough."
"Keep your eyes on the screen."	"Don't look away."

Modern spirometers may also give coaching tips such as "blow harder" or "blow longer" based on the final curves produced on the recorded graphs on the spirometer. Computerized spirometers also provide the incentive to blow hard and continuously by displaying a tree with hidden monkeys behind the leaves that must be blown away, or a cake with candles, for example. Instruct the patient to stay focused on the progress seen on the screen and help the patient verbally by counting down "5-4-3-2-1" to keep the patient exhaling for the full 6 seconds without inhaling or coughing. NOTE: You should look at the patient, not the screen, to make sure the procedure is being performed correctly (e.g., mouth position, body position, signs of fatigue).

Most spirometers will also let you know when there was a successful maneuver by reporting "Good test!" See Figure 10-18, which illustrates a computerized spirometer confirmation of a successful maneuver, along with the two graphs and predictors. The patient may need to attempt up to eight maneuvers, with 1 minute of rest in between each attempt, in order to produce the required two maneuvers with "Good test!" results. NOTE: If the patient has an obstructed airway, he or she may not be able to produce a "Good test" result. If this occurs, let the patient know there is still enough information to help with the diagnosis. Be sure to note any difficulties or issues during the maneuver on the patient's chart to help the physician with the final analysis.

Post-bronchodilator Response

When adults demonstrate airway obstruction (COPD) with their FEV_1/FVC ratio less than 70% of predicted or when children with asthma show a FEV_1/FVC ratio less than 80%, the physician may order a post-bronchodilator test. This consists of administering a prescribed bronchodilator dosage and then retesting the patient 20 minutes later to see if the patient's results are improved. Improved results after the bronchodilator may indicate the patient is a candidate for the medication.

You are now ready to perform a spirometer test. You will need to view the Spirometer video on the Evolve website before lab, and review Procedure 10-2 at the end of this section.

✳ PROCEDURE 10-1 Electrocardiograph (Three Channel and Computerized with Interpretation)

A, Place the three-channel ECG instrument on the patient's left side and enter demographic data as prompted into the electrocardiograph: patient name, age, sex, height, weight, medications.

B, If using a computerized ECG, enter the patient's demographic data and digital vital signs into the patient's electronic record.

C, The computerized ECG will also ask for the following vital signs: temperature from the digital thermometer, blood pressure from the digital BP cuff, pulse rate and percent saturated oxygen from the pulse oximeter.

D, Prepare lower limb electrode sites by shaving hair if necessary followed by rubbing with an alcohol swab. Allow the alcohol to completely dry while preparing the limb and chest electrode sites.

(Continued)

10-1

PROCEDURE 10-1 **Electrocardiograph (Three Channel and Computerized with Interpretation—cont'd**

E, Visualize and palpate the skeletal landmarks on the patient's chest. The key landmarks are: lead I at the fourth intercostal space to the right of the patient's sternum (with lead II directly across from it). Then lead IV on the fifth intercostal space is in line with the middle of the clavicle bone on the patient's left side. Lead III is placed midway between leads II and IV. Leads V and VI wrap around the chest in line with lead IV (on anterolateral line and the midaxillary line).

F, Palpate the first three intercostal spaces with your right hand and rub the alcohol swab on the next fourth intercostal space on the patient's right side of the sternum as seen in the illustration. Then rub alcohol directly across the sternum to the fourth intercostal space on the patient's left side of the sternum followed by a diagonal down to the fifth intercostal space at the midclavicular line. Continue rubbing the alcohol around the chest intersecting the anterior lateral line and the mid axillary line. Be aware of the patient's modesty when locating female chest sites.

G, Return to the limbs and firmly press the sticky, tabbed electrodes with tabs up on the legs and tabs down on the arms.

H, Attach each of the alligator clips located on the four color-coded, limb lead wires starting with the **green RL** on the leg across from you. Then the **red LL** on the patient's left leg (closest to you) completes "Christmas". Find the **black LA** wire and clip it to the arm close to you (red LL is when funds are down, and black LA means you are up in funds). Then **white LA** goes to the opposite arm away from you (which is the opposite of black).

10-1

PROCEDURE 10-1 Electrocardiograph (Three Channel and Computerized with Interpretation—cont'd

I, Return to the chest where the initial alcohol has dried. Repalpate for the fourth intercostal space on the side away from you and press the electrode with the tabs down followed by placing the electrode for V2 directly across the sternum on your side. Clip on the V1 and V2 wires.

J, After locating the V4 site and applying the electrode at the fifth intercostal space in line with the middle of the clavicle, apply V3 electrode on the diagonal line between V2 and V4. Then place V5 electrode at the anterior lateral line and V6 electrode in line with the middle of the armpit (midaxillary line). These four leads and their respective lead wires may all be applied with the female's gown carefully lifted up just enough to expose the sites.

K, On the male, all the chest electrodes may be placed on the bare chest followed by the lead wires. Note the following: V1 and V2 are parallel; V2, V3, and V4 are diagonal; V4, V5, V6 are around the chest.

L, Clip the chest lead wires (V1 through V6) to the electrodes, taking care to note the proper numbered wire is attached to the proper site. The patient is now ready to have his or her ECG recorded.

(Continued)

10-1

PROCEDURE 10-1 Electrocardiograph (Three Channel and Computerized with Interpretation—cont'd

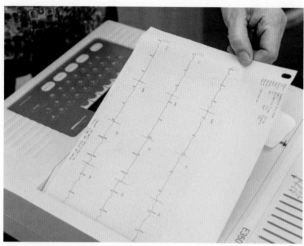

M, If running the three-channel ECG, examine the print-out for any artifacts. If artifacts are present, run another recording.

N, Alternatively, as the computerized ECG is running, make sure all 12 leads are stable with no artifacts, and then "freeze" the recording, followed by "analyze" and "print."

Procedure

Equipment and Supplies

The two most common ECG analyzers are the three-channel type seen in Figure A and the computerized ECG (Figure B). Both are placed on the patient's left side of the exam table, and both share the following supplies (not pictured):

- Razor
- Alcohol
- 10 disposable electrodes
- Patient cable
- Power cord
- Graph paper or printer connected to computer

Preanalytical

1. Cleanse hands and prepare room with clean table paper, pillow, gown, and drape.
2. Greet the patient and confirm identity while entering demographic data (e.g., patient's name, number, age, address) (see Figures A and B).
3. Explain procedure and how to disrobe (from the waist up with the gown opening in the front). Provide the patient with privacy.
4. After returning, obtain the patient's vital signs (Figure C). Enter the vital signs into the computer.
5. Prepare the 10 sites in a routine order to avoid errors when stressed.
6. Prepare the lower limbs by dry shaving the inner calf muscles if necessary (Figure D), and then rub the areas with the alcohol swab to encourage circulation at the sites.

7. While the lower limbs are drying, prepare the upper outer limbs with the alcohol swab followed by locating the general areas for the chest leads and rubbing the areas with the alcohol swab. See Figure E to help visualize the skeletal landmarks for V1 and V4 and their relationships with the other leads (as demonstrated in Figure 10-10 of the text). Figure F shows the three-finger method of locating V1 using three fingers for the first three intercostal spaces. Use the alcohol swab to cleanse the fourth intercostal area, and then swab across the sternum for V2. Next, swab a diagonal line from V2 to V4. Finally, swab a line from V4 around the chest to the midaxillary area.
8. Return to the legs and arms, and firmly press the electrode sensors with the tabs up on the legs (Figure G) and the tabs down on the arms. NOTE: It is important to let the alcohol dry completely before placing the electrodes on the prepared sites.
9. Connect the color-coded limb lead wires (Figure H) in the following order:
   - Start with the **green RL = right leg** for "go" and "ground" wire. (NOTE: You should always be working on the patient's left side, so this will always be on the leg farthest away.)
   - Next, the **red LL = left leg** is placed. NOTE: Green and red are always the "Christmas colors" on the legs.
   - After the LL comes the **black LA = left arm** on the same side closest to you. This wire is always coded black. (*Hint:* Red and black are the two

PROCEDURE 10-1 Electrocardiograph (Three Channel and Computerized with Interpretation—cont'd

colors used in accounting—red is in the hole (at the feet) and black is on top of finances (at the arm).

- The only limb lead left is the **white RA = right arm,** which is the opposite of black. So the arms are black and white!

10. The chest leads have been prepared with alcohol, but it is now necessary to relocate the actual sites and place the electrodes in the following order:

- Palpate to locate the fourth intercostal space across the right side of the patient's sternum and then place the **V1 electrode** with the tab down followed by the **V2 electrode** directly across the sternum on the patient's left side (closest to you) (Figure I).
- Next, locate the V4 lead location by following the fifth intercostal space to the mid-clavicular line and place the **V4 electrode** on the site followed by the **V3 electrode** midway between V2 and V4.
- The last two leads follow a horizontal line based on V4's location around the ribs, with the **V5 electrode** being placed on the anterior-lateral line of the chest and the **V6 electrode** being placed at the midaxillary line of the chest (Figure J).
- After all the electrodes are placed on the chest (Figure K), methodically connect the numbered **V lead wires** to each of their designated electrode locations (Figure L).

Analytical

11. The ECG is now ready to start recording. Before starting the recording, let the patient know that he or she needs to be very still and relaxed for about 15 seconds while the ECG is monitoring heartbeats. The patient should not talk or chew gum or do any muscular activity during the testing because the ECG instrument will pick up any patient movement.

12. When you are sure the patient understands the instructions and the patient is comfortable and still, start the recording.

Postanalytical

13. Observe the three-channel ECG printout (Figure M) and/or the computer results (Figure N) for the following:

- Check the inserted 1-millivolt standard pulse for an upward rise of 10 mm (little squares) and a sideways line of 2 mm, and then back down to the baseline.
- Check each lead in the tracing for unwanted artifacts and correct them if possible (e.g., AC interference, muscle tremors, wandering or interrupted baseline). If artifacts are seen, re-record another tracing if necessary.
- Allow the physician to see the final product before disconnecting the patient from the ECG.

14. Remove and dispose the electrodes and help the patient to a sitting position. Instruct the patient to get dressed and that the physician will be sharing the findings with him or her.

15. The ECG procedure is documented in the patient's chart or the electronic medical record, noting any variables due to artifacts or patient issues.

10-1

✴ PROCEDURE 10-2 Spirometry

10-2

A, Enter patient demographic data and current height and weight, plus the patient's gender, race, and age.

B, Fully inflate your lungs and then hold your breath while sealing your lips around the mouthpiece. Note the tree on the computer screen is filled with leaves.

C, Fully exhale into the mouthpiece **as fast and as hard as possible.** Note most of the leaves are gone, exposing the monkeys on the tree within the first second.

D, Give full effort to exhale the remaining air in your lungs for another 5 seconds if possible without inhaling until time has expired. Note all the leaves are off the tree.

PROCEDURE 10-2 Spirometry—cont'd

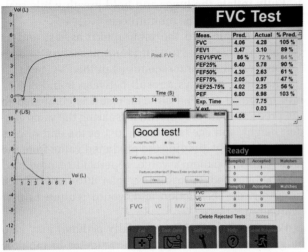

E, Spirometer results on computer showing "Good test" maneuver. NOTE: The upper left time/volume curve shows a sharp rise within the first second and then a slight steady rise for the next 2 to 6 seconds. In addition, the lower left volume/flow curve shows a fast rise in the beginning of the graph with a gradual curve downward that ends on the baseline.

Instrument and Supplies

Prepare the testing area with the following:
- Spirometer instrument or computer connected to a printer
- A disposable sterile mouthpiece connected to the plastic tubing on the spirometer. (Take care not to touch the area where the patient's mouth will be placed.)
- A nose clip (based on the physician's preference)
- A chair available for the patient to sit if he or she becomes fatigued during the maneuver
- Disposable gloves to be worn during and after the patient's test to avoid the transmission of possible respiratory viruses and other respiratory pathogens
- 3-L syringe for calibrating the spirometer

Preanalytical

1. Call the patient into the room and sanitize your hands while confirming the patient's name using three identifiers: have the patient spell his or her last name, give his or her date of birth, and provide one more identifiers such as phone number or address, or show a driver's license.
2. Enter the following data into the spirometer or into the computer's spirometer patient record: name, ID number, age, height, weight, gender, and race. NOTE: All this information is critical for the spirometer to produce the appropriate "predicted" results that compare the patient's performance with others in his or her demographic pool (Figure A).

3. Confirm when the patient last took bronchodilator medication and if the patient has smoked and note it on the chart. Also, if appropriate, check to make sure the patient does not have loose dentures that will interfere with the breathing maneuver.
4. Explain and demonstrate the three steps of the maneuver using a mouthpiece that is not connected to the spirometer:
   - **Fully inflate** your lungs and then hold your breath while sealing your lips around the mouthpiece (Figure B).
   - **Fully exhale** into the mouthpiece as fast and as hard as possible (Figure C).
   - Give **full effort** to exhale the remaining air in your lungs for another 5 seconds without inhaling until the time has expired (Figure D).
5. Show and explain the importance of standing upright during the maneuver and that the patient will have 1 minute to rest and sit between a minimum of three attempts.

Analytical

6. Coach the patient as he or she performs the maneuver. Watch the patient, making sure he or she performs all three steps: inspiration, rapid exhalation, extended exhalation. Praise what the patient did well and communicate positive ways to improve the next maneuver. Do not give negative feedback.
7. Observe the two graph results and the spirometer feedback after each maneuver (Figure E) and have the patient rest for 1 minute.
   - The time/volume curve should show a sharp rise within the first second and then a slight steady rise for the next 2 to 6 seconds.
   - The volume/flow curve should show a fast rise in the beginning of the graph with a gradual curve downward that ends on the baseline.
8. Repeat at least three maneuvers, until the patient is able to perform two reproducible results.

Postanalytical

9. Discard the patient's mouthpiece and your gloves in a biohazard container. Sanitize hands.
10. Chart the procedure and any difficulties or issues during the maneuver.
11. If the physician orders a post-bronchodilator test, administer the prescribed bronchodilator dosage and then retest the patient 20 minutes later to see if the patient responds well and is a candidate for the medication.

10-2

Advanced Concepts

This section covers ambulatory pulmonary testing using **peak flow rate** meters. It then presents two pulmonary treatments commonly performed in offices when dealing with asthmatic and COPD patients: nebulizer use and oxygen administration.

Preparing the patient for ambulatory ECG monitoring using a **Holter monitor** and a Zio patch will also be discussed followed by a brief overview of cardiac arrhythmias seen on ECG tracings. An atlas showing seven classic cardiac arrhythmias the physician will be interpreting is provided at the end of this section.

Peak Expiratory Flow Screening and Monitoring

The three common causes for COPD—bronchitis, asthma, and emphysema—were presented under Fundamental Concepts. Each has a distinct spirometry pattern seen during the initial in-office spirometry screening test and the post-bronchodilator test as presented in the previous diagnostic section. Peak expiratory flow (**PEF**) may also be measured with a peak flow meter (**PFM**), a portable, hand-held device (Figure 10-19). These inexpensive devices only test the initial "peak expiratory flow" (PEF) segment of the FVC (forced vital capacity).

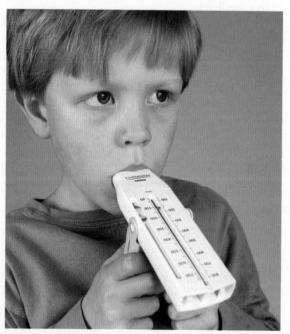

Fig. 10-19 Patient using a peak flow meter. The patient was instructed to (1) fully inflate the lungs and hold his breath while sealing his lips around the mouthpiece, and (2) then fully exhale into the mouthpiece as fast and as hard as possible.

In this screening test, the patient performs the first two steps of the FVC maneuver:
1. **Fully inflate** the lungs and hold breath while sealing lips around the mouthpiece.
2. **Fully exhale** into the mouthpiece as fast and as hard as possible. NOTE: It is not necessary to continue exhaling for 6 seconds as in the FVC test.

The meter displays a result between 0 and 800 L/min of forced exhaled air. The result is compared to the predicted rate of individuals sharing the same gender, height, and age (see Table 10-1 at the end of procedure 10-3). By dividing the predicted value from the table into the patient's value, a percent of predicted may be obtained. A result less than 80% may be due to an airway obstruction and would require further evaluation.

Patients with COPD (especially asthma) may also be given the hand-held peak flow meter to monitor their lung health daily in order to predict and prevent an asthmatic attack. Figure 10-20 shows the anatomy, symptoms, and physical findings seen in a child experiencing an asthmatic attack and respiratory distress.

Daily peak flow monitoring, when used properly, may reveal the narrowing of the airways well in advance of an asthma attack. Peak flow meters will help determine the following:
- When the patient needs to seek emergency medical care
- The level of effectiveness of the patient's asthma management and treatment plan
- When to stop or add medication as directed by a physician
- What triggers an asthma attack (such as exercise-induced asthma)

Before receiving the portable peak flow meter, the asthmatic patient performs three peak expiratory flow maneuvers using the peak flow meter. The highest of three readings, showing the patient's "best effort," is then used as the recorded value of the patient's specific peak expiratory flow rate (rather than using the predicted flow chart seen in Table 10-1). The peak flow meter is then classified into three zones of measurement according to the American Lung Association: green, yellow, and red.

Peak flow zones are based on the traffic light concept: red means danger, yellow means caution, and green means safe. The zones are different for each person. The goal of the peak flow zones is to recognize early symptoms of uncontrolled asthma.
- **Green**—This is the **go** zone. The green zone is from 80% to 100% of the patient's highest peak flow reading, or personal best. Measurements in this zone signal that air is moving well through the airways and that the patient should continue to follow the asthma plan as directed by the physician.
- **Yellow**—This is the **caution** or **slow down** zone. The yellow zone is from 50% to 80% of the patient's

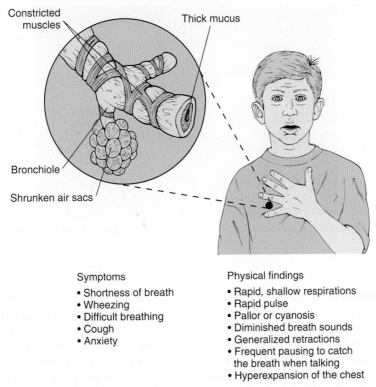

Constricted muscles

Thick mucus

Bronchiole

Shrunken air sacs

Symptoms
- Shortness of breath
- Wheezing
- Difficult breathing
- Cough
- Anxiety

Physical findings
- Rapid, shallow respirations
- Rapid pulse
- Pallor or cyanosis
- Diminished breath sounds
- Generalized retractions
- Frequent pausing to catch the breath when talking
- Hyperexpansion of the chest

Fig. 10-20 An asthma attack with respiratory distress. *Symptoms:* Shortness of breath, wheezing, difficult breathing, cough, anxiety. *Physical findings:* Rapid, shallow respirations, rapid pulse rate, pallor or cyanosis, diminished breath sounds, generalized retractions, frequent pausing to catch the breath when talking, hyperexpansion of the chest. *(From Frazier M:* Human diseases and conditions, *ed 5, St Louis, 2013, Saunders.)*

personal best. Measurements in this zone are a clue that the large airways are starting to narrow. The patient may begin to have mild symptoms, such as feeling short of breath, coughing, or feeling like the chest is tightening. The patient should notify the physician at this time.

- **Red**—This is the **stop** zone. The red zone is less than 50% of the patient's personal best. Readings in this zone indicate severe narrowing of the large airways has occurred. This is a medical emergency, and requires immediate attention. The patient may experience coughing, shortness of breath, and wheezing when breathing. There may be problems walking and talking. The patient should take his or her rescue medication immediately and call the physician.

See Procedure 10-3: Peak Expiratory Flow Monitoring at the end of this section for ways to screen patients as well as instruct them in the daily monitoring of their peak expiratory flow.

Asthma Therapies: Inhalers, Nebulizers, and Oxygen

When an asthmatic patient's breathing reaches the yellow and red zones, and the patient is experiencing respiratory distress, relief may be obtained in the following three ways:

- Inhale the prescribed bronchodilator medication using the correct inhaler.
- Breathe in a prescribed therapeutic dosage of medications via a nebulizer.
- Receive metered oxygen by nasal cannula.

The two basic types of drug therapies used in asthma treatment are as follows:

- **Anti-inflammatory medications** (e.g., steroids) are the most important treatment for most people with asthma. These work by reducing the production of mucus and swelling in the airways. As a result, the airways are less likely to become constricted, and they will be less sensitive to asthma "triggers" such as allergens and/or emotional or exercise stressors.

- **Bronchodilators** relieve the respiratory distress symptoms of asthma by further relaxing the muscles that can tighten around the airways. Short-acting bronchodilators are referred to as rescue inhalers because they relieve the cough, wheeze, chest tightness, and shortness of breath caused by an asthmatic attack. They may also be used before exercise for people with exercise-induced asthma. These should **not** be used daily in the routine treatment of asthma. Long-acting bronchodilators, on the other hand, are used in combination with inhaled steroids for control of asthma symptoms.

Fig. 10-21 Nebulizer and disposable supplies: *a,* nebulizer; *b,* reservoir tube; *c,* supply tubing; *d,* T tube; *e,* mouthpiece; *f,* medication jar.

The following two delivery systems are used by patients at home:

- **Meter dosed inhalers** are the most common. They are an effective way to deliver asthma drugs to the lungs. They are available in different types of devices that require different techniques for use. Some inhalers deliver one medication and others contain two different medications. They are generally hand-held devices and deliver a preset dosage of aerosol medication when activated and inhaled.
- **Nebulizers** are known as "breathing machines." The nebulizer forces air through the liquid medication, creating a mist that is then inhaled via a mouthpiece or mask. This method of asthma medication can be more easily inhaled into the lungs. Its use takes a few more minutes than an inhaler to take effect.

Ambulatory settings may also administer the inhaled dosage medications via nebulizers and/or oxygen to patients who are in respiratory distress. It is therefore important to have a basic foundation of these two in-office treatments.

Nebulizer Procedure

1. Sanitize your hands.
2. Gather and assemble the sterile disposable supplies and nebulizer as seen in Figure 10-21.
3. Place the prescribed solution into the nebulizer jar after checking the label three times, and connect firmly to the T tube.
4. Connect the mouthpiece to the T tube.
5. Connect the reservoir tube to the T tube.
6. Attach the supply tubing between the medication jar and the nebulizer as seen in Figure 10-22.
7. Ask the patient to place the mouthpiece into the mouth and make a seal with the lips, without biting the mouthpiece. Instruct the patient to breathe normally during the treatment, occasionally taking a deep breath.
8. Turn the machine on using the on/off switch. Set

the gas flow rate to 8 LPM (liters per minute), or according to the manufacturer's instructions. The medication in the jar will become a fine mist. Check for aerosol mist exiting out of the reservoir tube: if necessary, tap the device until it begins to nebulize.

9. Before, during, and after the breathing treatment, take and record the patient's pulse rate.
10. When the treatment is over and the medication is gone from the cup, turn the machine off and have the patient remove the mouthpiece.
11. During treatment, periodically tap the nebulizer to minimize residual volume.
12. Disconnect the disposable treatment setup and dispose all parts into a biohazard container.
13. Sanitize your hands and document the procedure, including the patient's pulse rate before, during, and after the treatment.

Fig. 10-22 The left hand is holding the medication jar (with green lid) that connects to the T tube where the mouthpiece and reservoir tube are also attached. The right hand is connecting the supply tubing to the nebulizer.

Administering Oxygen by Nasal Cannula

Oxygen therapy is a treatment that provides extra oxygen to the patient with obstructed airways. When a patient arrives at your facility with severe respiratory distress, the patient may be in critical need of oxygen. It is important to be familiar with how oxygen may be administered to the patient from an oxygen tank, a metal cylinder as seen in Figure 10-23, *A*.

The steps to take when preparing the oxygen tank are as follows:

1. Open the cylinder one full turn, counterclockwise. Check the pressure gauge (see Figure 10-23, *B*).
2. Attach the nasal cannula to the tubing and then to the flow meter.
3. Adjust the flow rate according to the physician's order (common standing order is 2 L per minute). Check to see if there is air flowing out of the nasal cannula.

4. Place the tips of the cannula into the nares no more than 1 inch.
5. As the patient holds the cannula, adjust the tubing around the patient's ears and secure it under the chin using the slider (Figure 10-24).
6. Answer patient's questions while making sure the patient is comfortable.

Ambulatory ECG Monitoring

The in-office ECG is a "snap shot" picture of the heart's electrical activity when the patient is at rest on the exam table. Often times, the physician needs to see the heart's reaction to a variety of conditions the patient experiences outside of the office (e.g., after eating, after exercising, during the stress of work, while sleeping). There are now very sophisticated, portable, ECG monitors that the patient may wear home and be monitored for 1 to 14 days.

The first ambulatory ECG monitor was invented by Norman J. Holter and Dr. W. R. Glasscock in 1961, thus the name "Holter monitor." Since then, Holter monitors have become smaller and capable of monitoring and recording increasing amounts of valuable data.

The medical assistant is usually the person to set up and instruct the patient with the ambulatory ECG monitor. See the Evolve site for a video of one method, and refer to Procedure 10-4: Holter Monitoring at the end of this section for the steps involved in the instruction and preparation of the patient for ambulatory ECG monitoring.

Zio Patch Wireless ECG Monitoring

The Zio® patch is the most recent development in cardiac rhythm monitoring that provides continuous wireless monitoring. A single patch is applied to the

Fig. 10-23 **A,** Compressed oxygen cylinders. **B,** Oxygen cylinder with regulator and flow meter attached. *(From Bonewit-West K: Clinical procedures for medical assistants, ed 9, St Louis, 2015.)*

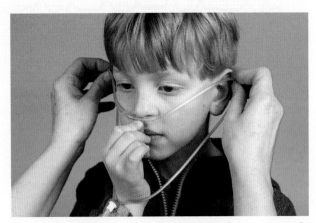

Fig. 10-24 While the patient is holding the two cannula tubes in his nose, bring the tubing from the front around each ear (creating a heart shape with the lower point at the chin). After the tubes are secure around the ears, tighten the lower tip under the chin with the white slider seen at the patient's wrist.

chest and records the heart's activity for up to 14 days, after which the patch is returned by mail for interpretation. See Procedure 10-4: Holter Monitoring for a picture demonstrating this new wireless method of ambulatory cardiac monitoring.

Cardiac Arrythmias and the ECG
Acute Myocardial Infarction

At the top of an interpretive ECG and/or the physician's interpretation, the term **sinus rhythm** means the normal pattern of waves and the rate of beats per minute are as expected. In contrast, when the neurological pattern and/or rhythm is not as expected, it is referred to as *arrhythmia*. One possible cause of an arrhythmia is when a coronary artery on the heart becomes blocked. A portion of the heart muscle becomes damaged from lack of oxygen and it becomes a *myocardial infarct* or *heart attack*. The damaged cardiac muscle disrupts the flow of electricity and changes the ECG tracing. See the Evolve website for an animation of how myocardial infarcts in various locations affect ECG tracings.

Bradycardia and **tachycardia** were discussed earlier. They both have normal PQRST waves but their beats (distance between the cardiac cycles) per minute occur slowly (far apart) in bradycardia and rapidly (close together) in tachycardia. Refer to the Atlas of Atrial Arrhythmias showing four additional arrhythmias that are caused by atrial dysfunction, and the Atlas of Ventricular Arrhythmias showing three additional ventricular arrhythmias. It should be noted that the ECG technician is not qualified to interpret these examples. But, an awareness of serious arrhythmias (i.e. ventricular fibrillation) should be brought to the physician's attention immediately.

Atlas of Atrial Arrhythmias

Fig. 10-25 Premature atrial contraction (**PAC**) seen between the fourth and fifth ECG cycle causing a premature heartbeat. *(From Huang SH et al: Coronary care nursing, St Louis, 1989, Saunders.)*

Atlas of Atrial Arrhythmias—cont'd

Fig. 10-26 Paroxysmal (sudden) atrial tachycardia (PAT) seen as rapid heartbeats initiated by atria. *(From Huang SH et al: Coronary care nursing, St Louis, 1989, Saunders.)*

Fig. 10-27 Atrial flutter seen here has 2 to 3 P waves for every QRS complex. *(From Johnson R, Swartz MH: A simplified approach to electrocardiography, St Louis, 1986, Saunders.)*

Fig. 10-28 Atrial fibrillation (A-fib) seen in this chest lead shows no P waves between the QRS complexes because the atria are not contracting in a coordinated way. *(From Huang S et al: Coronary care nursing, St Louis, 1989, Saunders.)*

Atlas of Ventricular Arrhythmias

Fig. 10-29 Premature ventricular contractions (**PVC**) are seen as the QRS firing on its own without any P wave preceding (see the fifth ECG cycle). It is usually followed by a recovery pause and then regular beats. *(From Huang S et al:* Coronary care nursing, *St Louis, 1989, Saunders.)*

Fig. 10-30 Ventricular tachycardia (V-tach) is seen as rapid QRS complexes with no P waves because the ventricles are rapidly firing on their own. *(From Huang S et al:* Coronary care nursing, *St Louis, 1989, Saunders.)*

Fig. 10-31 Ventricular fibrillation (V-fib) is seen as an uncoordinated irregular line of jagged spikes. There are no recognizable P waves, QRS complexes, or T waves because the ventricles are twitching irregularly. Consequently, there is no circulation of the blood. This is a medical emergency requiring cardiopulmonary resuscitation (CPR) and a defibrillator to return the heart to a coordinated effective rhythm. *(From Huang S et al:* Coronary care nursing, *St Louis, 1989, Saunders.)*

Becoming Proficient at ECG and Spirometry Diagnostic Tests

Now that you have learned about the significance of performing accurate cardiopulmonary diagnostic tests, take the time to complete the following:

1. Answer the text questions at the end of this chapter and do all of the exercises in Chapter 10 of the workbook using your structured notes, and PowerPoint slides on the Evolve website.

2. View the animations and videos on Evolve to see the anatomy and physiology of the heart and lungs, and to observe how to interact with patients when performing ECG and spirometry procedures.

3. Perform the Chapter 10 on-line exercises, which are designed to reinforce your terminology, theory, and testing techniques for measuring the the heart and lung function.

4. Study Procedures 10-3 and 10-4 at the end of this section before performing your lab procedures on peak expiratory flow monitoring and Holter monitoring.

✳ PROCEDURE 10-3 Peak Expiratory Flow Monitoring

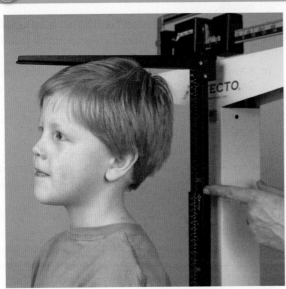

A, Before performing the peak flow screening test, accurately determine the child's height, age, and gender (all three are needed to compare the result against the predicted normal for the child's group).

B, The patient is instructed to (1) fully inflate the lungs and hold his breath while sealing the lips around the mouthpiece, and (2) fully exhale into the mouthpiece as fast and as hard as possible.

(Continued)

10-3

PROCEDURE 10-3 Peak Expiratory Flow Monitoring—cont'd

C, Peak flow result on the left registers 200 L/min. The preset green, yellow, and red indicators on the right indicate the patient is in the yellow zone.

Instrument and Supplies

- Height/weight scale
- Peak flow meter, new or sterilized
- Peak flow meter for demonstrating maneuver
- Daily monitoring chart

Preanalytical

1. Call the patient into the room and sanitize your hands while confirming the patient's name using three identifiers: have the patient spell his or her last name, give his or her date of birth, and provide one more identifier such as phone number or address, or show a driver's license.
2. Confirm when the patient last took his or her bronchodilator medication and if the patient has ingested a heavy meal in the last 4 hours.
3. Measure the patient's height in inches, and confirm the patient's age (to compare with the proper demographic group if it is a screening test) (Figure A).
4. Explain and demonstrate the two steps of the maneuver using a demo peak flow meter.
   - **Fully inflate** your lungs and then hold your breath while sealing your lips around the mouthpiece.
   - **Fully exhale** into the mouthpiece as fast and as hard as possible (Figure B).
5. Show and explain the importance of standing upright during the maneuver and that the patient will have 1 minute to rest and sit between a minimum of three attempts to determine "personal best."

Analytical

6. Test and teach the patient through the following steps:
   a. Before each use, make sure the sliding pointer on the PFM is reset to the zero mark. See Figure C showing the red sliding pointer on the left after a maneuver.
   b. Stand up straight.
   c. Remove chewing gum or any food from your mouth.
   d. Take a deep breath and put the mouthpiece in your mouth. Seal your lips and teeth tightly around the mouthpiece.
   e. Blow out as hard and as fast as you can. Remember, a "fast blast" is better than a "slow blow."
   f. Note the number where the sliding pointer has stopped on the scale. See Figure C result.
   g. Reset the pointer to zero.
   h. Repeat this routine three times. You will know you have done the technique correctly when the three readings are close together.
   i. If you cough during a measurement, you should repeat it.
   j. Record the highest of the three readings on a graph or in a notebook. This is called your *"best effort."* Do not average the numbers together.
   k. Use the peak flow meter once a day, or as directed by your physician. Measure peak flows about the same time each day. A good time might be when you first wake up or at bedtime.
7. Coach the patient as he or she performs the maneuver. Make sure the patient performs both steps: inspiration and rapid exhalation. Praise good techniques to the patient and communicate positive ways to improve the next maneuver. Do not give negative feedback.

10-3

PROCEDURE 10-3 Peak Expiratory Flow Monitoring—cont'd

Postanalytical

8. If the patient is taking a screening test, locate his or her predicted value on Table 10-1 based on the patient's age, gender, and height. Divide the predicted value into the patient's result. If the result is less than 80%, the patient may need further evaluation.

9. If the patient has been prescribed daily peak flow monitoring, determine his or her "best effort" reading from three attempts. The personal best value will be used as a baseline for the patient's routine measurements. Show the patient the peak flow chart where he or she will be entering daily results. See Figure D above showing a completed patient chart.

10. Document the procedure.

Quality Control

Be aware of and correct the following issues that will prevent accurate readings:
- Coughing during the maneuver
- Forming a poor seal around the mouthpiece while performing the procedure
- Taking asthma medication before the PFM (especially the bronchodilator medication because it opens the airways and gives a false high reading)
- Using a dirty meter
- Blocking the mouthpiece with the tongue
- Using a different type or brand of PFM, as the measurements may vary among brands and types of meters

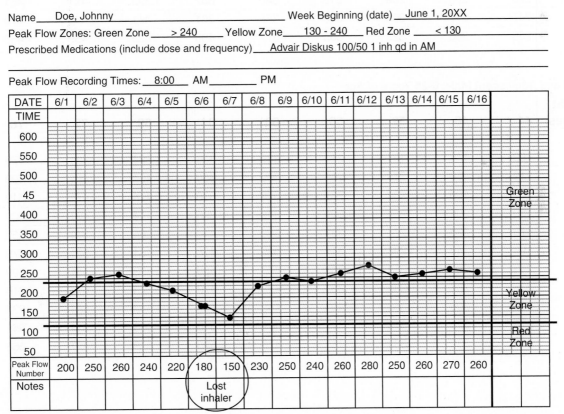

Name____Doe, Johnny_____ Week Beginning (date) ___June 1, 20XX_____
Peak Flow Zones: Green Zone ____> 240_____ Yellow Zone____130 - 240___ Red Zone _____< 130_____
Prescribed Medications (include dose and frequency)___Advair Diskus 100/50 1 inh qd in AM_____

Peak Flow Recording Times: __8:00__ AM_____ PM

DATE	6/1	6/2	6/3	6/4	6/5	6/6	6/7	6/8	6/9	6/10	6/11	6/12	6/13	6/14	6/15	6/16		
Peak Flow Number	200	250	260	240	220	180	150	230	250	240	260	280	250	260	270	260		
Notes						Lost inhaler												

D, Peak flow chart showing daily monitoring results. Notice the readings that fell in the yellow zone on the days the patient was not using his inhaler.

Table 10-1 Peak Expiratory Flow Rates*

Child and Adolescent Female: 6-20 Years of Age

Height (inches)	42	46	50	54	57	60	64	68	72
Age									
6	134	164	193	223	245	268	297	327	357
8	153	182	212	242	264	287	316	346	376
10	171	201	231	261	283	305	335	365	395
12	190	220	250	280	302	324	354	384	414
14	209	239	269	298	321	343	373	403	432
16	228	258	288	318	340	362	392	421	451
18	247	277	306	336	358	381	411	440	470
20	266	295	325	355	377	400	429	459	489

Child and Adolescent Male: 6-25 Years of Age

Height (inches)	44	48	52	56	60	64	68	72	76
Age									
6	99	146	194	241	289	336	384	431	479
8	119	166	214	261	309	356	404	451	499
10	139	186	234	281	329	376	424	471	519
12	159	206	254	301	349	396	444	491	539
14	178	226	274	321	369	416	464	511	559
16	198	246	293	341	389	436	484	531	579
18	218	266	313	361	408	456	503	551	599
20	238	286	333	381	428	476	523	571	618
22	258	306	353	401	448	496	543	591	638
24	278	326	373	421	468	516	563	611	658
25	288	336	383	431	478	526	573	621	668

| Table 10-1 | Peak Expiratory Flow Rates—cont'd |

Adult Female: 20-80 Years of Age

Height (inches)	58	60	62	64	66	68	70
Age							
20	357	372	387	402	417	432	446
25	350	365	379	394	409	424	439
30	342	357	372	387	402	417	431
35	335	350	364	379	394	409	424
40	327	342	357	372	387	402	416
45	320	335	349	364	379	394	409
50	312	327	342	357	372	387	401
55	308	320	334	349	364	379	394
60	297	312	327	342	357	372	386
65	290	305	319	334	349	364	379
70	282	297	312	327	342	357	371
75	275	290	304	319	334	349	364
80	267	282	297	312	327	342	356

Adult Male: 25-80 Years of Age

Height (inches)	63	65	67	69	71	73	75	77
Age								
25	492	520	549	578	606	635	664	692
30	481	510	538	567	596	624	653	682
35	471	499	528	557	585	614	643	671
40	460	489	517	546	575	603	632	661
45	450	478	507	536	564	593	622	650
50	439	468	496	525	554	582	611	640
55	429	457	486	515	543	572	601	629
60	418	447	475	504	533	561	590	619
65	408	436	465	494	522	551	580	608
70	397	426	454	483	512	540	569	598
75	387	405	444	473	501	530	559	587
80	376	405	433	462	491	519	5	

From www.sh.lsuhsc.edu/fammed/outpatientmanual/PeakFlowTables.htm. Accessed January 2, 2014.

*Note that the values are the average normal values for healthy persons of a given age and height (Knudson, 1976). There will always be a range of normal values; not everyone can be expected to have exactly the same value. Men can have peak flow values as low as 100 L/min less than the average value shown and still fall within the normal range. Women can have peak flow values as low as 80 L/min less than the average value shown and still fall within the normal range.

✳ PROCEDURE 10-4 Holter Monitoring

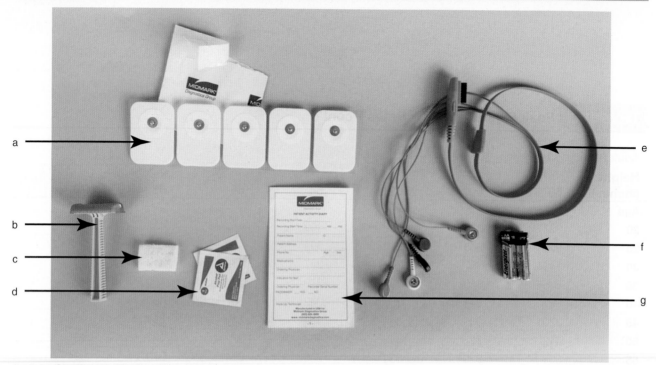

A, Supplies for Midmark Holter monitor: *a,* five electrodes to be placed on chest landmarks; *b,* sterile razor for removing hair from sites; *c,* abrasive pad to increase circulation; *d,* alcohol swabs for removing oil and sweat; *e,* patient cable with four lead wires and a green ground wire; *f,* new batteries for the monitor; *g,* patient log for recording cardiac "events."

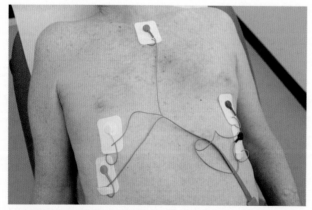

B, Midmark Holter monitor's recommended placement for the five color-coded lead and ground wires that snap onto the white electrodes. Note the looping of the wires to prevent tension during the 24 hours of monitoring.

Instrument and Supplies

There are a variety of Holter monitoring systems in use. Most systems provide patient packets with all the supplies for patient preparation. See Figure A showing the following supplies for the Midmark monitor:

a. Five white electrodes to be placed on chest landmarks
b. Sterile razor for removing hair from sites
c. Abrasive pad to increase circulation at the sites
d. Alcohol swabs for removing oil and sweat
e. Patient cable with four lead wires and a green ground wire
f. New batteries for the monitor
g. Patient log for recording cardiac "events"

10-4

PROCEDURE 10-4 Holter Monitoring—cont'd

Preanalytical

1. Greet the patient and confirm identity while sanitizing your hands.
2. Explain procedure and how to disrobe (from the waist up with the gown opening in the front). Provide the patient with privacy.
3. After returning to patient's room, prepare the electrode sites by:
   - Dry shaving hair (if necessary)
   - Applying alcohol to remove lotions, oils, and dirt
   - Rubbing the abrasive pad over the sites to increase circulation
   - Note, there are different configurations of where to place the electrodes and the color-coded wires as seen in Figure B. Be sure to follow the manufacturer's diagram of the site locations and/or the physician's preference.
4. While the sites are drying from the alcohol, snap the color-coded wires to their electrodes.
5. Then, one at a time, peel the backing off of each sticky electrode with its colored lead wire and firmly press it on to its designated prepared site. Remember, each Holter system will provide its own diagram showing where each colored lead wire belongs. The latest Holter system, seen at the bottom of this procedure (Figure C), is wireless and only needs one kidney-shaped "patch" that is placed on the upper left side of the patient's chest.
6. The wires coming from each electrode must then be looped and taped down with surgical tape, or looped and held down by the lower sticky tab at the bottom of the electrode as seen in Figure B. This alleviates any tension on wires and prevents them from being accidentally pulled off during the monitoring.
7. Insert the digital flashcard or tape into the recorder.
8. Place the new batteries (provided in the supply kit) into the monitor, and connect the lead cable to the monitor.

Analytical

9. Turn on the monitor and follow the manufacturer's directions for data input and quality control. Note the start time on the monitor and write it on patient's log.
10. Show the patient his or her log book and explain how the monitor works and is stored in its pouch. Emphasize that **the monitor and wires should not get wet.**

11. Then instruct the patient to do the following in the log book (diary):
    - Record the activities you do and exactly what time you do them using the clock on the Holter monitor screen. Activities include:
    - when you exert yourself.
    - when you are at rest.
    - when you eat.
    - when you take medications.
    - bowel movements.
    - Record any symptoms you have while you are wearing the monitor, such as:
    - chest pain.
    - shortness of breath.
    - Lightheadedness.
    - skipped heartbeats.
    - The physician will be comparing the data from the Holter monitor recorder with your diary, which will help diagnose your condition.
12. Explain how long the patient needs to wear the monitor. (It may vary from 12 hours to 14 days based on the physician's order.)
13. Document in the patient record that all the above steps were performed and the patient was informed when to return for a follow-up visit.

Postanalytical

15. When the monitoring period is over, the patient returns with the Holter monitor and their diary. Perform the following steps:
    - Check to ensure entries were made in the log (diary).
    - Turn off and disconnect the monitor per manufacturer's instructions.
    - Disconnect the cable from the monitor.
    - Remove the monitor from the pouch.
    - Carefully remove the electrodes from patient and from the lead wires and discard.
    - Clean the patient's chest of any residual gel from the electrodes.
    - Remove and discard the batteries from the monitor.
    - Remove the flashcard/tape from the monitor and submit it along with the patient's diary for interpretation.
    - Clean the Holter monitor and patient cable with its lead wires for next patient.
16. Document completed procedure.

10-4

Alternative Wireless Ambulatory ECG Monitoring System by ZIO

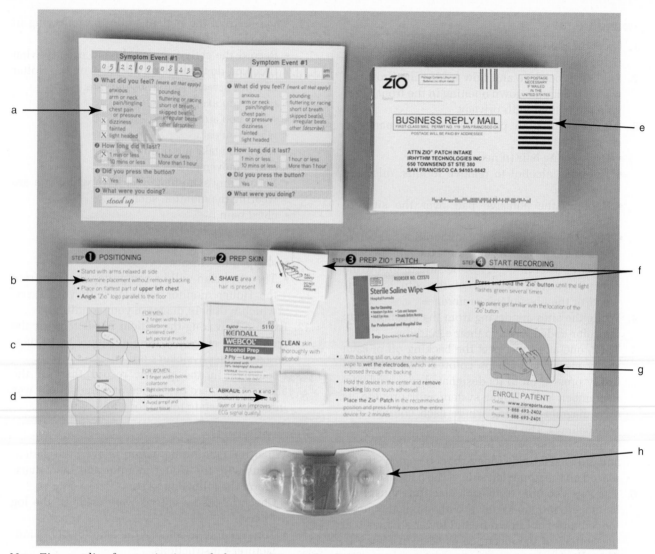

New Zio supplies for monitoring ambulatory ECGs wirelessly for up to 14 days: (a) patient log for marking cardiac events; (b) packet with directions and all the supplies needed for setting up the ZIO monitor; (c) alcohol pad; (d) abrasive pad; (e) mailer to send in the monitor after 14 days; (f) shaver and sterile gauze for preparing site; (g) picture showing placement of the kidney-shaped, wireless monitor on the patient's left side under the left collar bone; (h) the sticky gel side of the wireless monitor that is pressed against the chest as seen in the picture.

Review Questions

ECG Questions

1. Which chamber of the heart contracts to send oxygenated blood through the aortic valve and out to the body's cells?
   a. Left atrium
   b. Left ventricle
   c. Right atrium
   d. Right ventricle

2. Which of these tissues is known as the body's "natural pacemaker"?
   a. SA node   c. Bundle of His
   b. AV node   d. Purkinje fibers

3. Which component of the ECG cycle shows ventricular depolarization?
   a. P
   b. QRS
   c. T
   d. U

4. After the first precordial electrode is placed, what is the correct order for the next three electrodes?
   a. V2, then V3, then V4.
   b. V3, then V2, then V4.
   c. V2, then V4, then V3.
   d. There is no recommended order.

5. Match the leads with their codes and circle the leads that form Einthoven's triangle.
   a. Augmented unipolar limb leads
   b. Precordial chest leads
   c. Standard limb leads

   (1) V1 through V6
   (2) aVL, aVF, and aVR
   (3) I, II, III

6. Which of these items are placed on the patient's limbs and chest in an ECG to detect impulses?
   a. Amplifier
   b. Electrodes
   c. Galvanometer
   d. Stylus

7. Which limb electrode is used as a reference point and is not part of the ECG recording?
   a. right arm (RA)
   b. left arm (LA)
   c. right leg (RL)
   d. left leg (LL)

8. If ECG artifacts are seen on leads I and II, what is the likely source of interference?
   a. Left arm electrode
   b. Left leg electrode
   c. Right arm electrode
   d. Right leg electrode

9. What should the assistant do after seeing an urgent problem on an ECG tracing?
   a. Share the information with the patient right away.
   b. Notify the physician immediately.
   c. Look in the patient's chart for an explanation.

10. How many leads does a Holter monitor have?
    a. 2
    b. 3
    c. Up to 5
    d. Up to 12

11. What is the purpose of the patient diary in Holter monitoring?
    a. Reminds the patient about heart-healthy behaviors.
    b. Supplies a link to patient activity at the time of any abnormal results.
    c. Provides a place to document the results of the test.
    d. Informs the patient of what items to avoid during the test.

Spirometry Questions

12. Spirometry is used in primary care to:
    a. Determine the cause of lung diseases
    b. Screen and monitor pulmonary obstruction and/or restriction
    c. Determine exposure to pollutants
    d. Monitor how many cigarettes a patient has smoked.

13. Match the respiratory structure with its possible obstructive disorder:
    a. Terminal bronchioles
    b. Alveoli
    c. Upper respiratory tract
    d. Lower respiratory tract

    (1) emphysema
    (2) flu and colds
    (3) bronchitis
    (4) asthma

14. Spirometry is a pulmonary function test that measures:
    a. airway inflammation.
    b. how much and how fast air is exhaled.
    c. how long you can hold your breath.
    d. how fast you can inhale and exhale.

15. A healthy person exhales what percentage of his or her total exhaled volume in the first second?
    a. 25-30%
    b. 75%
    c. 80-90%
    d. 100%

16. When looking at the volume/time curve, what indicates a good patient effort?
    a. A quick rise in the beginning
    b. A FET (forced expiratory time) of 6 seconds
    c. A plateau of the curve at the end
    d. All the above

17. How often should the spirometer be checked with the calibrated syringe?
    a. Daily
    b. Weekly
    c. Monthly
    d. Not necessary if stable

Websites

Information on Peak Flow Monitoring:
www.hopkinsmedicine.org/healthlibrary/test_procedures/pulmonary/peak_flow_measurement_92,P07755/

Peak expiratory flow (PEF) charts for predicted normal:
www.sh.lsuhsc.edu/fammed/outpatientmanual/PeakFlowTables.htm

Peak flow rate measurement on Medscape:
http://emedicine.medscape.com/article/1413347-overview#aw2aab6b4aa

U-Tube news article on ZIO patch for ECG monitoring:
www.youtube.com/watch?v=Cjx6H9PdkSY

Answers to Review Questions

Chapter 1
1. pathologist
2. venipunctures, blood draws
3. POLs (physician's office laboratories) and reference laboratories
4. doctor of medicine or osteopathy
5. honesty, communication skills, efficiency, organizational skills, good eyesight, and dexterity
6. d, a, c, b
7. mL, dL, cm, mcm, cc
8. biohazards, chemical hazards, and physical hazards
9. fire, tornado, bomb, and electrical dangers
10. acids, caustics, flammables, inhalants
11. 10% solution of 1 part bleach and 9 parts water, or 70% alcohol
12. False
13. True

Chapter 2
1. All laboratories performing tests on specimens must register with CMS for permission to perform CoW, moderately complex, or highly complex tests based on the qualifications of the laboratory personnel and the difficulty of the tests performed to improve the accuracy and reliability of patient testing.
2. Laboratories performing moderately complex and complex tests must prove their proficiency by testing specimens from an outside accreditation agency twice a year and obtaining the correct results.
3. low
4. 10×
5. condenser
6. nosepiece
7. oil immersion
8. objective
9. c, a, b

Chapter 3
1. c
2. b
3. d
4. d
5. b
6. d
7. b
8. c
9. d
10. b
11. C
12. C
13. I—This would contaminate the urethral opening with bacteria from the rectal area.
14. I—Besides contaminating the urethral opening with bacteria from the rectal area, this step would also contaminate the opening with organisms from the other side.
15. C
16. C

Chapter 4
1. c
2. d
3. b
4. c
5. c
6. a
7. a
8. d
9. c
10. Light blue, red plastic (has clot activator—should not be drawn before the light blue), green, and lavender

Chapter 5
1. b
2. plasma, erythrocytes, granulocytes, anticoagulant, platelet, EDTA, megakaryocyte
3. g, h, b, e, c, d, f, a
4. prothrombin, fibrin
5. K
6. d, a, b, e, c
7. b, c, a
8. b, a, d, c, e
9. e, d, a, c, b

Chapter 6
1. whole blood from a fingerstick; serum from a red clot tube or gold SST of marbled red-gray rubber-topped SST tube
2. insulin
3. 90% to 95%
4. glucosuria
5. d
6. It provides a picture of average glucose levels over a 3-month period and helps determine whether the patient is keeping glucose levels under control.
7. f, d, c, e, a, b
8. from the diet (exogenous); from the liver (endogenous)

337

9. LDL adheres to the arteries, causing plaque, whereas HDL removes the plaque.
10. To check the instrument's optical performance and ensure quality results
11. poor specimen processing or technique; reagents stored at wrong temperature or expired; instrument dirty or faulty
12. less than 200 mg/dL; 200 to 240 mg/dL; greater than 240 mg/dL
13. To determine if bleeding is present within the colon or GI tract, which might indicate possible carcinoma:
    1. ColoScreen
    2. ColoCARE
    3. iFob—immunoassay Fecal Occult Blood
14. b, d, c, e, a

Chapter 7

1. b
2. c
3. d
4. a
5. b
6. a and c
7. d
8. b
9. d
10. B and Rh antigens
11. Blood; oral swab of the gums

Chapter 8

1. d
2. c
3. c
4. b
5. a
6. d
7. d
8. c
9. specimen—direct smear using swabbed specimen; colony growing on a solid medium; liquid medium with growth
10. d

Chapter 9

1. T
2. F (It is the mechanism of the drug's action in the body from introduction to elimination.)
3. Liberation
4. absorption
5. distribution
6. metabolism
7. kidney, liver
8. half-life
9. lead, arsenic, mercury, iron
10. alcohol
11. crank, speed
12. morphine, codeine, heroin
13. c
14. c

Chapter 10

1. b
2. a
3. b
4. c
5. a-2, b-1, c-3 (c-3 is Einthoven's triangle)
6. b
7. c
8. c
9. b
10. c
11. b
12. b
13. a-4, b-1, c-2, d-3
14. b
15. c
16. d
17. a

Index

Page numbers followed by "f" indicate figures, "t" indicate tables, and "b" indicate boxes.